# Chemotherapy and Immunotherapy in Urologic Oncology

Edouard J. Trabulsi • Costas D. Lallas
Anne E. Lizardi-Calvaresi
Editors

# Chemotherapy and Immunotherapy in Urologic Oncology

## A Guide for the Advanced Practice Provider

Springer

*Editors*
Edouard J. Trabulsi
Department of Urology
Sidney Kimmel Medical College
at Thomas Jefferson University
Philadelphia
PA
USA

Costas D. Lallas
Department of Urology
Sidney Kimmel Medical College
at Thomas Jefferson University
Philadelphia
PA
USA

Anne E. Lizardi-Calvaresi
Sidney Kimmel Medical College
at Thomas Jefferson University
Philadelphia
PA
USA

ISBN 978-3-030-52020-5 ISBN 978-3-030-52021-2 (eBook)
https://doi.org/10.1007/978-3-030-52021-2



This Springer imprint is published by the registered company Springer Nature Switzerland AG
The registered company address is: Gewerbestrasse 11, 6330 Cham, Switzerland

# Foreword

The front lines of genitourinary (GU) oncology have shifted over the past decade with growing awareness of the benefit of a multidisciplinary approach. Additionally, physician shortages and emphasis on continuity of care and survivorship have led to an increased role of the advanced practice provider (APP). Out of these two concepts has emerged the defined position of an APP in Genitourinary Oncology. We long ago recognized the value of this model and have promoted it in our practice for the last 10+ years. We firmly believe that this gives optimal care to our patients.

The idea for this book was created out of the ongoing collaboration between urologic oncologists, genitourinary oncologists, GU radiation oncologists, and advanced practice providers at our institution and others. Each chapter is a result of team effort by field experts and an APP, who works closely with them, helping them communicate with and manage their patients. These teams represent the new face of care in GU oncology and provide a prime example of stewardship, scholarship, and comprehensive care. Each team not only focuses on the science behind their tumor of choice but the individual patient concerns that are seen in everyday practice and how to best recognize and manage them. Key concepts, denoted as clinical pearls, are highlighted at the end of each chapter. The book represents the culmination of interprofessional bidirectional mentorship, hard work, and unfaltering comradery.

It is our hope that this book provides useful information and guidance to comprehensively care for our genitourinary cancer patients in order to obtain the best outcomes.

Edouard J. Trabulsi, MD, MBA, FACS
Department of Urology
Sidney Kimmel Medical College at
Thomas Jefferson University
Philadelphia, PA, USA

Costas D. Lallas, MD, FACS
Department of Urology
Sidney Kimmel Medical College at
Thomas Jefferson University
Philadelphia, PA, USA

Anne E. Lizardi-Calvaresi, DNP, CRNP, RNFA
Sidney Kimmel Medical College at
Thomas Jefferson University
Philadelphia, PA, USA

# Contents

# Contributors

**Courtney C. Anderson, MPA, PA-C** Department of Urology, Eastern Virginia Medical School, Norfolk, VA, USA

**Betsy M. Avinash, CRNP** The Pennsylvania State University, College of Medicine, Department of Surgery, Division of Urology, Hershey, PA, USA

**Demetrius Bagley, MD, FACS** Department of Urology, Thomas Jefferson University, Philadelphia, PA, USA

**Suzanne Barron, CRNP** Thomas Jefferson University Hospital, Department of Urology, Philadelphia, PA, USA

**Janice Carsello, DNP** Department of Medical Oncology, Thomas Jefferson University, Philadelphia, PA, USA

**Adele Marie Caruso, DNP, CRNP, FAANP** Urology Division, Department of Surgery, University of Pennsylvania, Philadelphia, PA, USA

**Erik P. Castle, MD, FACS** Department of Urology, Mayo Clinic, Phoenix, AZ, USA

**Kara R. Cossis, MPH, PA-C** Chesapeake Urology, Owings Mills, MD, USA

**Robert Den, MD** Thomas Jefferson University Hospital, Philadelphia, PA, USA

**Sara Dennin Johney, MSPAS, PA-C** Chesapeake Urology, Owings Mills, MD, USA

**Ann E. Donnelly, MSN, RN, CRNP, ANP-BC, OCN** Department of Radiation Oncology, Thomas Jefferson University Hospital, Philadelphia, PA, USA

**Elena Dreyzin, PA-C, MMS** Department of Surgical Oncology, Fox Chase Cancer Center, Philadelphia, PA, USA

**Mary W. Dunn, MSN, RN, OCN, NP-C** Department of Urology, University of North Carolina Chapel Hill, Chapel Hill, NC, USA

**Kassem S. Faraj, MD** Department of Urology, Mayo Clinic, Phoenix, AZ, USA

**Rachel Lin Flanagan, PA** Department of Surgery, MD Anderson Cancer Center at Cooper, Camden, NJ, USA

**Robert Given, MD** Urology of Virginia, LLC, Virginia Beach, VA, USA

**Leonard G. Gomella, MD, FACS** Department of Urology, Sidney Kimmel Cancer Center, Thomas Jefferson University/Thomas Jefferson University Hospital, Philadelphia, PA, USA

**Javaughn Corey R. Gray, MS, MHS, RN, PhD, FNP-BC, PNP-BC, CUNP, CCCN, FAANP, FAAN** The Greenberg Bladder Cancer Institute, Sidney Kimmel Comprehensive Cancer Center at Johns Hopkins, Baltimore, MD, USA

**Mikel Gray, PhD, FNP, PNP, CUNP CCCN, FAANP, FAAN** University of Virginia, Department of Urology, Charlottesville, VA, USA

**Carla Groshel, PA-C** Urology of Virginia, Schellhammer Cancer Center, Virginia Beach, VA, USA

**Laura P. Gurten, MSN, CRNP, CUNP** Department of Urology, St. Mary Medical Center, Langhorne, PA, USA

**Thomas Joseph Guzzo, MD, MPH** Urology Division, Department of Surgery, University of Pennsylvania, Philadelphia, PA, USA

**Waleed Hassen, MD** Department of Urology, Cleveland Clinic Abu Dhabi, Abu Dhabi, UAE

Cleveland Clinic Lerner College of Medicine, Cleveland, OH, USA

**Thai H. Ho, MD, PhD** Department of Hematology and Oncology, Mayo Clinic, Phoenix, AZ, USA

**Jean Hoffman-Censits, MD** The Greenberg Bladder Cancer Institute, Sidney Kimmel Comprehensive Cancer Center at Johns Hopkins, Baltimore, MD, USA

**Mark D. Hurwitz, MD, FASTRO, FACRO** Department of Radiation Oncology, Thomas Jefferson University Hospital, Philadelphia, PA, USA

**Joseph K. Izes, MD, FACS** Department of Urology, Sidney Kimmel Cancer Center, Sidney Kimmel Medical College, Thomas Jefferson University/Thomas Jefferson University Hospital, Philadelphia, PA, USA

**Jamison S. Jaffe, DO, FACS** Department of Urology, St. Mary Medical Center, Langhorne, PA, USA

**Matthew G. Kaag, MD** The Pennsylvania State University, College of Medicine, Department of Surgery, Division of Urology, Hershey, PA, USA

**Alexander Kutikov, MD, FACS** Department of Surgical Oncology, Fox Chase Cancer Center, Philadelphia, PA, USA

**Anne E. Lizardi-Calvaresi, DNP, CRNP, RNFA** Sidney Kimmel Medical College at Thomas Jefferson University, Philadelphia, PA, USA

**Benjamin Lowentritt, MD, FACS** Chesapeake Urology, Owings Mills, MD, USA

**Tara Mahan, MMS, PA-C** Chesapeake Urology, Owings Mills, MD, USA

**Mark J. Mann, MD** Thomas Jefferson University Hospital, Department of Urology, Philadelphia, PA, USA

**J. Ryan Mark, MD** Department of Urology, Sidney Kimmel Cancer Center, Thomas Jefferson University, Philadelphia, PA, USA

**Jessica Matande, MMS, PA-C** Department of Urologic Oncology, Temple University Hospital, Philadelphia, PA, USA

**Thomas Patrick McBride, PA-C** Urology, Adirondack Health, Adirondack Medical Center, Saranac Lake, NY, USA

**Kurt A. McCammon, MD, FACS, FPM-RS** Department of Urology, Eastern Virginia Medical School, Norfolk, VA, USA

**Patrick Mille, MD** Department of Medical Oncology, Thomas Jefferson University, Philadelphia, PA, USA

**Matthew I. Milowsky, MD** Department of Medicine, University of North Carolina Chapel Hill, Chapel Hill, NC, USA

**Laura Motherway, RGN, PgDip** Department of Urology, Cleveland Clinic Abu Dhabi, Abu Dhabi, UAE

**Seungeun Oh, CRNP** Department of Urology, Thomas Jefferson University, Philadelphia, PA, USA

**Jay D. Raman, MD** The Pennsylvania State University, College of Medicine, Department of Surgery, Division of Urology, Hershey, PA, USA

**Adam C. Reese, MD** Department of Urologic Oncology, Temple University Hospital, Philadelphia, PA, USA

**Charlene Reyes, PA-C** Department of Oncology, Urology of Virginia, Virginia Beach, VA, USA

**Terran W. Sims, RN, MSN, ACNP-BC, CNN-BC, COCN** University of Virginia, Department of Urology, Charlottesville, VA, USA

**Katherine Smentkowski, MD** Department of Urology, Thomas Jefferson University Hospital, Philadelphia, PA, USA

**Danielle Squadrito, MSN, BSN** Department of Urology, Thomas Jefferson University, Philadelphia, PA, USA

**Jeffrey John Tomaszewski, MD** Department of Surgery, MD Anderson Cancer Center at Cooper, Cooper Medical School of Rowan University, Camden, NJ, USA

**Miranda L. Tsang, MSN, CRNP, FNP-BC** Sidney Kimmel Cancer Center – Jefferson Health, Thomas Jefferson University Hospital, Philadelphia, PA, USA

**Mark D. Tyson, MD, MPH** Department of Urology, Mayo Clinic, Phoenix, AZ, USA

**Brooke Zilinskas, MMS, PA-C** Department of Urology, UT Southwestern Medical Center, Dallas, TX, USA

# Chapter 1
# Introduction: Integration of APP into Urologic Oncology Practice

**Leonard G. Gomella**

Improvements in the management of all stages and types of cancer have occurred at a rapid pace. Perhaps, where this is most apparent is in the area of advanced disease states. The traditional approach in the development of cancer therapeutics was to identify an active compound that worked in one type of cancer and then perform Phase 2 trials in a variety of other malignancies to determine its effect. Today's therapeutic development programs rely upon the identification of precise alterations in the structure and/or function of the malignant cell and specifically targets those abnormalities. This concept is broadly known as precision medicine where the delivery of the intervention is targeted to the right patient at the right time.

The field of urologic oncology has benefited greatly from this new approach to the discovery of new agents then the treatment of prostate, bladder, kidney, and other genitourinary specific cancers. Advanced prostate cancer is a shining example of how the treatment landscape of this disease has changed through the introduction of many new agents. The number of available treatment options for patients with advanced prostate cancer (e.g., metastatic at initial diagnosis, recurrent after local therapy, or metastatic and castration-resistant) has increased considerably in recent years. Before 2004, the treatment metastatic castration-resistant prostate cancer was considered palliative until two key clinical trials demonstrated that docetaxel could benefit these men. In 2010, immunotherapy entered the prostate care continuum with the FDA approval of sipuleucel-T. In rapid succession, other agents such as abiraterone, enzalutamide, cabazitaxel, and radium Ra 223 dichloride received approval. Immunotherapy using the tumor agnostic agent, pembrolizumab, is bringing the anti PD-1 agents into the next phase of metastatic prostate cancer therapeutics. Next on the horizon for prostate cancer are clinical trials combining

L. G. Gomella (✉)
Department of Urology, Sidney Kimmel Cancer Center, Thomas Jefferson University/Thomas Jefferson University Hospital, Philadelphia, PA, USA
e-mail: Leonard.gomella@jefferson.edu



E. J. Trabulsi et al. (eds.), *Chemotherapy and Immunotherapy in Urologic Oncology*, https://doi.org/10.1007/978-3-030-52021-2_1

immunotherapeutic agents with other agents and using genomic studies to identify men with advanced disease who may respond to a completely new class of medications known as PARP inhibitors.

These new medications are redefining what we are prescribing and how we treat our patients with advanced urologic oncology diseases; we are also increasingly relying on multidisciplinary care models. The traditional multidisciplinary care combines the collective skills of surgeons, radiation and medical oncologists to offer our patients the best care possible. Today, that multidisciplinary care is increasingly engaging advanced care providers such as nurse practitioners and physicians' assistants to help manage the complexities of these new agents. While the precision medicine model is based on basic science discoveries, many other factors are considered in this process. Beyond an individual's genomics, biomarkers, and molecular characterization of the tumor to be most effective, precision medicine should take into account lifestyle, patient preferences, health history, socioeconomic factors, and other unique patient characteristics that cannot be determined by any laboratory test. Often, the skillset of the advanced practice provider can help integrate these complex patient factors into effective and compassionate care.

Common areas where nurse practitioners and physicians assistants provide important assistance in patient care in the setting of urologic oncology diseases include patient counseling about the disease state and medications that are being administered, assisting with laboratory and imaging monitoring, administration of the agents, identification and management of toxicity, and perhaps most importantly, providing a knowledgeable resource for patient questions or concerns.

The advanced practice providers' role can vary widely based on the particular practice setting. Some may work as independent providers or more commonly as physician extenders working alongside the various urologic oncology specialists. They may be integrated into multidisciplinary clinics or tumor boards where key treatment decisions may be made. In the modern busy practice, they are often viewed as resources and educators for other members of the staff or students who they may be working with.

This book takes a unique approach with each major section partnering an experienced physician with an advanced practice provider. This approach closely replicates the real-world contemporary approach to advanced urologic diseases that in many cases are based on this strong interaction in the continuum of clinical care. Where appropriate, the chapters discuss the practical aspects of surgical and radiation management that are essential elements in many urologic oncology diseases that use a multidisciplinary management approach.

The editors of *Chemotherapy and Immunotherapy in Urologic Oncology: A Guide for the Advanced Practice Provider* are all participants of our well-developed multidisciplinary genitourinary oncology care team at the Sidney Kimmel Cancer Center at Jefferson. We have been engaged in a weekly real-time multidisciplinary clinic at our center since 1996, long before the concept became more widely adopted. We and others have demonstrated this approach improves outcomes in particular for more complicated and high-risk disease states. Other benefits of a multidisciplinary approach include improved patient and family satisfaction, education of a variety of trainees, and enhanced clinical trials recruitment critical to maintain our NCI Cancer Center designation. Our ongoing clinical cancer care relies heavily on the expertise and support of our advanced practice providers.

Although written with the advanced care provider in mind, this book serves as an up-to-date reference for the spectrum of modern urologic oncology. Others who work in genitourinary oncology including physicians, fellows, nurses, and students will find the subject matter and style of presentation of these chapters a useful and practical reference.

# Part I
# Prostate Cancer

# Chapter 2
# Overview and Active Surveillance of Prostate Cancer

**Joseph K. Izes and Thomas Patrick McBride**

## Introduction

Adenocarcinoma of the prostate is the most common noncutaneous cancer among American men and the second leading cause of cancer death after lung cancer. Over the past decades, our understanding of this disease has continued to evolve. We have faced a dramatic increase in the incidence of prostate cancer secondary to an expanding population of older men, the development of increasingly sensitive techniques for prostate cancer detection such as prostate-specific antigen, ultrasound-directed needle biopsy techniques, and advanced imaging. As such, prostate cancer has been a target of special concern from the medical and socioeconomic standpoint and the disease has attracted much popular interest.

Almost 30 years into the prostate-specific antigen (PSA) era, our understanding of this ubiquitous malignancy continues to develop. While great strides have been made, meaningful outcomes data may take several more decades to gather, given the generally slow progression rate and relatively glacial natural history of this disease. While it seemed intuitively reasonable to urologists three decades ago that prostate cancer screening for early-stage disease would reduce morbidity and mortality secondary to this malignancy, a clear survival benefit from all of our diagnostic and therapeutic research effort is only beginning to emerge.

Prostate cancer is a heterogeneous disease of varying aggressiveness. While the 5-year survival rate for early localized prostate cancer is close to 100%, survival is less than 30% for patients presenting distant metastatic disease [1]. While multiple measures of tumor aggressiveness have been developed, these are each somewhat

J. K. Izes
Department of Urology, Sidney Kimmel Cancer Center, Sidney Kimmel Medical College, Thomas Jefferson University/Thomas Jefferson University Hospital, Philadelphia, PA, USA
e-mail: Joseph.izes@Jefferson.edu

T. P. McBride (✉)
Urology, Adirondack Health, Adirondack Medical Center, Saranac Lake, NY, USA



E. J. Trabulsi et al. (eds.), *Chemotherapy and Immunotherapy in Urologic Oncology*, https://doi.org/10.1007/978-3-030-52021-2_2

limited and imperfect. Multiple treatment options exist for both localized and advanced disease. As such, the counseling of affected patients, toward the end of educated shared decision-making will occupy a significant percentage of the treating professional's time and energy for the foreseeable future.

## Epidemiology

It is estimated that 191,930 new cases of prostate cancer will be diagnosed in the United States in 2020. It is predicted to be the leading visceral site of new cancer cases in the male body at 21%. Prostate cancer will cause an estimated 33,330 deaths, accounting for 10% of male deaths from cancers, second only to malignancies of lung and bronchus which will comprise 23% [2]. The disease may be less common in developing countries; however, its incidence and mortality have been on the rise internationally as well [3].

Overall prostate cancer death rates have declined by 52% from a peak of 39.3 deaths per 100,000 men in 1993 to a low of 18.8 per 100,000 men in 2017. This substantial decrease occurred during a time of increased male life expectancy, a circumstance under which prostate cancer mortality would be expected to increase. The explanation is likely multifactorial, reflecting more extensive screening as well as improved treatment. It is controversial; however, in that the number of prostate cancer deaths is far outweighed by the number of diagnoses annually. Critics of PSA-based screening suggest that these improvements in mortality are achieved at the cost of substantial overdiagnosis and overtreatment.

The age-adjusted incidence rate of prostate cancer in African-American men is more than 30% higher than white men and historically, mortality rates have been higher and survival substantially shorter [4]. A genetic versus socioeconomic explanation for this is favored as these findings are consistent in patients within the same large health maintenance organization and in the military [4], where there is an expectation of identical screening and postdiagnosis care. A higher incidence of lymph node versus bone or other metastasis has been identified among African-Americans based on a national review of hospitalized patients with metastatic disease [5].

## Risk Factors

Multiple risk factors for prostatic adenocarcinoma have been identified to be both endogenous and exogenous. Awareness of these is critical to assessing which patients are best served increased screening vigilance, lowered threshold for recommending biopsy, and intensity/timing of therapy.

Endogenous risk factors include family history, race, and age. As above, racial disparities exist affecting the incidence, stage at diagnosis, and mortality.

African-American men have the highest rates of prostate cancer in the world. This may partially be related to access to care and differences in the decision-making process, but appear to also reflect genetic differences including allelic frequencies of microsatellites of androgen receptor locus and polymorphic variation [6].

The incidence of prostate cancer is clearly related to advancing age, and unlike other cancers which have a peak age incidence, the risk of prostate cancer continues to increase throughout a man's lifetime. After 50 years of age, mortality and incidence rates from prostate cancer increase almost exponentially. In interpreting this data, it is critical to distinguish between incidentally discovered cancers that are clinically insignificant and indolent versus those that are more aggressive and possibly lethal if left untreated. Autopsy studies have shown histologic evidence of prostate cancer and more than 40% of men dying in their 80s [7]. The lifetime risk of a 50-year-old man for a cancer detected at autopsy not related to the cause of death is 40%. The risk of diagnosis of prostate cancer while alive is roughly 15% whereas the risk of death from prostate cancer is 2.9% [8]. Clinicians must remain mindful that the goal in diagnosing prostate cancer is decreasing of risk of progression to symptomatic disease, which generally takes many years. As such, detection of disease in the elderly with competing comorbidities is of limited benefit.

Familial clustering of prostate cancer has been observed in studies dating back to the 1960s. Relative risk estimates associated with a history of prostate cancer in a first-degree relative range from 1.7 to 3.7. Younger ages at diagnosis and multiple relatives with prostate cancer are associated with even higher relative risks [9, 10]. Two highly penetrant genes that predispose individuals to breast cancer (BRCA1 and BRCA2) are known to confer an increased risk of prostate cancer of about threefold and sevenfold, respectively [11]. Lynch Syndrome is another risk factor for prostate cancer. Mutations of DNA mismatch repair (MMR) genes, which are associated with Lynch syndrome, also confer a twofold increase in the risk of prostate cancer, amounting to a 30% lifetime risk. It is appropriate to consider earlier and more frequent prostate-specific antigen (PSA) screening for men with known personal or familial mutations of BRCA2, HOXB13, or MMR genes linked to Lynch syndrome [12]. There is some evidence of increased aggressiveness associated with these germline mutations. A full family history should be obtained and genetic counseling should be offered to patients with familial prostate cancers.

Exogenous risks factors have also been reported. Fatal prostate cancer has been associated with smoking history, height, obesity, and a high-fat Western diet [13]. Migrant studies demonstrate that when men from a low-risk country move to United States and adopt a Western diet, their rates of prostate cancer increase dramatically. A variety of dietary elements have been studied. Tomato sauce intake has been correlated with a lower incidence and decreased stage of prostate cancer [14]. To date, no dietary supplement study has shown significant benefits. Previous vasectomy had been suggested as a risk factor [15], but this association could not be validated in enlarged studies [16].

## Signs and Symptoms

Most patients with early-stage prostate cancer are asymptomatic. Because this is a disease that occurs in the same demographic as BPH, some level of voiding complaints and erectile dysfunction is commonplace. While bladder outlet obstruction and irritative voiding complaints can result from local growth of cancer, in most cases these symptoms reflect coincident benign prostatic hypertrophy and age-related changes. Early-stage prostate cancer is rarely associated with hematuria. Constitutional symptoms are rare. Metastatic disease, however, may present with bone pain and symptoms of spinal cord impingement.

In addition to a complete history, with attention to risk factors described above, a physical exam including digital rectal exam (DRE) should be performed. Careful attention should be paid to overall gland consistency which should be homogeneous and will range from spongy to rubbery in texture. Abnormalities in the digital rectal exam may include obvious nodularity, a localized decrease in compressibility or induration and loss of normal landmarks including the midline and lateral sulci. Tenderness or bogginess of the gland suggests underlying prostatitis which may spuriously increase prostate-specific antigen. The abdomen should be palpated for suprapubic fullness and bladder distention can be confirmed with office ultrasound. Advanced prostate cancer may present with palpable lymphadenopathy or edema of the lower extremities and scrotum. A neurologic examination may suggest findings consistent with spinal cord compression.

While the digital rectal exam is significantly less sensitive than other modalities [17, 18] and there is some intra- as well as interexaminer variability of the examination [19], it should be routinely performed. DRE is not recommended as the sole evaluation of the patient for prostate cancer and should be combined with PSA testing. The positive predictive value of DRE is 28% with a sensitivity of 59% and a specificity of 95%, according to one meta-analysis [20]. A significant proportion of prostate cancers detected by digital rectal exam at low PSA levels have features associated with clinically aggressive tumors [21]. This inexpensive and minimally invasive physical examination will also provide information on the staging and fixation of cancers that are diagnosed [22].

## PSA and Screening

Prostate-specific antigen (PSA) was initially developed as a tumor marker to assess the extent of disease and response to therapy. Initially isolated from the semen, it was first described in the forensic literature as a tool for identifying seminal fluid in sexual assault investigations [23]. It was subsequently identified in prostatic tissue [24] and is organ-specific, and presents only in the cytoplasm of benign and malignant prostate epithelial cells. It is important to recognize that this glycoprotein is prostate-specific but not prostate cancer-specific. Ultimately, a technique was developed to measure level in the serum using a variety of antibody-based assays.

Toward the goal of allowing early detection of prostate cancer for curative therapy, PSA was incorporated into prostate cancer screening in the early 1990s. PSA was initially approved by the United States FDA using a threshold of 4 ng/mL as the upper limit of normal [25]. The use of this tumor marker in screening leads to a dramatic increase in newly detected prostate cancer. A substantial percentage of detected cancers were low risk and early stage. At the time, clinically insignificant carcinoma was a revolutionary concept and these patients were often aggressively treated. In the subsequent decades, a better understanding of the clinical importance of low-risk disease has led to significant controversy and somewhat disparate recommendations for screening amongst organizations formulating clinical guidelines. It is important to remember that the use of PSA as a tumor marker to assess disease response and progression, remains noncontroversial and generally well accepted.

PSA levels are increased in malignancy because of increased production by cancer epithelial cells and secondary to cancer-related disruption of vasculature. PSA elevation has been shown to proceed the development of clinically apparent prostate cancer by 5–10 years, but can also be caused by a number of benign conditions. Prostate enlargement can also cause elevated PSA [26] as can prostatic inflammation, trauma, and sexual activity. Using a cut off value of 4 ng/mL, the sensitivity of this test is 21% for detecting any prostate cancer and 51% for high-grade cancer. The negative predictive value of a PSA less than four is 85% [27].

Because of concern that widespread screening has led to an excessive number of biopsies and to the diagnosis of clinically insignificant cancers, numerous strategies to refine PSA for cancer detection have been explored. Toward this end, the rate of rise or PSA velocity has been explored. A serum PSA increase of 0.75 ng/mL per year is indicative of an increased risk of an occult prostate cancer. It is critically important to interpret PSA values only after they have been confirmed by the same laboratory. Very rapidly rising PSAs or outlier values may reflect prostatic inflammation or even laboratory error. The PSA doubling time is frequently used in the post-treatment setting to determine the need for intervention among patients with biochemical recurrence after treatment [28].

Larger prostate glands tend to produce more PSA and the concept of PSA density has been described. PSA levels average approximately to 0.12 ng/mL/g of tissue. Some have advocated prostate biopsy based on excessive PSA density. This approach is problematic for a variety of reasons beyond the scope of this discussion [29]. It is important, however, to consider the impact of significant BPH, especially in the setting of a relatively mildly elevated PSA [30]. Further, PSA has been shown to increase with normal aging, and tables for age-specific PSA values have been published. These increase the sensitivity of the marker in younger patients and increase its specificity in older men.

Free and total PSA measurement is an assay comparing molecular forms of PSA bound to large serum proteins. Statistically important only for patients with PSAs between 4 and 10 ng/mL, the risk of a positive biopsy can be stratified [31] to some extent by the percentage of free PSA. A free PSA greater than 25% is consistent with benign disease whereas a value under 10% is quite worrisome. A variety of commercially available molecular tests have been developed to augment the specificity and sensitivity of PSA screening. These are both serum and urine based, and are generally proprietary and expensive.

Special consideration must be given to patients on 5-alpha reductase inhibitors including finasteride (both the 1 and 5 mg dosages) and dutasteride. These drugs are marketed for the treatment of benign prostatic hypertrophy and male pattern baldness. Clinicians must be mindful that PSA will decrease by approximately 50% by these medications. A rising PSA in a patient on these drugs raises suspicion for underlying prostate cancer [32].

The overall efficacy of PSA screening has been investigated in multiple studies, many of which are ongoing. Guideline agencies including the United States Preventative Service Task Force, the American Urologic Association, the American Cancer Society, the American Society of Clinical Oncology, and the National Comprehensive Cancer Network have each offered clinical guidance, which has been published elsewhere. Common features of these recommendations are for shared decision-making regarding prostate cancer screening in men with average risk between the ages of 55 and 69. PSA screening is not recommended in men with a less than 10–15-year life expectancy. An individualized approach is recommended, especially with regard to high-risk patients including those with family history, genetic predisposition, and African-Americans and those with previously elevated PSAs or abnormal findings on digital rectal exam.

## Diagnostic Evaluation

Definitive diagnosis of prostate cancer requires tissue diagnosis by prostate biopsy. As above, the decision to proceed to biopsy must be made with full consideration of both prostate-related worrisome findings as well as the patient's overall health. Life expectancy, risk tolerance, and special considerations such as chronic anticoagulation must be considered. Prostate biopsy is generally performed using a transrectal approach. The prostate is visualized ultrasonically using a biplanar rectal probe. Because of a significant risk of sepsis with transrectal biopsies, patients are prepared with enemas and broad-spectrum antibiotic coverage. Usually, a fluoroquinolone and/or third-generation cephalosporin are used for antibiotic prophylaxis. Local anesthesia is injected adjacent to the prostate at the junction of prostate and seminal vesicles under ultrasound guidance. Topical anesthesia may also be employed. The procedure is generally performed in the office or outpatient setting. The majority of patients will tolerate this without sedation or general anesthesia.

Prostate biopsy is performed under ultrasound guidance using a spring-loaded biopsy device coupled to the imaging probe. In general, 12 cores are taken in a systematic geographic. The ultrasonic zonal anatomy of the prostate has been well described [33]. The peripheral zone, where the majority of tumors are located is systematically sampled. On occasion, biopsies of the transition zone are taken as well as biopsies of the anterior commissure, both areas that are important to sample in patients with rising PSA who present for second biopsy.

Patients must be counseled thoroughly regarding the complications and sequelae transrectal ultrasound with biopsy. Prostate biopsy is frequently associated with minor bleeding and urinary symptoms that did not require intervention. Hematospermia may persist for several months. Roughly 25% of men have transient worsening of lower urinary tract symptoms <2% after biopsy percent have frank urinary retention. Hematuria and hematochezia may occur and these are exacerbated by coagulopathy, resumption of anticoagulant medication, possibly with prostate size, and the number of biopsies taken [34]. Serious complications including urosepsis may be life-threatening. There was a significant increase in hospitalizations for sepsis from 1991 to 2007, likely as a consequence of increasing fluoroquinolone resistance in the community [35, 36].

There is increasing interest in, and use of, a transperineal biopsy approach under ultrasound guidance, which avoids perforation of the rectal mucosa. The technique employs a perineal template affixed to a transrectal ultrasound probe in a manner similar to the placement of transperineal brachii therapy. This approach requires additional equipment and a bit of a learning curve but has the advantage of affording better access for anterior biopsies and a significant decrease in the incidence of biopsy-related sepsis.

Increasingly, multiparametric MRI of the prostate is used for more precise imaging. The MRI is effective at identifying higher risk and clinically relevant prostate cancers that may not be seen by ultrasound. Eighty-seven percent of tumors detected by MRI are clinically significant [37]. While the information obtained from MRI can be used to direct traditional prostate biopsies, a "cognitive" technique, commercially available technologies exist to combine MRI and ultrasound images in real time. Such MRI-ultrasound fusion technologies consist of passive mechanical components for guiding and tracking position of an end-fire ultrasound transducer and software to reconstruct the images so that the operator can take biopsies using ultrasound outside of the MRI bore. The use of this technology, initially limited to patients required re-biopsy for rising PSA, is growing. The expense of equipment and availability of technology are the limiting factors.

## Pathology

The vast majority of prostate cancers and the focus of this chapter are adenocarcinomas. Less than 5% of prostate cancers are urothelial or squamous, arising from the urothelium. Rarely, tumors arising from supportive structures including sarcomas, lymphoma, etc., are seen. Neuroendocrine or small-cell carcinomas sometimes occur after prolonged androgen deprivation. A variety of special stains are helpful to the pathologist in differentiating these. Most prostate cancers originate in the peripheral zone and these tumors are generally multifocal.

The aggressiveness of a prostatic adenocarcinoma is reflected in the appearance of the glandular architecture under the low-power microscope. The most commonly used grading system is the Gleason system. A grade from 1 to 5, is assigned to describe the pattern of cancer that is most predominant and a secondary grade is assigned to describe the next most predominant pattern. The total of these two gives the Gleason score. If the specimen is entirely uniform, two scores are reported as the same grade, for example, 4 + 4 = 8. In current practice, grades 1 and 2 are rarely used. Gleason pattern 5 corresponds with high-grade disease with no gland formation, pattern 4 is cribriform and of intermediate aggressiveness. Gleason pattern 3 is low-grade comprised of variable-sized but individual glands. Occasionally, a tertiary grade is assigned. Modifications of this system, which is somewhat historical and entrenched, continue to be proposed [38]. Gleason scores of 7, considered intermediate grade may be 3 predominant and favorable (3 + 4 = 7) or pattern 4 predominant and unfavorable (4 + 3 = 7). The percentage core positivity seen at biopsy is also an important prognostic factor.

The Gleason score correlates well with long-term prognosis, likelihood of positive margins at surgery, and long-term risk of recurrence [39, 40]. In addition, multiple commercially available proprietary gene and biomarker panels may be used to further stratify risk. These are tissue-based tests performed on biopsy or radical prostatectomy specimens. These include the following:

- Decipher™, which predicts 5-year metastasis risk, is used to help determine the need for adjuvant radiation after surgical resection.
- Oncotype DX™ which predicts the likelihood of favorable pathology at radical prostatectomy.
- Prolaris™ which predicts 10-year mortality risk and biochemical recurrence risk.
- ProMark™ which helps identify indolent versus aggressive cancer.

## Staging

The 2017 American Joint Committee on Cancer TMN clinical staging system is presented below. A distinction must be made between clinical staging based on exam and imaging and pathologic stage which requires surgical excision. Modalities to assess lymph nodes, bony and distant metastasis include axial imaging by CT or MRI and bone scan. The primary tumor, T stage, is assessed by digital rectal exam, transrectal ultrasound, and possibly MRI. Guidelines exist to avoid overuse of modalities, for example, bone scan and low-risk disease. In general, staging by imaging is not performed if the Gleason grade is less than 7, and the PSA less than 10 in clinically localized disease.

There is a growing, but undefined role for PET/CT with various prostate and prostate-cancer-targeted radionuclides. These have no defined role in the initial staging of prostate cancer. They are often used to determine if a biochemical recurrence is localized to the prostatic bed and might be amenable to salvage treatments versus widely metastatic and better treated with systemic agents.

## Risk Stratification

The Gleason score, clinical stage, and PSA together are strong predictors of clinical outcomes. These are used in combination to estimate risk and to determine the need for selection of choice of aggressive therapy. There are several available models and nomograms that are used to estimate risk. These include the Partin tables [41], CAPRA score, and the D'Amico classification [42, 43]. These nomograms are helpful to assess the risk of clinical or biochemical treatment failure and the likelihood of surgical margin positivity. Importantly, they are all essentially a graphic based on regression analysis of a specific cohort of patients, and while useful must be applied judiciously. Individual treatment decisions may be influenced by what is felt to be likely on these nomograms, but should not be solely based on the results. They are designed to stratify risk as summarized on the table from the national comprehensive cancer network below.

## Active Surveillance

While treatment options for localized and advanced prostate cancer are discussed in other chapters, it seems fitting to include a brief discussion of active surveillance (AS) here following our discussion of risk stratification. Active surveillance (AS) can be defined as a treatment paradigm offered to certain prostate cancer patients, based on very low, low, or favorable intermediate-risk prostate cancer, who will continue to have screening with PSA, DRE, and MRI, along with subsequent prostate biopsy, in lieu of immediate progression to, or conversion to, more active therapies like surgery or radiation therapy. The numerous techniques for risk assessment including nomograms genetic testing must be combined and individualized before a decision to embark on a program of active surveillance is made.

It should be emphasized that active surveillance is not the absence or avoidance of treatment. AS is a specific protocol for a very close and ongoing patient follow-up to determine the timing of active treatment. While a sizable subset of patients on AS may never require active treatment, the intent is to provide intervention when it is clearly needed and to avoid that treatment while the disease remains low risk. AS must be distinguished from "watchful waiting," which is designed to avoid curative therapy and to ultimately treat symptomatic disease with palliation. Patients on active surveillance are candidates for curative therapy and are monitored to determine when and if that therapy is necessary.

It must be emphasized to patients that low-risk prostate cancer is a progressive, albeit slowly progressive disease. The aim of AS is to avoid overtreatment while preserving options. Strict compliance with follow-up is absolutely essential and AS should not be offered to unreliable patients.

Data on a cohort of 993 patients with low-risk prostatic adenocarcinoma followed in Toronto demonstrated the development of metastatic disease in 2.8% of patients, 1.5% of whom died of prostate cancer. At 5, 10, and 15 years, 75.7%, 63.5%, and 55% of patients, respectively, remained untreated on surveillance [44]. Similar results have been reported by other centers and the national cancer database has reflected a dramatic increase in the use of AS for the initial management of low-risk prostate cancer [45].

Active surveillance typically involves PSA testing every 6 months. A confirmatory biopsy is recommended within 1 year and then no more than annually. Digital rectal exam is recommended every 12 months.

Follow-up prostate biopsies, use of multiparametric MRI, and genomic profiling are used to monitor disease. Regular discussions should be carried out with patients to review options. Triggers for active treatment include significant progression in grade, increase in tumor volume, or the development of palpable disease. PSA elevation is a softer indication but should certainly provoke reevaluation by MRI, biopsy, and, if dramatic, imaging for metastatic disease [46].

There are controversial aspects of active surveillance. Patients with germline mutations, African-American men, patients with a component of Gleason 4 disease, relatively larger volume of disease on biopsy, or high-risk features on multiparametric MRI, are all particularly worrisome. Closer than usual surveillance and shared decision-making are critical in these cases.

**Clinical Pearls**

- The most sensitive test is not always the best. The development of PSA, which allowed early detection of life-threatening cancers and decreased prostate cancer mortality, came at the price of subjecting low-risk prostate cancer patients to diagnostic and therapeutic interventions that may have been unnecessary.
- There is prostate cancer and prostate cancer. Some of your patients will die from this disease. Adenocarcinoma of the prostate is a heterogeneous disease, which varies in aggressiveness from indolent to lethal. A biopsy can be lifesaving in many cases.
- Use your tools. The diagnosis of prostate cancer is still often clinical. A good history and physical will alert you to risk factors for high-risk disease such as race and family history. Think about PSA in the context of PSA history and take the time to dig up old PSA values, which might indicate that a PSA in the normal range is *abnormal* for an individual patient.
- Use the technology. Make best use of newer imaging techniques and understand the newly available serum and tissue markers.

- There is no substitute for good judgment. Decisions to biopsy and decision to treat are difficult. Make use of new technology and molecular markers. Confer with colleagues regarding difficult cases.
- Share decision-making. Try to educate your patients to understand the complexity and uncertainty of many prostate-related issues. Patients are more compliant when they understand that we are doing our best for them in the face of finite knowledge.

## Bibliography


1. Siegel RL, Miller KD, Jemal A. Cancer statistics, 2016. CA Cancer J Clin. 2016;66(1):7–30. https://doi.org/10.3322/caac.21332.
2. Siegel RL, Miller KD, Jemal A. Cancer statistics, 2020. CA Cancer J Clin. 2020;70(1):7–30. https://doi.org/10.3322/caac.21590.
3. Delongchamps NB, Singh A, Haas GP. Epidemiology of prostate cancer in Africa: another step in the understanding of the disease? Curr Probl Cancer. 2007;31:226.
4. Miller BA, Kolonel LN. Racial/ethnic patterns of cancer in the United States, 1988–1992. 1996. books.google.com.
5. Stolzenbach LF, Rosiello G, Deuker M, et al. The impact of race and age on distribution of metastases in patients with prostate cancer. J Urol. 2020; https://doi.org/10.1097/JU.0000000000001131.
6. Bostwick DG, Burke HB, Djakiew D, et al. Human prostate cancer risk factors. Cancer. 2004;101(10 Suppl):2371–490. https://doi.org/10.1002/cncr.20408.
7. Thompson IM. Overdiagnosis and overtreatment of prostate cancer. Am Soc Clin Oncol Educ Book. 2012:e35–9. https://doi.org/10.14694/EdBook_AM.2012.32.98.
8. Chan JM, Jou RM, Carroll PR. The relative impact and future burden of prostate cancer in the United States. J Urol. 2004;172(5 Pt 2):S13–6; discussion S17. https://doi.org/10.1097/01.ju.0000142068.66876.53.
9. Stanford JL, Ostrander EA. Familial prostate cancer. Epidemiol Rev. 2001;23(1):19–23. https://doi.org/10.1093/oxfordjournals.epirev.a000789.
10. Grönberg H, Damber L. Familial prostate cancer in Sweden: a nationwide register cohort study. Cancer. 1996;77:138.
11. Gayther SA, de Foy KAF, Harrington P, Pharoah P. The frequency of germ-line mutations in the breast cancer predisposition genes BRCA1 and BRCA2 in familial prostate cancer. Cancer Res. 2000;60:4513.
12. Crumbaker M, Chan EKF, Gong T, et al. The impact of whole genome data on therapeutic decision-making in metastatic prostate cancer: a retrospective analysis. Cancers (Basel). 2020;12(5):1178. https://doi.org/10.3390/cancers12051178.
13. Giovannucci E, Liu Y, Platz EA, Stampfer MJ, Willett WC. Risk factors for prostate cancer incidence and progression in the health professionals follow-up study. Int J Cancer. 2007;121(7):1571–8. https://doi.org/10.1002/ijc.22788.
14. Wu K, Hu FB, Willett WC, Giovannucci E. Dietary patterns and risk of prostate cancer in U.S. men. Cancer Epidemiol Biomark Prev. 2006;15(1):167–71. https://doi.org/10.1158/1055-9965.EPI-05-0100.
15. Giovannucci E, Tosteson TD, Speizer FE, Ascherio A, Vessey MP, Colditz GA. A retrospective cohort study of vasectomy and prostate cancer in US men. JAMA. 1993;269(7):878–82.
16. Stanford JL, Wicklund KG, McKnight B, Daling JR, Brawer MK. Vasectomy and risk of prostate cancer. Cancer Epidemiol Biomark Prev. 1999;8(10):881–6.

17. Lee F, Littrup PJ, Torp-Pedersen ST, Mettlin C. Prostate cancer: comparison of transrectal US and digital rectal examination for screening. Radiology. 1988;168:389.
18. Schroder FH, Kruger AB, Rietbergen J, et al. Evaluation of the digital rectal examination as a screening test for prostate cancer. J Natl Cancer Inst. 1998;90(23):1817–23. https://doi.org/10.1093/jnci/90.23.1817.
19. Smith DS, Catalona WJ. Interexaminer variability of digital rectal examination in detecting prostate cancer. Urology. 1995;45(1):70–4.
20. Hoogendam A, Buntinx F, de Vet HC. The diagnostic value of digital rectal examination in primary care screening for prostate cancer: a meta-analysis. Fam Pract. 1999;16(6):621–6.
21. Okotie OT, Roehl KA, Han M, Loeb S, Gashti SN, Catalona WJ. Characteristics of prostate cancer detected by digital rectal examination only. Urology. 2007;70(6):1117–20. https://doi.org/10.1016/j.urology.2007.07.019.
22. Flanigan RC, Catalona WJ, Richie JP, et al. Accuracy of digital rectal examination and transrectal ultrasonography in localizing prostate cancer. J Urol. 1994;152(5 Pt 1):1506–9.
23. Sensabaugh GF. Isolation and characterization of a semen-specific protein from human seminal plasma: a potential new marker for semen identification. J Forensic Sci. 1978;23:10659J.
24. Wang MC, Papsidero LD, Kuriyama M, Valenzuela LA, Murphy GP, Chu TM. Prostate antigen: a new potential marker for prostatic cancer. Prostate. 1981;2(1):89–96. https://doi.org/10.1002/pros.2990020109.
25. Loeb S, Carter HB, Schaeffer EM, Kettermann A. Distribution of PSA velocity by total PSA levels: data from the Baltimore Longitudinal Study of Aging. Urology. 2011;77:143.
26. Wright EJ, Fang J, Metter EJ, et al. Prostate specific antigen predicts the long-term risk of prostate enlargement: results from the Baltimore Longitudinal Study of Aging. J Urol. 2002;167(6):2484–7; discussion 2487.
27. Gann PH, Hennekens CH, Stampfer MJ. A prospective evaluation of plasma prostate-specific antigen for detection of prostatic cancer. JAMA. 1995;273(4):289–94.
28. Wu Z-Y, Yang C, Luo J, Deng S-L, Wu B, Chen M. Establishment of reference intervals for serum [-2]proPSA (p2PSA), %p2PSA and prostate health index in healthy men. Onco Targets Ther. 2019;12:6453–60. https://doi.org/10.2147/OTT.S212340.
29. Djavan B, Zlotta A, Kratzik C, et al. PSA, PSA density, PSA density of transition zone, free/total PSA ratio, and PSA velocity for early detection of prostate cancer in men with serum PSA 2.5 to 4.0 ng/mL. Urology. 1999;54(3):517–22. https://doi.org/10.1016/S0090-4295(99)00153-3.
30. Seaman E, Whang M, Olsson CA, Katz A, Cooner WH, Benson MC. PSA density (PSAD). Role in patient evaluation and management. Urol Clin North Am. 1993;20(4):653–63.
31. Catalona WJ, Southwick PC, Slawin KM, et al. Comparison of percent free PSA, PSA density, and age-specific PSA cutoffs for prostate cancer detection and staging. Urology. 2000;56(2):255–60. https://doi.org/10.1016/S0090-4295(00)00637-3.
32. Thompson IM, Chi C, Ankerst DP, et al. Effect of finasteride on the sensitivity of PSA for detecting prostate cancer. J Natl Cancer Inst. 2006;98(16):1128–33. https://doi.org/10.1093/jnci/djj307.
33. Lee F, Torp-Pedersen ST, McLeary RD. Diagnosis of prostate cancer by transrectal ultrasound. Urol Clin North Am. 1989;16(4):663–73.
34. Loeb S, Vellekoop A, Ahmed HU, et al. Systematic review of complications of prostate biopsy. Eur Urol. 2013;64(6):876–92. https://doi.org/10.1016/j.eururo.2013.05.049.
35. Loeb S, Carter HB, Berndt SI, Ricker W, Schaeffer EM. Complications after prostate biopsy: data from SEER-Medicare. J Urol. 2011;186(5):1830–4. https://doi.org/10.1016/j.juro.2011.06.057.
36. Nam RK, Saskin R, Lee Y, et al. Increasing hospital admission rates for urological complications after transrectal ultrasound guided prostate biopsy. J Urol. 2010;183(3):963–8. https://doi.org/10.1016/j.juro.2009.11.043.
37. Hoeks CMA, Barentsz JO, Hambrock T, et al. Prostate cancer: multiparametric MR imaging for detection, localization, and staging. Radiology. 2011;261(1):46–66. https://doi.org/10.1148/radiol.11091822.

38. Epstein JI, Zelefsky MJ, Sjoberg DD, et al. A contemporary prostate cancer grading system: a validated alternative to the Gleason score. Eur Urol. 2016;69(3):428–35. https://doi.org/10.1016/j.eururo.2015.06.046.
39. Egevad L, Granfors T, Karlberg L, Bergh A, Stattin P. Prognostic value of the Gleason score in prostate cancer. BJU Int. 2002;89(6):538–42. https://doi.org/10.1046/j.1464-410x.2002.02669.x.
40. Chan TY, Partin AW, Walsh PC, Epstein JI. Prognostic significance of Gleason score 3+4 versus Gleason score 4+3 tumor at radical prostatectomy. Urology. 2000;56(5):823–7.
41. Partin AW. Commentary RE: contemporary update of prostate cancer staging nomograms (Partin Tables) for the new millennium & Updated Nomogram to Predict Pathologic. Urology. 2020.
42. Zelic R, Garmo H, Zugna D, et al. Predicting prostate cancer death with different pretreatment risk stratification tools: a head-to-head comparison in a nationwide cohort study. Eur Urol. 2019;77:180. https://doi.org/10.1016/j.eururo.2019.09.027.
43. Sargos P, Leduc N, Giraud N, Gandaglia G. Predicting biochemical recurrence after prostatectomy: can machine learning beat CAPRA score? Results of a multicentric retrospective analysis on 4,700 patients. J Clin Oncol. 2020;38:343.
44. Klotz L, Vesprini D, Sethukavalan P, et al. Long-term follow-up of a large active surveillance cohort of patients with prostate cancer. J Clin Oncol. 2015;33(3):272–7. https://doi.org/10.1200/JCO.2014.55.1192.
45. Chipollini J, Pollock GR. National trends in the management of low-risk prostate cancer: analyzing the impact of Medicaid expansion in the United States. Int Urol Nephrol. 2020; https://doi.org/10.1007/s11255-020-02463-5.
46. Albers P, Wiegel T, Schmidberger H, et al. Termination rates and histological reclassification of active surveillance patients with low- and early intermediate-risk prostate cancer: results of the PREFERE trial. World J Urol. 2020; https://doi.org/10.1007/s00345-020-03154-7.
47. Marks L, Young S, Natarajan S. MRI-ultrasound fusion for guidance of targeted prostate biopsy. Curr Opin Urol. 2013;23(1):43–50. https://doi.org/10.1097/MOU.0b013e32835ad3ee.

# Chapter 3
# Monitoring and Managing Men Following Initial Treatment of Prostate Cancer

**Terran W. Sims and Mikel Gray**

## Introduction

In 2018, approximately 174,650 men will be diagnosed with prostate cancer and 31,620 will die because of prostate cancer [1]. Research has shown that men with prostate cancer are living longer following initial treatment. Comparison of cancer-free survival among men undergoing surgery versus radiotherapy is challenging because recurrence is defined differently based on treatment modality. For men undergoing radical prostatectomy as definitive therapy 28–35% will experience a rising prostate-specific antigen (PSA)/biochemical recurrence within 10 years [2, 3]. Similarly, among men managed with radiotherapy for initial treatment, 28–39% will develop a rising PSA/biochemical recurrence within 5 years [4]. Regardless of initial treatment or PSA/biochemical recurrence, 10-year cancer-specific survival rates are 92% for men treated with radical prostatectomy and 92% for radiotherapy with androgen deprivation therapy (ADT), versus for 88% for radiotherapy alone [5].

Monitoring men with prostate cancer may take multiple forms based on the patient's pathology at diagnosis, stage, and primary treatment. Advanced practice providers (APPs) are increasingly playing a key role in the monitoring, management, and treatment of men with prostate cancer following primary intervention. In addition, APPs are providing care for men experiencing recurrence of prostate cancer, and they are using evidence-based guidelines for surveillance of these patients. This chapter will provide an overview of evidence and guideline-based approaches for monitoring and managing men who have completed initial staging and definitive treatment of prostate cancer, including those with recurrent prostate cancer. We will not discuss active surveillance prior to primary therapy or men who are not candidates for primary local therapy due to N1 or widely metastatic disease at initial diagnosis.

T. W. Sims (✉) · M. Gray
University of Virginia, Department of Urology, Charlottesville, VA, USA
e-mail: tws4m@virginia.edu



E. J. Trabulsi et al. (eds.), *Chemotherapy and Immunotherapy in Urologic Oncology*, https://doi.org/10.1007/978-3-030-52021-2_3

## Monitoring Categories

Following the initial treatment of prostate cancer, men can be divided into one of three categories: no evidence of disease, disease status unknown (biochemical recurrence), and evidence of recurrence (measurable disease). Men categorized as having no evidence of disease have undergone surgery or radiation therapy for organ-confined disease, have a serum PSA that is deemed undetectable following surgery, or have a PSA within acceptable limits following radiotherapy over a defined period. Men with persistence or recurrence of cancer after radical prostatectomy have a detectable PSA increasing on two or more measurements [6]. In contrast, men with persistent or recurrence of cancer following radiotherapy have a PSA rise of 2 ng/ml above the nadir achieved after radiation. The Phoenix Consensus goes further and states that men with a rise in PSA above nadir, even if it has not risen 2 ng/ml, should be characterized as recurrent or persistent prostate cancer [4]. Men with a measurable disease have radiographic or biopsy-proven evidence of recurrence.

We searched the literature and identified two evidence-based, national guidelines for surveillance and management of men in these three categories. The National Comprehensive Cancer Network guidelines provide guidance for monitoring after initial management (definitive therapy) and for patients with recurrence [6]. In addition, 2017 guidelines from the American Urological Association (AUA), American Society for Radiation Oncology (ASTRO), and Society of Urologic Oncology (SUO) provide recommendations similar to the NCCN for monitoring men with recurrent disease in their combined guideline on clinically localized prostate cancer [7].

## Monitoring for Biochemical Recurrence

Regardless of definitive treatment, monitoring for persistence or recurrence begins with the measurement of serum PSA. The timing of the first PSA after prostatectomy is based on the knowledge that its half-life is 2.5–3 days [8, 9]. Men with a higher pretreatment PSA may require a longer time period to achieve an undetectable level. The NCCN guidelines do not specify a time frame for measurement of the baseline PSA after initial treatment [6]. Nevertheless, a majority of clinicians obtain a serum PSA 4–6 weeks after surgery, although some delay as long as 12 weeks [8, 9].

Identifying persistence or recurrence of prostate cancer is more challenging following radiotherapy. Unlike men managed with surgery, the PSA will slowly fall to a nadir over a period of as long as 2–3 years, but it rarely falls to an undetectable level and ultimate treatment success is defined as a stable PSA $\geq$1.0 ng/ml [10]. Digital rectal examination (DRE) is also used to monitor for recurrence or persistence unless the PSA value is undetectable. In addition, 10–30% of men will experience a temporary elevation in PSA levels, without evidence of disease recurrence [11, 12]. This bounce in PSA may take up to 18 months to normalize or reach a new nadir. Because of this variability, NCCN guidelines suggest PSA measurement every 3–6 months. However, practice patterns vary widely based on expert opinion and patient's risk factors.

Men defined as having no disease after radical prostatectomy, will undergo PSA measurement every 6–12 months for 5 years, then annually thereafter [6]. In men who are treated with radiotherapy and have an undetectable PSA, the DRE may be omitted. Some providers choose to monitor PSA every 3 months for 1 year following definitive therapy based on surgical pathology or other pretreatment risk factors. These include a pretreatment PSA >10 ng/ml, Gleason score ≥ 8, positive margins, perineural invasion, or positive lymph nodes on surgical pathology.

As noted earlier, differentiation of persistence versus recurrence is influenced by the initial treatment. For men undergoing radical prostatectomy (RP), *biochemical recurrence* is defined as an undetectable PSA after surgery that becomes detectable and subsequently rises on two or more measurements [8, 9]. In contrast, *persistence* is defined as failure of PSA to reach undetectable levels after radical prostatectomy. For men who underwent radiation therapy, persistent and recurrence are often used interchangeably when the PSA rises above nadir following radiation therapy versus failure to reach an acceptable nadir [3].

Men with rising PSA levels following initial surgery or radiation are the second largest group of men with prostate cancer [13]. Prostate-specific antigen doubling time (PSADT) is defined as the number of months needed for serum PSA to increase twofold [13]. It is used as first-line monitoring for recurrence because a change in PSA levels, rather than the absolute baseline value, may be the only manifestation indicating biochemical recurrence. Of the factors used to predict local versus systemic progression, PSADT is essential because it enables providers to differentiate a local disease that may still be curable from a systemic disease that may not. There are multiple nomograms and techniques for measuring PSADT. Nevertheless, all require measurement of more than two PSA values, preferably over a time period of 12 months or greater. A diagnosis of recurrence is not only based on PSADT, it also incorporates findings from chest imaging (chest X-ray or computerized tomography [CT]), abdominopelvic CT or magnetic resonance imaging (MRI), bone imaging (whole-body bone scan), and/or transrectal ultrasound (TRUS) for recurrence [6]. If imaging studies suggest recurrence, prostate bed biopsy may be considered. This principle is based on evidence that a doubling time <12 months is a key indicator for obtaining further diagnostic testing for metastatic disease [13–15].

## Risk Stratification and Additional Testing

Approximately, 15% of men with prostate cancer are considered as high risk for disease progression and metastases [16]. Multiple criteria have been used to identify this subgroup of men. Many providers use the D'Amico et al. taxonomy which has been adopted by the American Urological Association (AUA) [17, 18]. These criteria are clinical T stage ≥cT2c, Gleason score 8–10, or a PSA >20 ng/ml at the time of diagnosis. The NCCN defines high risk as T3a, Gleason score ≥ 8, or PSA ≥ 20 ng/ml, and very high risk as T3b or T4 disease [19]. The Cancer of the Prostate Risk Assessment (CAPRA) score is similar but it incorporates the percentage of positive biopsy scores in its assessment of risk. The shortcoming of these taxonomies is their potential for inaccurate determination of T stage [16].

Patients with biochemical progression and concerning PSADT require further evaluation to detect metastases. This evaluation includes imaging and/or tissue biopsy. The goal of imaging is to detect and characterize metastatic disease in order to select treatment or guide a change in management. Imaging techniques are used to evaluate anatomic or functional parameters. The selection of a specific test is based on risk level, PSADT, age, and general health. While prostate cancer can metastasize anywhere in the body, the most common sites are the lymph nodes, bones, lungs, and liver. The following tests may be used to identify and localize distant metastases in the face of PSA persistence/recurrence: chest X-ray or CT, bone imaging (whole-body bone scan), abdominopelvic CT or MRI, TRUS, C-11 choline or F-18 fluciclovine PET-CT or PET-MRI, molecular assay, or prostate bed biopsy [6]. Understanding the patient's risk level is useful because it helps the clinician to decide which test and in which order to proceed when evaluating disease progression or metastatic disease.

Chest imaging begins with a chest X-ray; it is cost-effective and provides a reasonable screening strategy before considering CT. Findings from the chest X-ray are considered definitive only when it is read as entirely normal. Any abnormality (bone lesions or fractures, concern for nodules, fluid collections, and opacities in the lungs) provides a basis for obtaining a chest CT. In the presence of abnormalities on a chest X-ray, the CT is obtained because it provides definitive cross-sectional imaging needed to identify lesions of concern for metastatic disease. These findings are essential for determining the need for potentially morbid biopsy for histologic confirmation of metastatic disease. Nevertheless, patients at high risk may proceed to chest CT as the initial study.

In addition to chest imaging, abdominopelvic CT or MRI should be performed because they provide a high level of detail for the detection of gross extracapsular disease, nodal disease, or visceral metastases. Typically, providers choose a CT, but an MRI is a viable alternative because of its ability to provide high soft-tissue contrast/characterization and multiparametric image acquisition.

The initial test used for the detection of bony metastases is the whole-body bone scan [6]. A radionuclide tracer (technetium-99-MDP) is injected to identify areas of increased uptake in the bones, implying increased osseous turnover and possible metastatic disease. If the bone scan is negative, but clinical suspicion of bone metastases persists, an F-18 sodium fluoride PET-CT is considered. Similarly, PET-CT or PET-MRI with C-11 choline of F-18 fluciclovine radionuclides may be performed when chest imaging and abdominopelvic CT-MRI do not identify suspected recurrent disease in the nodes, bones, or viscera.

Molecular assays may be completed such as the Decipher Prostate RP® used in treatment decision-making in men who have detectable levels of PSA after radical prostatectomy [20]. Its use is a 2B recommendation from the NCCN Guidelines for postoperative patient treatment decision-making [6]. The tissue obtained from RP is evaluated for active genes that express levels of 22 RNA biomarkers linked to an increased risk for metastatic prostate cancer at 5 years [20]. Decipher® proved robust in differentiating men with an increased risk of metastasis from those without metastasis 5 years after surgery, but its use did not improve outcomes when guiding postoperative treatment planning. Nevertheless, the use of a genomic assay enables providers to engage in shared decision-making of adjuvant versus salvage radiation therapy. Shared decision-making is clinically relevant, given the potential adverse side effects of additional therapy on sexual function, continence, and overall health-related quality of life.

Histologic confirmation is obtained via nodal, soft tissue, or bone biopsy based on findings from cross-sectional imaging suggesting a target for biopsy. Nodal biopsies are usually performed under ultrasonic or CT guidance by an interventional radiologist. Soft tissue biopsy can be performed by an interventional radiologist or pathologist, or a pathology biopsy team based on local resources and institutional practice. Bone biopsies are usually performed by a musculoskeletal radiologic team with expertise in this area.

Transrectal ultrasound or prostate MRI is occasionally used when local recurrence in the prostate bed is suspected. Transrectal ultrasound is a lower cost alternative to MRI; however, its diagnostic accuracy is based on the availability of a skilled ultrasonographer and urologist familiar with this procedure. One or more tissue samples, guided by TRUS, are typically obtained under local anesthesia.

## Evidence of Recurrence

When evidence of persistent (measurable) disease is present in men who underwent radical prostatectomy as definitive therapy, monitoring or treatment is based on evidence of local recurrence versus distant metastases. Local recurrence is defined as evidence of disease in the prostate bed or surrounding tissue. Based on a process of shared decision-making, management options include observation and salvage external beam radiation therapy with or without androgen deprivation therapy (ADT) [6]. In postsurgical patients evaluated for persistent or recurrent PSA whose studies are positive for distant metastasis, choices include observation or ADT with or without external beam radiation therapy to the site of metastases (symptomatic and/or weight-bearing bones). Refer Chap. 10 for a more detailed discussion of salvage therapy.

Unlike patients managed with surgery, PSA levels are not expected to be undetectable following definitive radiation therapy [6]. In this case, biochemical recurrence is defined as PSA persistence/recurrence with or without a positive DRE. Recurrence is defined as an increase in PSA of 2 ng/ml or more above PSA nadir. Evaluation for recurrence should be considered when PSA is increasing, even if the rise above nadir is less than 2 ng/ml, especially for candidates who can be considered for salvage local therapy (otherwise young and healthy men). The initial evaluation is the same as for patients who underwent surgery and have persistent PSA or recurrence. Shared decision-making for treatment is based on candidacy for local therapy (original clinical stage T1/T2, N × N0, life expectancy >10 years, PSA < 10 ng/ml) versus continued observation.

Candidates for local therapy are further categorized based on a positive result of TRUS biopsy or negative findings of imaging studies for distant metastases [6]. Shared decision-making options for this group are observation, radical prostatectomy and pelvic lymph node dissection, cryosurgery, high intensity focused ultrasound, or brachytherapy. Based on the decision to pursue a specific intervention, they are again monitored for progression as described earlier. Alternatively, patients with a negative TRUS biopsy or absence of distant metastases on imaging studies will travel a different pathway. Management options for this group are observation, ADT, or participation in a clinical trial. Observation includes individualized PSA monitoring based on PSADT. Serial cross-sectional or bone imaging intervals are determined based on PSADT and symptoms.

For candidates deemed ineligible for local therapy, their pathway is based on results of cross-sectional CT or MRI and bone imaging, along with PSADT. Treatment options for this group are observation, ADT, or participation in a clinical trial [6]. Treatment varies based on several factors including patient choice and access to community-based resources such as a urologist who offers systemic therapy. Others may receive treatment from a medical oncologist. Refer Chap. 10.

## Conclusion

Men with recurrent prostate cancer are living longer. Since progression occurs over a period of 10 years or more, long-term monitoring is essential. Monitoring men for biochemical or recurrent disease is based on interval measurement of PSA and PSADT. Further diagnostic evaluation is considered when PSADT raises concerns. Additional diagnostic testing allows the patient and the provider to understand when PSA monitoring alone is inadequate because of measurable disease. Monitoring is based on building a trusting relationship and reaching consensus on a plan of care within a framework of shared decision-making. Shared decision-making is based on the need to seek additional diagnostic information that determines the timing of evaluation and treatment ensuring mutually established goals for care.

**Pearls for the Advanced Practice Provider**

- Men with recurrent prostate cancer are living longer and require long-term monitoring.
- Men can be divided into three monitoring categories: no evidence of disease, disease status unknown (biochemical recurrence/persistence), and evidence of recurrence (measurable disease).

- Irrespective of initial treatment, monitoring is based on interval measurement of serum prostate-specific antigen (PSA).
- After RP, serum PSA should be undetectable (often reported as ≤0.01 ng/ml).
- After radiation, serum PSA should reach a nadir of ≤1.0 ng/ml.
- Concern for biochemical recurrence or recurrent disease is based on PSADT.
- Diagnostic testing for metastatic disease includes CT, MRI, bone scan, and PET-CT or PET-MRI.
- Shared decision-making and establishing a trusting, working relationship enhance the patients' experience as they traverse this pathway.

## References

1. American Facts and Figures 2019. https://www.cancer.org/content/dam/cancer-org/research/cancer-facts-and-statistics/annual-cancerfacts-and-figures/2019/cancer-facts-and-figures-2019.pdf accessed July 13,2020.
2. Freedland SJ, Humphreys EB, Mangold LA, Eisenberger M, Dorey FJ, Walsk PC, et al. Risk of prostate cancer-specific mortality following biochemical recurrence after radical prostatectomy. JAMA. 2005;294:433–9.
3. Zaorsky NG, Raj GV, Trabulsi EJ, Lin J, Den RB. The dilemma of a rising prostate-specific antigen level after local therapy: what are our options? Semin Oncol. 2013;40(3):322–36.
4. Roach M 3rd, Hanks G, Thames H Jr, et al. Defining biochemical failure following radiotherapy with or without hormonal therapy in men with clinically localized prostate cancer of the RTOG-ASTRO Phoenix Consensus Conference. Int J Radiat Oncol Biol Phys. 2006;65(4):965–74.
5. Boorjian SA, Karnes RJ, Viterbo R, et al. Long–term survival after radical prostatectomy versus external-beam radiotherapy for patients with high-risk prostate cancer. Cancer. 2011;117(13):2883–91.
6. National Comprehensive Cancer Network Clinical Practice Guidelines in Oncology (NCCN Guidelines) Prostate Cancer, Version 4.2018-August 15, 2018. Accessed 11 Nov 2018. PROS C. PROS F, PROS 10Y, 12s, 11 hh.
7. Sanda MG, Chen RC, Crispoino T, Freedland S, Greene K, Klotz LH et al. Clinically Localized Prostate cancer: AUA/ASTRO/SUO Guideline. Journel of Urology. 2018;199(3):683–90. https://www.auajournals.org/doi/10.1016/j.juro.2017.11.095.
8. Partin AW, Oesterling JE. The clinical usefulness of prostate specific antigen: update 1994. J Urol. 1994;152(5 Pt 1):1358–68.
9. Lange PH, Ercole CJ, Lightner DJ, et al. The value of serum prostate specific antigen determinations before and after radical prostatectomy. J Urol. 1989;141(940):873–9.
10. Sandler HM, Dunn RL, Mclaughlin PW, et al. Overall survival after prostate-specific-antigen-detected recurrence following conformal radiation therapy. Int J Radiat Oncol Biol Phys. 2000;48(3):629–33.
11. Critz FA, Williams WH, Benton JB, et al. Prostate specific antigen bounce after radioactive seed implantation followed by external beam radiation for prostate cancer. J Urol. 2000;163(4):1085–9.
12. Cavanagh W, Blasko JC, Grimm PD, Sylvester JE. Transient elevation of serum prostate-specific antigen following (125)I/(103) Pd brachytherapy for localized prostate cancer. Semin Urol Oncol. 2000;18(920):160–5.

13. Vickers AJ, NIH Public Access, et al. PSA velocity and doubling time in diagnosis and prognosis of prostate cancer. Br J Med Surg Urol. 2012;5(4):162–8. https://doi.org/10.1016/j.bjmsu.2011.08.006.
14. Slovin SF, Wilton AS, Heller G, Scher HI. Time to detectable metastatic disease in patients with rising prostate-specific antigen values following surgery or radiation therapy. Clin Cancer Res. 2005;11(24):8669–71.
15. Klayton TL, Ruth K, Buyyounouski MK, Uzzo RG, Wong YN, Chen DY, et al. PSA doubling time predicts for the development of distant metastases for patient who fail 3DCRT or IMRT using the phoenix definition. Pract Radiat Oncol. 2011;1(4):235–42.
16. Chang AJ, Autio KA, Roach M III, Scher IS. "High-risk" prostate cancer: classification and therapy. Nat Rev Clin Oncol. 2014;11(8):308–23.
17. D'Amico AV, et al. Biochemical outcome after radical prostatectomy, external beam radiation therapy or interstitial radiation therapy for clinically localized prostate cancer. JAMA. 1988;280:969/74.
18. Thompson I, Thrasher JB, Aus G, Burnett AL, Canby-Hagino ED, Cookson MS, et al. Guideline for the management of clinically localized prostate cancer: 2007 update. J Urol. 2007;177(6):2106–31. https://doi.org/10.1016/j.juro.2007.03.003.
19. Cooperberg MR, Pasta DJ, Elkin EP, The University of California, San Francisco, et al. Cancer of the prostate risk assessment score: a straightforward and reliable preoperative predictor of disease recurrence after radical prostatectomy. J Urol. 2005;173:1938–4.
20. Marrone M, Potosky AL, Penson D, Freedman AN. A 22 gene –expression assay, Decipher ® (GenomeDX Biosciences) to predict five-year risk of metastatic prostate cancer in men treated with radical prostatectomy. PLoS Curr. 2015;7. https://doi.org/10.1371/currents.eogt.761b81608129ed61b0b42c04f92ae.

# Chapter 4
# Radical Prostatectomy and Survivorship After Radical Prostatectomy

**Courtney C. Anderson and Kurt A. McCammon**

## Radical Prostatectomy

The optimal approach to prostate cancer treatment has been and continues to be debated in the field of medicine based on the plethora of variables that are factored into the treatment equation. Grade and stage of tumor, patient age and life expectancy, treatment success rates and associated complications, as well as patient and clinician preferences all contribute to treatment decisions. Clinically localized prostate cancer may be treated with radical prostatectomy (RP); radiation therapy (external beam radiation therapy and/or brachytherapy); cryotherapy; or, potentially, active surveillance. Weighing the patient characteristics and preference, tumor classification, and surgeon experience will yield different approaches for different patients. Occasionally, a combined modality approach is recommended.

In order to engage in a discussion about RP, it is important to first understand the difference between active surveillance and observation (or watchful waiting). This is an important distinction to make, as many of the clinical trials researching the efficacy of RP compare it to observation, as opposed to another active treatment approach or active surveillance. Simply stated, active surveillance is considered a treatment strategy offered to men with low-risk prostate cancer wherein the patient is not initially treated with definitive therapy but rather is monitored for disease progression and, if detected, offered definitive therapy at that time. Any treatment undertaken is usually aimed to cure the cancer. The benefit of this delayed treatment approach is minimization of treatment-related morbidity. Observation/watchful waiting, on the other hand, is a way of monitoring prostate cancer with the aim of any potential treatment being to control, not cure, the cancer. This approach is usually suitable for men with other comorbidities, who may be less able to cope with surgical treatments or who have a decreased life expectancy. When RP was

C. C. Anderson (✉) · K. A. McCammon
Department of Urology, Eastern Virginia Medical School, Norfolk, VA, USA
e-mail: anderscc@evms.edu; MccammKA@evms.edu



E. J. Trabulsi et al. (eds.), *Chemotherapy and Immunotherapy in Urologic Oncology*, https://doi.org/10.1007/978-3-030-52021-2_4

compared with watchful waiting, it was found to afford patients an improved overall survival (lower incidence of death from all causes as well as death from prostate cancer) and/or decrease local, regional, or systemic disease progression. The benefits were more pronounced in patients younger than 65 at the time of diagnosis as well as in those with intermediate risk. As such, radical prostatectomy has been the reference standard for treatment of localized prostate cancer for several decades.

Hugh Hampton Young performed the first radical perineal prostatectomy in 1904 at Johns Hopkins Hospital in Baltimore, Maryland. Forty-one years later, in 1945, Terence Millin described the first retropubic approach. Yet, despite the fact that surgeons had successfully found a way to access the prostate, the open procedure remained an unpopular choice for treatment due to its complication rates. It was not until the early 1990s that the new era of prostate surgery emerged, and over the past three decades, we have seen momentous advances in prostatectomy techniques. The first laparoscopic prostatectomy was performed in 1991 and the use of robotic assistance followed a short time thereafter in 2000. At present, various surgical approaches for RP are utilized, namely, open versus minimally invasive techniques. Open RPs can be approached retropubically or perineally. Minimally invasive approaches involve laparoscopy and often include robotic assistance nowadays. The last three decades have also yielded significant enhancement in our understanding of prostate anatomy, which, in turn, has led to additional changes in surgical dissection techniques, thereby improving postoperative functional outcomes. Specifically, preservation of prostate vascular supply and neurovascular bundle anatomy have been emphasized in the context of post-RP outcomes. A wide range of nerve-sparing techniques are described and, at present, several dissection planes are recognized, contributing to varying "degrees" of nerve-sparing procedures (incremental nerve-sparing approaches) [1].

Currently in the United States, robotic-assisted laparoscopic and open retropubic approaches are the most commonly performed RP procedures. It is estimated that 75% of all prostatectomies performed in the United States are currently done so robotically [2]. The American Urological Association (AUA), American Society for Radiation Oncology (ASTRO), and Society of Urologic Oncology (SUO) jointly sponsored a practice guideline in 2017, which considered open and robotic-assisted radical prostatectomy (RARP) similar in terms of cancer control, continence recovery, and sexual function. In addition to these functional outcomes, surgical-related complications have also been studied. Intraoperative complications for RP include blood loss, rectal/bowel injury, ureteral/bladder injury, and damage to the obturator nerve. Perioperative risks associated with RP include deep venous thrombosis, pulmonary embolism, urethrovesical anastomotic leak, lymphocele formation, and wound infection. Late complications are considered to be urinary incontinence and erectile dysfunction, both of which are discussed below. Initial research suggested that minimally invasive techniques do not confer any lower risk of complications as compared to the open approach, but more recent studies have found a statistically significant reduction in cardiac and respiratory events in laparoscopic RP and RARP patients, suggesting perhaps that increased surgeon experience with minimally invasive techniques is a

**Table 4.1** Disease-free survival rates based on Gleason score following RP

| Gleason score | 10-year disease-free survival rates |
|---|---|
| 2–6 | >70% |
| 7 | 50% |
| >8 | 15% |

contributing factor [3]. Although RARP is also associated with decreased blood loss and postoperative length of hospital stay, positive surgical margin rates and short-term biochemical progression-free rates appear similar with the open technique. In terms of cost, RARP remains the most expensive surgical approach to treat prostate cancer.

Overall disease-free survival rates following RP are correlated with the extent and grade of the tumor itself. Those patients with organ-confined disease have a 10-year disease-free survival rate of 70–85% following RP. Those with focal extracapsular extension had disease-free survival of 85% at year 5 and 75% at year 10 postoperatively. As expected, patients with more extensive extracapsular extension have worse results (70% 5-year disease-free survival and 40% 10-year disease-free survival). Higher grade tumors (Gleason score > 7) are associated with faster risk of progression (Table 4.1) [4].

Determining whether or not pelvic lymph node dissection needs to occur in conjunction with RP is driven by the risk of regional lymph node involvement, which is gauged by T stage, serum PSA, and Gleason score. Nomograms exist for determining the likelihood of lymph node involvement and can guide patient discussion. Significant variation exists in pelvic lymph node dissection practice patterns by surgeons and institutions. Although the overall impacts of lymph node dissection on perioperative complications and postoperative functional outcomes are debated, patients should be made aware that there is a potential impact on urinary continence, erectile function, and increased risk for vascular injury and postoperative lymphoceles.

Patients treated with RP are restaged thereafter based upon the pathological extent of disease detected in the surgical resection specimen. This pathologic staging offers useful information for counseling a patient on his prognosis as well as guiding future therapy. Postoperative PSA levels should become and remain undetectable following RP. Biochemical recurrence identified by rising PSA warrants multimodal treatment.

## Survivorship after Radical Prostatectomy

Due to advanced screening practices, it is common for increasingly younger patients to be diagnosed with prostate cancer; as such, both urinary continence and erectile function are of growing importance in the postsurgical patient population. It is vital for members of the oncologic team to appropriately educate patients and their families preoperatively on reasonable expectations for short-term and long-term effects of surgery on activity level, continence, and sexual function so as to preserve patients' quality of life.

## *Urinary Recovery*

Assessing the incidence of postprostatectomy incontinence (PPI) has proven quite difficult, given the lack of standardized definition of "incontinence" as well as the varying reporting sources (surgeon reports vs patient self-reporting). To some, the term incontinence reflects any degree of leakage no matter how inconsistent or how small the quantity. To others, it is defined as leakage which requires the daily use of at least one pad or more, thereby eliminating those patients with sporadic or small volume leakage not necessitating pad use. As such, reported incontinence rates following RP range from <1% to 87% in the literature and may include stress urinary incontinence (SUI) as well as overactive bladder (OAB)/urge incontinence. Most often, the outcomes of interest are daily pad use and quality of life impact. Relying on surgeon- and institution-specific continence rates is useful when educating preoperative patients on the potential sequelae surrounding RP. Discussing both the natural history of incontinence after RP as well as contributing factors to poor continence recovery are essential in the weeks preceding surgery, as these topics provide the patient with realistic expectations regarding their postoperative status.

Prostatectomy candidates must be aware that the vast majority of RP patients experience mild to severe leakage immediately following catheter removal post-RP. The degree of leakage experienced varies based on several patient, surgeon, and procedural risk factors (Table 4.2). The older the patient, the larger the prostate size, and the shorter the membranous urethral length all increase a patient's risk for postoperative incontinence. The current literature suggests that open prostatectomy rates of SUI range from 7% to 40% and laparoscopic and RARP continence rates are similar at 4–34% [5]. In the case of salvage prostatectomy following radiation, 50% of the patients experience leakage.

Although incontinence can persist for months, there is a rapid decrease in leakage noted during the first 18 weeks following RP [6]. Thereafter, patients continue to improve up to 1 year, with greater than 90% having minimal leakage at that time. A small number of patients (1%) continued to note improvement in their continence status between 12 and 24 months postprostatectomy [7]. In the 5–10% of men who

**Table 4.2** Risk factors affecting continence rates following radical prostatectomy

| Preoperative factors | Intraoperative factors | Postoperative factors |
|---|---|---|
| Age | Surgical technique | Anastomotic stricture |
| Preoperative continence status | Surgeon's experience level | Postoperative radiation |
| | Membranous urethral length | |
| | Prostate size | |

continue to experience postprostatectomy incontinence at 12 months post-RP, there is a huge impact on quality of life.

Using analysis from the Cancer of the Prostate Strategic Urologic Research Endeavor (CaPSURE), patients tended to self-report better urinary function in the first year after open prostatectomy, as compared to those patients undergoing robot-assisted prostatectomy. However, there were no significant differences in urinary incontinence between the two techniques at 2 and 3 years postoperatively [8].

In the initial evaluation of post-RP incontinence, a thorough history can uncover various aspects, which contribute to the patient's leakage. Characterizing the aforementioned risk factors as well as the severity and type of the patient's incontinence is of paramount importance. Experts commonly use "pads per day" (PPD) nomenclature to define a patient's degree of leakage. Nitti et al. established that daily pad usage correlates well with the severity of incontinence, usually falling into one of three broad domains: mild (1–2 PPD), moderate (3–5 PPD), or severe (>5 PPD or requiring the use of an external catheter) [9]. Knowing whether the patient's leakage is activity-related (stress) or urgency-related (OAB) can be crucial in determining effective treatment options for the patient. Additionally, various psychometric tools can be used to assess degree of bother and provide a more objective framework for comparing the impact of incontinence both before and after treatment. Some examples of these assessments are International Consultation on Incontinence Questionnaire – Urinary Incontinence (ICIQ-UI); UCLA-Rand Health Survey; and Urogenital Distress Inventory (UDI).

In addition to a detailed history, the patient's post void residual (PVR) should be assessed. If consistently elevated, further evaluation via cystourethroscopy and UDS is warranted to rule out urethral obstruction from stricture disease and/or detrusor underactivity. Other indications for the use of UDS in the work-up of post-RP incontinence include those patients at risk for poor detrusor compliance, such as those with radiation cystitis or neurogenic lower urinary tract dysfunction.

The presence of bothersome OAB symptoms (urinary urgency, frequency, and urge urinary incontinence) should be identified and treated at any time following RP according to the AUA Guidelines on OAB [10]. Treatment options for postprostatectomy SUI span the spectrum from conservative therapy (including lifestyle interventions and physiotherapy) to surgical interventions (Table 4.3). In general, the more invasive the treatment, the higher the success rates, but the greater the adverse events. Conservative options for treatment include absorbent pads, penile

**Table 4.3** Postprostatectomy incontinence treatment options

| Intervention | Examples |
|---|---|
| Supportive devices | Clamps, external catheters, pads/briefs |
| Physiotherapy | Kegel exercises, PFMT, biofeedback |
| Medications | Approved for SUI: None |
| | For OAB: Antimuscarinics, B3 agonist, OnabotulinumtoxinA |
| Injectable bulking agents | Coaptite®, Macroplastique®, Durasphere® |
| Surgery | Artificial urinary sphincter (AUS), male slings |

compression devices (clamps), and appropriately sized external catheters. These options may be used in conjunction with pelvic floor muscle training (PFMT) efforts. No approved pharmacotherapy for SUI exists for treatment of PPI in the United States; however, OAB symptoms can be treated with antimuscarinics or a B3-agonist. The artificial urinary sphincter (AUS) has been the therapeutic gold standard for treatment of post-RP SUI for many years.

Typically, surgical treatment of SUI is recommended at 12 months post-RP if initial conservative treatment strategies fail [11]. In that 12-month interval following RP, most providers agree that patients should attempt PFMT. Various studies have sought to determine the efficacy of early PFMT post-RP. Unfortunately, the heterogeneity of these studies and the varying definition of incontinence make it extremely difficult to compare results. Currently, there is no compelling evidence as to the appropriate timeframe or specific modalities used to teach and reinforce PFMT. A randomized controlled trial of RP patients revealed no statistical difference in return to continence between the group that started PFMT 3 weeks before RP and the control group, which started PFPT postoperatively [12]. Despite that finding, many patients and physical therapists, alike, feel that preoperative education on PFMT is less arduous given the lack of leakage and enhanced sensation. What is clear, however, is that there is a faster return to continence in those patients who employ PFMT techniques in the early postoperative period (once the urethral catheter has been removed). After 1 year, there was no statistical significance between the continence rates of those patients who utilized PFMT and those who did not [13, 14]. Ultimately, there was an improvement in symptoms regardless of management.

The decision to progress to surgical treatment of post-RP SUI should be a combined decision made by the patient and treating urologist. Knowledge of the overall success rates, dry rates, and potential complication rates should be clearly communicated to the patient, thereby facilitating shared decision-making (Table 4.4).

Injectable bulking agents should not be considered a first-line treatment for PPI based on the low success rate. Their use is restricted to patients who cannot tolerate or refuse more invasive surgical options. However, in men with persistent, mild incontinence following sling placement, bulking agents can be utilized at the area of coaptation with relatively good results [15].

Mild to moderate incontinence (quantified at 1–4 pads per day) can effectively be treated with the male sling. Advantageous based on its safety profile and lack of mechanical components, the AdVance sling (Boston Scientific) is the most

**Table 4.4** Outcomes associated with surgical treatment of post-RP SUI

| | Injectable bulking agents | Male sling | AUS |
|---|---|---|---|
| Success rate | 15–23% | 75% | 90–94% |
| Dry rate | <10% after single injection | 45–50% | 60% |
| Infection rate | | 1% | 2–4% |
| Erosion rate | | <1% | 8.5% |
| Mechanical failure | n/a | n/a | 3–6% |

frequently used transobturator urethral sling worldwide for the treatment of PPI. Its mechanism of action involves relocating the posterior urethra and the sphincter region into its original (pre-RP) position, thereby increasing the venous sealing effect and increasing the functional urethral length. Patients note an immediate benefit following sling placement and subsequent catheter removal. Recent studies with follow-up 3 years post-sling revealed a cure rate of 60% and at least 50% improvement noted in another 13% of patients [16]. Cure rates vary between 9% and 63% up to 40 months [17]. Newer generation slings have been marketed outside the United States but are not currently available for use in the US (Advance XP). Adjustable male slings have also been introduced abroad, but there has been no evidence that adjustability of a sling offers any tangible benefit for the patient in terms of QOL outcomes or overall cure rate [11].

In patients with moderate to severe PPI, circumferential occlusion of the urethra is necessary in order to completely coapt the urethral lumen and prevent the undesired flow of urine. In the United States, the perineal artificial urinary sphincter (AUS) is the established standard in the treatment of moderate to severe PPI. First introduced in 1972, the AUS has been modified several times to create its current model. At present, the AMS 800 (Boston Scientific/American Medical Systems) is by far the most commonly used device, accounting for approximately 70–80% of the market. This implantable device consists of three components: an inflatable cuff, a pressure-regulating balloon, and a control pump. Once the device is surgically placed, the patient must squeeze the pump several times in order to transfer the fluid from the urethral cuff to the reservoir, thereby releasing the pressure on the urethra and allowing urine to flow. A refill-delay resistor keeps the cuff open, allowing sufficient time for voiding. Approximately 60–90 seconds after the initial cycling, the cuff will reinflate and compress the urethra. There is a deactivation button that allows the cuff to be locked in the open position, if needed. Published literature indicates the efficacy of the AMS 800 to approach 90% with high patient satisfaction rates [18].

Based on the recommendations from the AUS Consensus Group in 2015, an AUS should be "considered no earlier than 6 months after prostatectomy in patients presenting with sufficient dexterity and cognitive function to operate the device" [19]. Typically, placement is via the perineal approach. Patients will need to limit physical activity for 4–6 weeks postoperatively. The device is activated 4–6 weeks after its implantation. Complications can include infection (1–8%), urethral erosion (8.5%), urethral atrophy (7.9%), and mechanical failure (6.2%) [20]. The most common cause for urethral erosion is placement of an indwelling urethral catheter, usually for another reason, such as during an orthopedic procedure. If a catheter must be placed in a patient with an AUS, it should be done using the smallest possible catheter size for the shortest time possible (ideally less than 48 hours) with the artificial sphincter in the inactivated/open position. Prolonged bladder drainage in a post-AUS patient necessitates suprapubic tube placement to minimize the risk of urethral erosion [19].

In terms of the lifespan of an AUS, Linder et al. reported an AUS device survival rate of 90% at 1 year, 74% at 5 years, 57% at 10 years, and 41% at 15 years [21].

Radiated patients should be aware that they constitute a high-risk population with increased adverse outcomes and associated complications, such as an increased risk of erosion. Adjusted improvement rates for radiated patients approach 66% following AUS placement.

In the case of both the male sling and AUS, coexisting OAB should be treated preoperatively according to AUA guidelines and is not considered a contraindication for either procedure.

## *Sexual Recovery*

Much like post-RP incontinence, some degree of erectile dysfunction should be expected postoperatively but, with nerve-sparing approaches in younger patients with no pre-existing ED, the loss of sexual function should be temporary. Despite our advances in the realm of surgical anatomy of the prostate as well as development of minimally invasive surgical techniques, the incidence of patient-reported post-RP ED ranges from 65% to 85% with spontaneous recovery of baseline erectile function only occurring in 30% of patients following RP [22, 23]. Factors that influence the severity and duration of postoperative ED include type of surgery, patient age at time of surgery, and preoperative sexual function/satisfaction (including the presence of depression preoperatively). Additionally, overall vascular risk factors such as hypertension, hypercholesterolemia, DM, coronary disease, and cigarette smoking were deemed independent predictors of decreased erectile function at 3 years post-RP, regardless of nerve-sparing status and baseline erectile function [24].

CaPSURE data reveals no significant differences in sexual function at any time point based on open versus robotic-assisted techniques utilized. However, other studies indicate that there is a faster return to potency in RARP patients, as compared to patients undergoing open RP. Nerve-sparing approaches are known to influence postoperative sexual recovery. In the case of bilateral nerve-sparing techniques, potency rates approach 70–80%, as opposed to potency rates in unilateral nerve-sparing techniques, which are closer to 50–60% [25]. Neuropraxia and tissue injury can occur during RP regardless of a nerve-sparing approach; thus, it should be expected that there is an immediate postoperative period of absent penile response under all stimulatory conditions. When the cavernous nerves are spared, patients note a gradual recovery of erectile function over many months, ranging from 12 to 36 months after surgery [26]. Time of erection recovery does not uniformly occur in all cases. Studies have shown that patients able to achieve a spontaneous or PDE5-inhibitor-assisted functional erection within 3 months of RP have a favorable prognosis of return to potency [27]. With that being said, the older the patient at the time of RP, the less likely his potency will return to baseline status, especially over the age of 60. At 36 months postoperatively, 70% of men less than 60 years old at the time of surgery demonstrate recovered erectile function. That number declines to

45% of 60–65 year olds and only 30% of those men >65 years old [28]. When surgical techniques require a wide excision of locally advanced prostate cancer or nerve-sparing attempts are inadequate, the expectation should be unrecoverable loss of erectile function.

To facilitate in the assessment of degree of impact from ED, providers may use validated questionnaires such as the Erection Hardness Score (EHS), Sexual Health Inventory for Men (SHIM), or the more-detailed International Index of Erectile Function (IIEF) [29–31]. These instruments can also help gauge treatment effectiveness. As such, it can prove very useful to have preoperative RP patients complete one of these psychometric tools so as to establish baseline erectile function.

Treatment options for post-RP ED include psychosocial support (which has proven highly beneficial in the immediate postoperative period), oral phosphodiesterase 5 inhibitors, vacuum erection devices, intracavernosal injections, or penile prostheses. At the time of publication, low intensity extracorporeal shock wave therapy and intracavernosal stem cell therapy are considered investigational in the treatment of ED.

Penile rehabilitation strategies can be used to promote corporal circulation in the postoperative period. Typically, penile rehab protocols involve the use of oral phosphodiesterase 5 inhibitors (PDE5-i) postoperatively. Interestingly, however, randomized controlled clinical trials failed to demonstrate that PDE5-i use within the first 45 days post-RP improved unassisted erectile function. In fact, there was no difference in erectile function between men using PDE5-i and those taking a placebo in the early postoperative period; moreover, the use of PDE5-i did not increase the utility of on-demand erection medications in the future [32]. For these reasons, there is no clear indication for a particular post-RP penile rehabilitation protocol.

Just as in the general ED population, post-RP patients experience a similar efficacy between sildenafil, tadalafil, and vardenafil. Due to its more recent entry into the market, avanafil has limited data in the post-RP population. Despite the comparability between the various PDE5-inhibitors, the overall success rate in men using oral pharmacotherapy status post-RP is much lower than in the general population (30% and 60%, respectively) [33]. Interestingly, men post-RP reported higher rates of side effects than their counterparts in the general ED population. This was particularly the case with sildenafil in regards to headache and flushing. It is not known whether post-RP patients actually have more side effects from these medications or if they are simply more likely to report adverse events. Based on American Urological Association (AUA) Guidelines, treatment with PDE5-i is better than doing nothing but there is no solid evidence that a specific drug or even daily vs on-demand therapy is more advantageous [32].

Some patients may inquire about the risk of prostate cancer recurrence as a result of PDE5-i use. Initial studies did postulate that PDE5-i use was an independent risk factor for prostate cancer recurrence in men with localized disease who underwent RP, but subsequent studies have revealed no increased risk associated with recurrence in men who use PDE5-i post-RP [32].

In those patients who do not desire, do not respond to, or cannot tolerate oral pharmacotherapy, vacuum erection devices (VED), medicated urethral system for erections (MUSE), or intracavernosal injections (ICIs) can be considered. VEDs have been on the market since the 1960s and offer a noninvasive, non-pharmacologic option for treatment of ED. Studies on VED use in post-RP men indicate a high patient and partner satisfaction rate, with over 80% of users achieving an erection sufficient for intercourse [34]. The combined use of PDE5-i and VED further increased the ability to achieve a usable erection [35]. However, long-term use of a VED is low, as only 40% of users continue this modality as their primary form of treatment of ED after 1 year. Potential transient side effects associated with VED use include penile bruising, discomfort, loss of sensitivity, inhibited ejaculation, or difficulty with the device. Although more invasive, ICI use has higher outcome measures in observational studies, including satisfactory erections. Various injectable medications can be used, including combinations of the following: alprostadil, papaverine, phentolamine, and atropine. Once appropriately dosed in the office, a patient can then self-inject a specified amount of medication in the corpus carvernosa of the penis to produce an erection at that time in which it is desired. Despite the fact that different medications lead to similar rates of successful intercourse, their adverse profiles differ. Specifically, pain was greatest in men who used papaverine (pain with injection) and alprostadil (pain with erection) [32]. Other potential side effects of all ICI medications include priapism, injection site hematoma, penile fibrosis/plaque, or deformity.

Once other treatments for post-RP ED have been offered, implantation of a penile prosthesis may be discussed. Currently, there are several devices available including malleable (noninflatable options) as well as two- or three-piece inflatable prostheses. Inherent in any surgical procedure are risks. In addition to general surgical adverse events, placement of a penile prosthesis incurs the additional risks of infection (typically within the first 3 months after surgery), erosion, and mechanical failure. Once a penile prosthesis is placed, the likelihood of response to any of the aforementioned treatment options for ED is very low, even if the prosthesis is subsequently removed. Thus, this treatment option should be considered as one of last resort. However, satisfaction rates approach 95% in men with inflatable prostheses and 75% in men with malleable (noninflatable) prostheses. Partner satisfaction rates were similar [32, 36]. Moreover, 98% of patients with an inflatable penile prosthesis continue to find it suitable for intercourse after 5 years. Despite these high efficacy rates, only 0.78% of patients treated with either RP or radiation therapy eventually receive a penile implant [37].

In patients suffering from both PPI and post-RP ED who desire surgical intervention for both conditions, a combined surgical procedure involving placement of an AUS and penile prosthesis can be offered. Complication rates for these individual procedures are not increased for the combined surgical procedure and the cost of a combined procedure is significantly less than two separate procedures [38].

**Pearls for the Advanced Practice Provider**

- Open and robotic-assisted radical prostatectomies are similar in terms of cancer control, continence recovery, and sexual function.
- Overall disease-free survival rates following radical prostatectomy are correlated with the extent and grade of the tumor itself.
- The vast majority of radical prostatectomy patients experience mild to severe urinary leakage immediately following catheter removal postoperatively.

  Most patients note a rapid decrease in urinary incontinence during the first 4 months following surgery; thereafter, patients continue to improve up to 1 year.
- Daily pad usage correlates well with the severity of incontinence, usually falling into one of three broad domains: mild (1–2 PPD), moderate (3–5 PPD), or severe (>5 PPD or requiring the use of external catheter).
- Surgical treatment of urinary stress incontinence is recommended at 12 months postradical prostatectomy if initial conservative treatment strategies fail.
- Factors that influence the severity and duration of postoperative erectile dysfunction include type of surgery, patient age at the time of surgery, and preoperative sexual function/satisfaction (including presence of depression preoperatively).
- When the cavernous nerves are spared, patients note a gradual recovery of erectile function over many months, ranging from 12 to 36 months after surgery.
- Treatment options for postprostatectomy erectile dysfunction include psychosocial support, oral phosphodiesterase 5 inhibitors, vacuum erection devices, intracavernosal injections, or penile prostheses.

## Works Cited

1. Capogrosso P, Salonia A, Briganti A, Montorsi F. Postprostatectomy erectile dysfunction: a review. World J Mens Health. 2016;34(2):73–88.
2. Lowrance WT, Eastham JA, Savage C, et al. Contemporary open and robotic radical prostatectomy practice patterns among urologists in the United States. J Urol. 2012;187(6):2087–92.
3. Trinh QD, Sammon J, Sun M, et al. Perioperative outcomes of robot-assisted radical prostatectomy compared with open radical prostatectomy: results from the nationwide inpatient sample. Eur Urol. 2012;61:679–85.
4. Cooperberg MR, Presti JC Jr, Shinohara K, Carroll PR. Chapter 23. Neoplasms of the prostate gland. In: JW MA, Lue TF, editors. Smith and Tanagho's general urology. New York: McGraw-Hill; 2013.
5. Crivellaro S, Morlacco A, Bodo G, et al. Systematic review of surgical treatment of post radical prostatectomy stress urinary incontinence. Neurourol Urodynam. 2016;35:875–81.
6. Smither AR, Guralnick ML, Davis NB, See WA. Quantifying the natural history of post-radical prostatectomy incontinence using objective pad test data. BMC Urol. 2007;7:2.

7. Choo MS, Choi WS, Cho SY, Ku JH, Kim HH, Kwak C. Impact of prostate volume on oncological and functional outcomes after radical prostatectomy: robot-assisted laparoscopic versus open retropubic. Korean J Urol. 2013;54(1):15–21.
8. Herlemann A, Cowan JE, Carroll PR, Cooperberg MR. Community-based outcomes of open versus robot-assisted radical prostatectomy. Eur Urol. 2018;73(2):215–23.
9. Nitti VW, Mourtzinos A, Brucker BM. Correlation of patient perception of pad use with objective degree of incontinence measured by pad test in men with post-prostatectomy incontinence: the SUFU pad test study. J Urol. 2014;192(3):836–42.
10. Gormley EA, Lightner DJ, Faraday M, Vasavada SP, American Urological Association, Society Of Urodynamics FPM. Diagnosis and treatment of overactive bladder (non-neurogenic) in adults: AUA/SUFU guideline amendment. J Urol. 2015;193:1572–80.
11. Lucas MG, Bosch RJ, Burkhard FC, et al. EAU guidelines on surgical treatment of urinary incontinence. Eur Urol. 2012;62:1118–29.
12. Geraerts I, Van Poppel H, Devoogdt N, et al. Influence of preoperative and postoperative pelvic floor muscle training (PFMT) compared with postoperative PFMT on urinary incontinence after radical prostatectomy: a randomized controlled trial. Eur Urol. 2013;64:766–72.
13. Filocamo MT, Li Marzi V, Del Popolo G. Effectiveness of early pelvic floor rehabilitation treatment for post-prostatectomy incontinence. Eur Urol. 2005;48:734–8.
14. Anderson CA, Omar MI, Campbell SE, et al. Conservative management for postprostatectomy urinary incontinence. Cochrane Database Syst Rev. 2015;1:CD001843.
15. Chung ASJ, Suarez OA, McCammon KA. Advance male sling. Transl Androl Urol. 2017;6(4):674–81.
16. Kowalik CG, DeLong JM, Mourtzinos AP. The advance transobturator male sling for post-prostatectomy incontinence: subjective and objective outcomes with 3 years follow up. Neurourol Urodynam. 2015;34:251–4.
17. Kretschmer A, Hubner W, Sandhu JS, Bauer RM. Evaluation and management of post-prostatectomy incontinence: a systematic review of current literature. Eur Urol Focus. 2016;2:245–59.
18. Kim SP, Sarmast Z, Daignault S, Faerber GJ, McGuire EJ, Latini JM. Long-term durability and functional outcomes among patients with artificial urinary sphincters: a 10-year retrospective review from the University of Michigan. J Urol. 2008;179(5):1912–6.
19. Biardeau X, Aharony S, AUS Consensus Group, Campeau L, Corcos J. Artificial urinary sphincter: executive summary of the 2015 consensus conference. Neurourol Urodyn. 2016;35(Suppl 2):S5–7.
20. Van der Aa F, Drake MJ, Kasyan GR, et al. The artificial urinary sphincter after a quarter of a century: a critical systematic review of its use in male non-neurogenic incontinence. Eur Urol. 2013;63:681–9.
21. Linder BJ, Rivera ME, Ziegelmann MJ, et al. Long-term outcomes following artificial urinary sphincter placement: an analysis of 1082 cases at Mayo Clinic. Urology. 2015;86:602–7.
22. Kundu SD, Roehl KA, Eggener SE, Antenor JA, Han M, Catalona WJ. Potency, continence and complications in 3,477 consecutive radical retropubic prostatectomies. J Urol. 2004;172(6 Pt 1):2227–31.
23. Salonia A, Burnett AL, Graefen M, et al. Prevention and management of postprostatectomy sexual dysfunctions part 1: choosing the right patient at the right time for the right surgery. Eur Urol. 2012;62:261–72.
24. Teloken PE, Nelson CJ, Karellas M, et al. Defining the impact of vascular risk factors on erectile function recovery after radical prostatectomy. BJU Int. 2013;111:653–7.
25. Dubbelman YD, Dohle GR, Schröder FH. Sexual function before and after radical retropubic prostatectomy: a systematic review of prognostic indicators for a successful outcome. Eur Urol. 2006;50(4):711–20.
26. Rabbani F, Schiff J, Piecuch M. Time course of recovery of erectile function after radical retropubic prostatectomy: does anyone recover after 2 years? J Sex Med. 2010;7:3984–90.

27. Mulhall JP. Defining and reporting erectile function outcomes after radical prostatectomy: challenges and misconceptions. J Urol. 2009;181:462–71.
28. Tal R, Alphs HH, Krebs P, Nelson CJ, Mulhall JP. Erectile function recovery rate after radical prostatectomy: a meta-analysis. J Sex Med. 2009;9:2538–46.
29. Mulhall JP, Goldstein I, Bushmakin AG. Validation of the erection hardness score. J Sex Med. 2007;4:1626–34.
30. Rosen RC, Cappelleri JC, Smith MD, et al. Development and evaluation of an abridged, 5-item version of the International Index of Erectile Function (IIEF-5) as a diagnostic tool for erectile dysfunction. Int J Impot Res. 1999;11:319–26.
31. Cappelleri JC, Rosen RC, Smith MD. Diagnostic evaluation of the erectile function domain of the International Index of Erectile Function. Urology. 1999;54:346–51.
32. Burnett AL, Nehra A, Breau RH, et al. Erectile dysfunction: AUA guideline. J Urol. 2018;200:633–41.
33. McMahon CG, Samali R, Johnson H. Efficacy, safety and patient acceptance of sildenafil citrate as treatment for erectile dysfunction. J Urol. 2000;164:1192–6.
34. Nason GJ, McNamara F, Twyford M, et al. Efficacy of vacuum erectile devices (VEDs) after radical prostatectomy: the initial Irish experience of a dedicated VED clinic. Int J Impot Res. 2016;28:205–8.
35. Engel JD. Effect on sexual function of a vacuum erection device post-prostatectomy. Can J Urol. 2011;18:5721–5.
36. Levine LA, Becher E, Bella A, Brant W, Kohler T, Martinez-Salamanca JI, et al. Penile prosthesis surgery: current recommendations from the International Consultation on Sexual Medicine. J Sex Med. 2016;13(4):489–518.
37. Tal R, Jacks LM, Elkin E, Mulhall JP. Penile implant utilization following treatment for prostate cancer: analysis of the SEER-Medicare database. J Sex Med. 2011;8(6):1797–804.
38. Sellers CL, Morey AF, Jones LA. Cost and time benefits of dual implantation of inflatable penile and artificial urinary sphincter prosthetics by single incision. Urology. 2005;65(5):852–3.

# Chapter 5
# Multimodal Treatment Plans in Prostate Cancer

**Rachel Lin Flanagan and Jeffrey John Tomaszewski**

## Introduction

In Western nations, most patients with prostate cancer are diagnosed with localized disease (T1–T4N0M0), including >80% of patients in the USA [1]. Localized prostate cancer can present with a low, intermediate, or high risk of biochemical relapse, with ~15% of patients being classified as high risk at presentation [2, 3]. Prostate cancer is highly curable, and the choice between treatment options including surgery, radiotherapy, and/or androgen deprivation therapy (ADT) is dependent upon risk group. Since patients with a high-risk disease remain at increased risk for prostate cancer mortality [4], the establishment of an appropriate multimodal treatment strategy approach is particularly important for men with high-risk localized disease [5]. There is no consensus regarding the optimal treatment strategy for high-risk localized disease; both EBRT plus ADT and surgery administered within the confines of a multimodality setting are excellent treatment options. Given more precise pathological staging, avoidance of morbidity associated with ADT, and the ability to use postoperative PSA to guide the choice of adjuvant or salvage strategies, surgical resection is becoming the initial treatment modality of choice for high-risk and locally advanced prostate cancer [5–9].

Radical prostatectomy (RP) provides excellent local control for patients with organ-confined prostate cancer; however, the overall risk of biochemical recurrence, defined by a postoperative prostate-specific antigen (PSA) level of >0.2 ng/mL, is approximately 30% at 10 years following surgery [10]. Among patients with high-risk localized prostate cancer, including those with PSA > 20 ng/mL, Gleason

R. L. Flanagan
Department of Surgery, MD Anderson Cancer Center at Cooper, Camden, NJ, USA

J. J. Tomaszewski (✉)
Department of Surgery, MD Anderson Cancer Center at Cooper, Cooper Medical School of Rowan University, Camden, NJ, USA

 
E. J. Trabulsi et al. (eds.), *Chemotherapy and Immunotherapy in Urologic Oncology*, https://doi.org/10.1007/978-3-030-52021-2_5

score > 7, stage ≥ pT3, or an accompanying positive surgical margin [6], the risk of recurrence varies between 20% and 70% at 5 years following surgery [11]. To avoid overtreatment and unnecessary morbidity, measured and nuanced objective risk stratification is imperative prior to consideration and initiation of postoperative radiotherapy (RT) [12]. In addition to the aforementioned risk categories and traditional variables, the utilization of genomic biomarkers following RP can assist patients and physicians in their decision-making process regarding conservative management versus adjuvant RT and ADT [13].

## Postoperative Radiation Therapy

Several types of RT are available for use following RP. External beam radiation therapy (EBRT) is defined as the use of high-energy radiation directed to a localized area of the body in an attempt to kill or slow the growth of cancer cells and shrink tumors. In the setting of multimodal treatment of prostate cancer following RP, EBRT is directed at the pelvis. RT damages intranuclear DNA, which inhibits appropriate DNA transcription and protein translation, inhibits cellular replication, and ultimately induces apoptosis. Following RP, RT can be considered in patients at higher risk for biochemical recurrence secondary to the presence of positive surgical margins, stage ≥ pT3 disease, or a detectable PSA. Other commonly used RT modalities include three-dimensional conformal radiotherapy (3D-CRT), which incorporates the use of imaging technology such as MRI, CT scan, or PET in an effort to shape the radiation beams to match the targeted treatment area. This in turn helps limit collateral damage to adjacent healthy tissue. Intensity-modulated radiotherapy (IMRT) is an advanced form of 3D-CRT that allows for more precise delivery of concentrated radiation doses to a specific location, thereby sparing the surrounding healthy tissue [14].

The appropriate timing of RT following RP has been studied extensively and thoroughly debated. For patients with pT3 node-negative disease and an undetectable PSA following RP, two RT options exist: adjuvant radiation therapy directed at the prostatic fossa, and observation with routine PSA testing to monitor for biochemical recurrence followed by salvage radiation therapy once PSA levels rise to 0.2 ng/mL and ideally prior to PSA levels exceeding 0.5 ng/mL [15]. The notable differences between adjuvant and early salvage RT require close consideration and further exploration.

(a) *Adjuvant Radiation Therapy (ART)*: ART is indicated for the treatment of patients at high risk for biochemical recurrence, including those with adverse pathologic features such as seminal vesicle invasion, extracapsular extension, or positive surgical margins. In the adjuvant radiation treatment setting, the PSA is typically very low to undetectable (<0.1 ng/mL). The initiation of ART typically begins between 4 and 6 months after RP and is administered at an average dose between 60–64 Gy [14].

(i) *Efficacy*: Three large, high-quality randomized control trials have examined the efficacy of ART following RP. The Southwest Oncology Group (SWOG 8794) [16], European Organization for Research and Treatment (EORTC 22911) [17, 18], and Applied Radiation Oncology (ARO 96-02, [11]) trials evaluated the effect of ART following RP on metastasis-free survival, clinical progression-free survival, and biochemical progression-free survival, respectively. Overall, these studies demonstrated significant improvements in biochemical recurrence-free survival in patients with ≥pT3 disease treated with ART when compared to observation following RP [19, 20]. Further, the ARO trial reported an 18% benefit in biochemical progression-free survival in patients with pT3 disease with or without positive margins at 5 years following ART [11]. The SWOG and EORTC trials also demonstrated reduced rates of local recurrence and improved clinical progression-free survival in patients treated with ART. However, the SWOG trial was the only trial that found a significant improvement in overall survival (74% in ART vs 66% in RP) and metastasis recurrence-free survival (71% in ART vs 61% in RP) at >12 years of follow-up [20].

(b) *Salvage Radiation Therapy* (SRT): SRT is recommended in patients with a PSA-only recurrence (PSA of >0.2 ng/mL) following RP, and no evidence of distant metastatic disease. A second confirmatory PSA should be obtained prior to initiation of SRT to ensure PSA levels are >0.2 ng/mL. The average dosing for SRT starts around 66 Gy if PSA does not exceed 0.5 ng/mL [14].

(i) *Efficacy*: Outcomes following SRT vary greatly and are largely dependent upon PSA levels at the time of administration. Observational studies have demonstrated improved rates of local recurrence when compared to surgery alone, but the benefits may be specific to certain pathologic risk groups [20]. The highest efficacy rates are observed in patients with at least two high-risk pathologic features, including Gleason Grade 8 disease or greater, pT3b/pT4 stage, or negative margins when SRT was administered at the first detectable rise in PSA. Patients exhibiting more adverse traits demonstrated an increased risk of 5-year biochemical recurrence, with rates increasing by 10% for every 0.1 ng/mL rise in PSA. This is in stark contrast to the 5-year biochemical recurrence risk (0.5% per 0.1 ng/mL of PSA) for men who demonstrated one or no adverse risk features [10].

At present, the question regarding which modality of post-RP RT is superior remains unclear. Studies of SRT focus on patients who have already relapsed, and they cannot be directly compared to those treated with ART, thus it is not possible from the available evidence to conclude the superiority of one approach [20].

(c) *Risks and Side Effects of RT*: Both ART and SRT have the potential to negatively affect functional outcomes relating to urinary, erectile, and gastrointestinal symptoms [10]. RT toxicity varies dependent upon the modality of RT utilized. It is also understood that the decision to treat patients at higher risk for biochemical recurrence with ART will ultimately result in overtreatment for a number of patients, as a percentage of patients would never have gone on to develop recurrent disease, thus exposing them to unnecessary radiation [20].

The *World* Health Organization (WHO) uses a functional scale ranging from grade 0 to 4 to quantify patient-reported symptom severity. 0 = no change, 1 = slight disturbance, 2 = greater disturbance but no interference with daily life, 3 = symptoms require treatment and 4 = severe symptoms requiring higher-level treatment or hospitalization. Acute toxicity from RT typically occurs within 90 days of treatment. The most common acute genitourinary symptoms (totaling percentages as a whole for grades 1–4 on the WHO scale) are urinary frequency (65%), dysuria (49%), and hematuria (4%). The most common acute gastrointestinal symptoms reported include diarrhea (61%), nausea, and vomiting (4%). Late toxicity is defined as symptoms persisting or developing past 90 days and can last for many years following RT. In patients treated with SRT, the probability of developing grade 2–3 genitourinary toxicity rose from 12% at 24 months to 22% at 60 months. The most common grade 2 or greater late genitourinary side effects experienced 5 years following EBRT or 3d CRT include urinary frequency (14%), hematuria (8%), and urinary incontinence. Incontinence was more prominent in patients who underwent EBRT (7.5%) versus 3D CRT (4%). Urethral stricture requiring dilation was comparable between ART (5%) and SRT (3%) at 8 years following treatment. Late gastrointestinal side effects 5 years following RT are infrequent, with rectal bleeding occurring most commonly (12%). Rectal bleeding was significantly more common in patients treated with 3D CRT than EBRT (17% versus 8%, respectively) [20].

(i) *Effects on Erectile Function*: The effects of post-RP RT on erectile function are difficult to ascertain given limited available comparative studies and a lack of significant data in the post-prostatectomy setting. To appropriately analyze and interpret functional outcomes following RT, a number of variables must be accounted for, including consistent use of RT among all patients in a selected study, erectile function prior to RP, documentation of erectile function recovery following RP prior to RT, and the utilization and degree of nerve-sparing at the time of RP. In a study that thoroughly documented erectile function before and after RP and RT, 62% of patients had erectile dysfunction following RP but prior to RT; the rates of ED increased to 66% at 2 years post-RT. There were no changes over time in the number of men reporting problems with erectile strength, sexual performance, or anorgasmia [20]. Given the variation in the sequencing of therapy, incompletely reported outcomes, and the inability to differentiate the contribution of each treatment component on function, the true impact of postoperative RT on erectile function may be difficult to determine.

(ii) *Secondary Malignancies*: Due to the lack of available data, the impact of RT on the development of secondary malignancies is not known. There have been no trials focused on ART or SRT that have demonstrated significant secondary malignancy information. Other coexisting variables must be taken into consideration, such as tobacco abuse, family history, and environmental exposure. It is difficult to attribute the sole etiology of secondary malignancies to RT [20]. In the primary therapy setting, determining the risk of secondary pelvic malignancy following prostate cancer radiotherapy has been proved to be difficult due to several factors: long lag time, insufficient power in institutional databases to detect differences, lack of comparator populations, and lack of details regarding radiotherapy modalities in large database studies; there is a clear need for high-quality studies [21].

*Huang* et al. [22] found no significant increase in in-field secondary malignancy risk compared with prostatectomy. de Gonzalez et al. [23] found that the relative risk of bladder cancer was 1.16 (95% confidence interval [CI] 0.95–1.40) and that of rectal cancer was 0.59 (95% CI 0.4–0.88). When comparing BT with EBRT, they found that the risk was lower for all in-field cancers (bladder and rectal) with BT; however, when combining BT with EBRT, the relative risk of bladder cancer was 1.25 (95% CI 1.00–1.56) compared with EBRT alone [24]. Zelefsky et al. [25] reported on patients treated with IMRT (using a median prescribed dose of 81 Gy), and with BT alone or in combination therapy [24]. They found that 15% of EBRT patients and 10% of BT patients developed in-field and out-of-field secondary malignancies after a mean follow-up of 84–90 mo. However, compared with a population-matched cohort derived from the SEER tumor registry, they found that there was no excess risk of in-field malignancy [24, 25].

## Genomics

Extensive genomic studies and whole-genome mapping have greatly improved our understanding of prostate carcinogenesis. Prostate cancer is characterized by a high degree of pathological and genetic heterogeneity compared to other human cancers [26]. Recently, several studies have investigated the molecular basis of primary prostate cancer and have identified recurrent genomic alterations, including mutations, DNA copy-number changes, gene rearrangements, and gene fusions [26–28]. Heterogeneous genomic aberrations may lead to prostate cancer onset, disease progression, and metastatic potential [26]. This heterogeneity may also contribute to the variable drug responses observed among affected patients [26]. The most common gene fusion in prostate cancer is between the transmembrane protease serine 2 (TMPRSS2) and a transcription factor known as ERG, which is part of the erythroblast-transformation specific (ETS) gene family. The TMPRSS2-ERG fusion gene is present in 50% of prostate tumors. This finding along with other genetic studies has demonstrated combinations of gene expression, which may help determine prostate cancer aggressiveness [29]. Knowledge of TMPRSS2-ERG gene fusion status provides additional risk stratification information to patients and providers and can inform decisions regarding adjuvant therapy [30]. Prostate cancer is a disease that involves dynamic changes in the genome, and further risk stratification using molecular features could potentially help distinguish indolent from aggressive prostate cancer [26].

(a) *Hereditary Prostate Cancer*: There have been no known cloned hereditary prostate cancer genes; therefore, the diagnosis of hereditary prostate cancer is based on knowledge of a nuclear family with three cases of prostate cancer, a family with three generations of prostate cancer in either paternal or maternal lineages, and families with at least two cases of prostate cancer diagnosed prior to the age of 55. Further, brothers of men with the disease are at greater risk for the development of prostate cancer when compared to sons of men who have been diagnosed. In terms of early-onset disease, family history appears to play a significant role as hereditary prostate cancer is diagnosed 6–7 years earlier on average than sporadic prostate cancer [31]. As a result of earlier emergence, a larger number of men with hereditary prostate cancer die of the disease when compared to men with nonhereditary disease [31]. Studies have shown that dominantly inherited susceptibility genes with high penetrance cause 5–10% of all diagnosed prostate cancers and as high as 30–40% of early-onset disease [29]. No studies available to date have demonstrated a difference in tumor grade or pathologic stage at diagnosis between sporadic vs hereditary prostate cancer, and treatment strategies remain the same for both types [31].

    Men at high risk for prostate cancer should be offered screening at or before the age of 45, and in families with known hereditary disease, it is appropriate to start screening 5 years before the earliest age of diagnosis in the family and 10 years prior to the age of first metastatic development [31]. PSA and digital rectal exam are the generally accepted means of initial prostate cancer screening. If these measures are found to be abnormal, prostate biopsy typically ensues. Biopsy provides beneficial information regarding primary/secondary Gleason patterns, the number of positive biopsy cores, and the percentage of disease involved within each core, all of which may influence risk stratification and treatment. There are also several genomic biomarker tests available in the USA that utilize tissue obtained via biopsy or prostatectomy, which can further help to risk stratify patients. The three predominant genomic biomarker tests include Decipher® Prostate Cancer Test (GenomeDx Biosciences, San Diego, CA), Oncotype offered through Genomic Health, and the Prolaris test offered through Myriad Genetics [13].

(b) *Genomic Tests:*

    (i) *Decipher*: The Decipher Prostate Cancer Test is a genomic test that serves as a prognostic marker of cancer control outcomes in patients who have undergone RP [32]. Based on the expression pattern of 22 RNA markers in the RP specimen, it allows postsurgery risk stratification of patients to predict the likelihood of metastases and cancer-specific mortality, determine the need for adjuvant versus salvage therapy based on a discrete cut-off score, and, in patients who have already had a biochemical recurrence (BCR), guide the treatment decision for early/multimodal salvage therapy versus salvage therapy alone [32, 33]. The test can be performed with either prostate biopsy tissue from newly diagnosed men or micro-dissected tissue from RP patients demonstrating unfavorable pathologic features. The test utilizes a Genomic Classifier score ranging from 0 to 1, in which a higher score indicates a higher probability of clinical metastasis. For every 0.1 increase in the classifier score, there is a 10% increased risk for metastasis. The GC scores are stratified into three risk groups (GC < 0.45, GC 0.45–0.6, and GC > 0.6), based on the cumulative incidence of metastasis [32]. Novel biomarkers like the Decipher test can be used to improve patient selection for RT after surgery, and the results may influence decisions regarding the initiation of ART and SRT. Following RP, men with Decipher scores of >0.6 (high risk) displayed up to an 80% reduced rate of metastatic progression if they received ART [30]. Furthermore, men with two or more risk factors (including pT3b-pT4 disease, lymph node invasion, Gleason 8 or higher disease, or Decipher scores of >0.6) revealed over a quadruple reduction in metastasis at the 10-year mark if they underwent ART [11]. There was no significant risk reduction associated with ART in men who were classified as low genomic risk [31].

*Among* 188 PCa patients with pT3 disease and/or positive surgical margins who were treated with RP and postoperative RT, the cumulative incidence of metastasis at 5 years after RT was 0%, 9%, and 29% for low, average, and high Decipher scores, respectively ($P = 0.002$) [34]. Within the low Decipher score (<0.4), there were no reductions in the cumulative incidence of metastasis for patients who received aRT compared with sRT ($P = 0.79$) [34]. Conversely, for patients with higher Decipher scores (≥0.4), the cumulative incidence of metastasis at 5 years was 6% for patients treated with aRT compared with 23% for patients treated with sRT ($P = 0.01$) [34]. Cox regression modeling demonstrated an 80% reduction in metastasis risk in the Decipher high-risk patients who received aRT compared with sRT [34]. Compared to clinicopathologic characteristics alone, using the Decipher test can significantly improve the discrimination accuracy in predicting biochemical failure (improved by 8%) and distant metastasis (improved by 10%) [30, 35].

(ii) *Prolaris*: The Prolaris assay developed by Myriad Genetics evaluates the expression of 31 cell-cycle-related genes and 15 housekeeping genes. The results are represented as a cell-cycle progression (CCP) score (scale −3 to 7), which is a proliferative index that can be used to assess the risk of adverse outcomes [36]. The test attempts to predict the 10-year risk of biochemical recurrence or death from prostate cancer, and has been validated on tissue obtained from RP and prostate needle biopsies [36, 37]. For every unit increase in the Prolaris score, a patient's risk of prostate-cancer-specific mortality doubles. The CCP score has been shown to be a stronger predictor of 10-year PCa-specific mortality than PSA and Gleason Grade (HR of 1.65 for a one-unit change in CCP) [38]. Two studies have evaluated the role of

Prolaris to predict metastasis and recurrence following definitive therapy. Following RP (HR 1.55 per unit increase in CCP for diagnostic needle biopsy) [39] and EBRT (HR per unit increase in CCP = 2.11, [40]), CCP scores were able to predict BCR at 10 years posttreatment follow-up. While there is considerable heterogeneity in the uptake and impact of this test among physicians [41], the test may provide a useful objective way to stratify men considering adjuvant therapy [36].

(iii) *Oncotype Dx*: The Oncotype Dx assay (Genomic Health) is a tissue-based test that evaluates the expression of 17 genes and reports the results as a Genomic Prostate Score (GPS), ranging from 0 to 100 [42]. The test is currently included in the National Comprehensive Cancer Network (NCCN) guidelines and, combined with clinical risk group guidelines, can help predict the risk of discovering high-grade pathology after RP in patients who present with biopsy-confirmed low- to intermediate-risk disease. The genes evaluated are involved in tissue response, growth, androgen signaling, and cellular organization. A number of studies have validated the ability of the GPS to predict adverse pathology at RP. Among a cohort of nearly 400 men, a 20-point increase in GPS predicted adverse pathology (OR 1.9, 95% CI 1.3–2.9), as well as high-grade disease (OR 2.3, 95% CI 1.5–3.7), and non-organ confined disease (OR 1.9, 95% CI 1.3–3.0). Similar results were observed in a second validation study [43], with GPS associated with adverse pathology (OR 3.23, 95% CI 2.14–4.97 per 20 units), high-grade disease (OR 2.60, 95% CI 1.65–4.15), and non-organ confined disease (OR 3.55, 95% CI 2.33–5.54). The test has also been shown to predict BCR (HR 2.93, 95% CI 2.03–4.15) and metastasis (HR 3.83, 95% CI 1.13–12.6 per 20-unit increase) [44].

(c) *Disadvantages of Genomic Screening*: With any testing or treatment modality, there will always be drawbacks. Cost is typically the number one factor taken into consideration and is largely associated with the underutilization of these measures. The tests can range from $3400–$4250 per use, and many insurance companies provide no or only partial coverage, increasing patient's out-of-pocket expense. Estimates have shown that publicly funding Prolaris could result in a total net budget impact of $41.3 million in the first 5 years, which would not be offset by the $7.3 million in projected savings associated with the increased use of active surveillance [36]. At least one study estimated a cost savings of $2286 per patient with the use of OncotypeDx testing, likely arising from the decrease in interventions [16]. No studies to date have evaluated the cost-effectiveness of Decipher.

A *second* consideration prior to the utilization of genomic biomarker testing is whether the test will ultimately result in a change of clinical decision-making. There is always a chance that genomic biomarker tests may yield results that are non-informative, and thus be considered unnecessary. In an effort to determine if these measures were notably influential on clinical decision-making, multiple clinicians have been surveyed following the use of all three of the aforementioned tests, and the results appear to indicate increased confidence in clinical decision-making, reduced decisional conflict, and patient anxiety, as well as a change in conclusions regarding treatment in up to one-third of patients following Prolaris or Decipher [30, 36].

**Clinical Pearls for the APP**

- Prostate cancer may benefit from a multimodal treatment approach, with combination treatment for high-risk men, similar to other solid tumors where surgery, radiotherapy, chemotherapy, and hormonal therapy are combined (e.g., breast cancer, lung cancer, bladder cancer, colorectal cancer, etc.).
- Postoperative patients with adverse pathological features (extracapsular extension, positive surgical margins, seminal vesical invasion, or lymph node involvement) have a higher risk of recurrence and may benefit from additional therapy.
- There is a controversy of the timing of postoperative therapy between early adjuvant therapy based on risk features and early salvage therapy determined by persistent or rising PSA.
- A genomic evaluation may clarify which patients should get adjuvant therapy and which patients can safely be observed with PSA monitoring.

# Bibliography


1. Winter A, et al. Comparison of prostate cancer survival in Germany and the USA: can differences be attributed to differences in stage distributions? BJU Int. 2017;119(4):550–9.
2. Cooperberg MR, Broering JM, Carroll PR. Time trends and local variation in primary treatment of localized prostate cancer. J Clin Oncol. 2010;28(7):1117–23.
3. D'Amico AV, et al. Biochemical outcome after radical prostatectomy, external beam radiation therapy, or interstitial radiation therapy for clinically localized prostate cancer. JAMA. 1998;280(11):969–74.
4. Patrikidou A, et al. Who dies from prostate cancer? Prostate Cancer Prostatic Dis. 2014;17(4):348–52.
5. Pignot G, et al. Systemic treatments for high-risk localized prostate cancer. Nat Rev Urol. 2018;15(8):498–510.
6. Mottet N, et al. EAU-ESTRO-SIOG guidelines on prostate cancer. Part 1: screening, diagnosis, and local treatment with curative intent. Eur Urol. 2017;71(4):618–29.
7. Budaus L, et al. Inverse stage migration in patients undergoing radical prostatectomy: results of 8916 European patients treated within the last decade. BJU Int. 2011;108(8):1256–61.
8. Silberstein JL, et al. Reverse stage shift at a tertiary care center: escalating risk in men undergoing radical prostatectomy. Cancer. 2011;117(21):4855–60.
9. Tsai HK, et al. Androgen deprivation therapy for localized prostate cancer and the risk of cardiovascular mortality. J Natl Cancer Inst. 2007;99(20):1516–24.
10. Fossati N, et al. Assessing the optimal timing for early salvage radiation therapy in patients with prostate-specific antigen rise after radical prostatectomy. Eur Urol. 2016;69(4):728–33.
11. Wiegel T, et al. Phase III postoperative adjuvant radiotherapy after radical prostatectomy compared with radical prostatectomy alone in pT3 prostate cancer with postoperative undetectable prostate-specific antigen: ARO 96-02/AUO AP 09/95. J Clin Oncol. 2009;27(18):2924–30.

12. Herrera FG, Berthold DR. Radiation therapy after radical prostatectomy: implications for clinicians. Front Oncol. 2016;6:117.
13. Davis JW. Novel commercially available genomic tests for prostate cancer: a roadmap to understanding their clinical impact. BJU Int. 2014;114(3):320–2.
14. Heidenreich A, et al. EAU guidelines on prostate cancer. Part 1: screening, diagnosis, and treatment of clinically localised disease. Eur Urol. 2011;59(1):61–71.
15. Fossati N, et al. Long-term impact of adjuvant versus early salvage radiation therapy in pT3N0 prostate cancer patients treated with radical prostatectomy: results from a multi-institutional series. Eur Urol. 2017;71(6):886–93.
16. Swanson GP, et al. Predominant treatment failure in postprostatectomy patients is local: analysis of patterns of treatment failure in SWOG 8794. J Clin Oncol. 2007;25(16):2225–9.
17. Bolla M, et al. Postoperative radiotherapy after radical prostatectomy for high-risk prostate cancer: long-term results of a randomised controlled trial (EORTC trial 22911). Lancet. 2012;380(9858):2018–27.
18. Bolla M, et al. Postoperative radiotherapy after radical prostatectomy: a randomised controlled trial (EORTC trial 22911). Lancet. 2005;366(9485):572–8.
19. Valicenti RK, et al. Adjuvant and salvage radiation therapy after prostatectomy: American Society for Radiation Oncology/American Urological Association guidelines. Int J Radiat Oncol Biol Phys. 2013;86(5):822–8.
20. Thompson IM, et al. Adjuvant and salvage radiotherapy after prostatectomy: AUA/ASTRO guideline. J Urol. 2013;190(2):441–9.
21. Wallis CJ, et al. Second malignancies after radiotherapy for prostate cancer: systematic review and meta-analysis. BMJ. 2016;352:i851.
22. Huang J, et al. Analysis of second malignancies after modern radiotherapy versus prostatectomy for localized prostate cancer. Radiother Oncol. 2011;98(1):81–6.
23. Berrington de Gonzalez A, et al. Risk of second cancers according to radiation therapy technique and modality in prostate cancer survivors. Int J Radiat Oncol Biol Phys. 2015;91(2):295–302.
24. Matta R, et al. Pelvic complications after prostate cancer radiation therapy and their management: an international collaborative narrative review. Eur Urol. 2019;75(3):464–76.
25. Zelefsky MJ, et al. Secondary cancers after intensity-modulated radiotherapy, brachytherapy and radical prostatectomy for the treatment of prostate cancer: incidence and cause-specific survival outcomes according to the initial treatment intervention. BJU Int. 2012;110(11):1696–701.
26. Grizzi F, et al. Prostate cancer: from genomics to the whole body and beyond. Biomed Res Int. 2017;2017:8707690.
27. Lecarpentier J, et al. Prediction of breast and prostate cancer risks in male BRCA1 and BRCA2 mutation carriers using polygenic risk scores. J Clin Oncol. 2017;35(20):2240–50.
28. Grasso CS, et al. The mutational landscape of lethal castration-resistant prostate cancer. Nature. 2012;487(7406):239–43.
29. Witte JS. Prostate cancer genomics: towards a new understanding. Nat Rev Genet. 2009;10(2):77–82.
30. Loeb S, Ross AE. Genomic testing for localized prostate cancer: where do we go from here? Curr Opin Urol. 2017;27(5):495–9.
31. Bratt O, et al. Hereditary prostate cancer: clinical characteristics and survival. J Urol. 2002;167(6):2423–6.
32. Dalela D, et al. Contemporary role of the decipher(R) test in prostate cancer management: current practice and future perspectives. Rev Urol. 2016;18(1):1–9.
33. Freedland SJ, et al. Utilization of a genomic classifier for prediction of metastasis following salvage radiation therapy after radical prostatectomy. Eur Urol. 2016;70(4):588–96.
34. Den RB, et al. Genomic classifier identifies men with adverse pathology after radical prostatectomy who benefit from adjuvant radiation therapy. J Clin Oncol. 2015;33(8):944–51.
35. Den RB, et al. Genomic prostate cancer classifier predicts biochemical failure and metastases in patients after postoperative radiation therapy. Int J Radiat Oncol Biol Phys. 2014;89(5):1038–46.

36. Fine ND, et al. Genomic classifiers for treatment selection in newly diagnosed prostate cancer. BJU Int. 2019;124(4):578–86.
37. Cuzick J, et al. Prognostic value of an RNA expression signature derived from cell cycle proliferation genes in patients with prostate cancer: a retrospective study. Lancet Oncol. 2011;12(3):245–55.
38. Cuzick J, et al. Prognostic value of a cell cycle progression signature for prostate cancer death in a conservatively managed needle biopsy cohort. Br J Cancer. 2012;106(6):1095–9.
39. Bishoff JT, et al. Prognostic utility of the cell cycle progression score generated from biopsy in men treated with prostatectomy. J Urol. 2014;192(2):409–14.
40. Freedland SJ, et al. Prognostic utility of cell cycle progression score in men with prostate cancer after primary external beam radiation therapy. Int J Radiat Oncol Biol Phys. 2013;86(5):848–53.
41. Shore N, et al. Clinical utility of a biopsy-based cell cycle gene expression assay in localized prostate cancer. Curr Med Res Opin. 2014;30(4):547–53.
42. Knezevic D, et al. Analytical validation of the Oncotype DX prostate cancer assay - a clinical RT-PCR assay optimized for prostate needle biopsies. BMC Genomics. 2013;14:690.
43. Cullen J, et al. A biopsy-based 17-gene genomic prostate score predicts recurrence after radical prostatectomy and adverse surgical pathology in a racially diverse population of men with clinically low- and intermediate-risk prostate cancer. Eur Urol. 2015;68(1):123–31.
44. Klein EA, et al. A 17-gene assay to predict prostate cancer aggressiveness in the context of Gleason grade heterogeneity, tumor multifocality, and biopsy undersampling. Eur Urol. 2014;66(3):550–60.

# Chapter 6
# Radiotherapy for Prostate Cancer

**Ann E. Donnelly and Robert Den**

## Radiotherapy Techniques

### *External Beam Radiation Therapy*

External beam radiation therapy (EBRT) is a method of radiation therapy in which radiation is delivered by means of a beam of energy that passes into and out of a targeted body site. External beam radiation therapy is delivered in several fractions, or doses, over a prescribed number of days. Patients do not carry any radioactive material in their bodies after each dose of EBRT. There are several methods of delivering EBRT.

In 3D conformal radiation therapy, solid beams of radiation are targeted to the site of a tumor in the shape of that tumor. The shapes of the beams are designed to limit radiation dose to the surrounding tissues but are not generally as precise as some other forms of radiation therapy. The 3D conformal radiation can be given in multiple doses over a period of days or can be given as a single higher dose fraction, usually for palliation.

IMRT, or intensity-modulated radiation therapy, is a radiation therapy technique in which computers are used to aid in the modification of radiation beams to conform to the shape and location of a tumor using a CT scan simulation for planning. In IMRT, the radiation beam is made up of multiple smaller beamlets in which the intensity, or strength, of each beam can be altered so that a more precise dose of

A. E. Donnelly (✉)
Department of Radiation Oncology, Thomas Jefferson University Hospital,
Philadelphia, PA, USA
e-mail: ann.donnelly@jefferson.edu

R. Den
Thomas Jefferson University Hospital, Philadelphia, PA, USA
e-mail: Robert.Den@jefferson.edu

 
E. J. Trabulsi et al. (eds.), *Chemotherapy and Immunotherapy in Urologic Oncology*, https://doi.org/10.1007/978-3-030-52021-2_6

radiation is delivered to the tumor while decreasing the dose to the surrounding tissues. In IMRT, radiation is given in fractions over a period of days to weeks.

SBRT, or stereotactic body radiation therapy, is a method of radiation therapy that delivers a high dose per fraction, highly targeted radiation in five or fewer fractions. SBRT is only possible with image-guided delivery systems [3]. SBRT may cause more toxicities than IMRT due to the higher dose of each fraction given [22]. Most often, SBRT is used to target the prostate in patients with localized disease. Further studies are needed to look at the long-term effects of SBRT with prostate cancer patients [3].

Proton beam radiation therapy is a type of radiotherapy in which positively charged atomic particles are used to treat a precise area of the body [23]. Proton beam therapy has a more narrow range of delivery of energy to the surrounding tissues, which may deliver a more targeted dose of radiation therapy to the tumor and avoid injury to the surrounding healthy tissue [1]. Proton beam therapy can decrease the radiation dose to the surrounding tissues, such as bones, vasculature, and muscle, which do not usually contribute to the overall morbidity of radiation therapy to the prostate [3]. Evidence now indicates that the potentially high doses of radiation therapy to the bladder and rectum contribute most to the toxicities that patients experience in the long term after treatment [3]. Therefore, if a plan can limit the radiation dose to the bladder and rectum, it is more likely to have benefit in the long term for the patient than decreasing the dose to other surrounding structures that are likely getting a lower overall dose [3]. Several studies have looked at the differences in overall effectiveness and toxicities between proton beam therapy and photon beam radiotherapy. Costs associated with proton beam therapy are generally higher than for photon beam therapy. Overall, it is thought that more information is needed in order to determine if proton beam therapy is superior or inferior to photon beam therapy approaches. The position of the American Society for Radiation Oncologists (ASTRO) on proton therapy includes treatment with protons for nonmetastatic prostate cancer when a patient is enrolled in an IRB-approved clinical trial or as part of a registry [23]. According to the American Urological Association (AUA) guidelines, patients should be informed that proton therapy offers no advantages over other forms of treatment [4].

IGRT, or image-guided radiation therapy, uses daily imaging techniques prior to each dose of radiation to ensure that the patient is lined up in the exact same way each day of treatment in order to optimize accuracy. Often times, gold fiducials are placed into the prostate gland prior to starting radiation therapy as a way to track the patient's positioning and ensure accuracy during treatment. Other means of IGRT include cone beam CT scans, MRIs, and ultrasounds. IGRT can be incorporated with any of the previously discussed external beam techniques.

## *Brachytherapy*

Brachytherapy is a radiation technique in which a radiation source is delivered directly into the targeted area of treatment. Certain factors may make brachytherapy more difficult for some patients, such as those with a very small or very large prostate gland [3]. Patients may have more side effects if they have evidence of bladder outlet obstruction or a history of previous transurethral resection of the prostate (TURP) [3]. Occasionally, androgen deprivation therapy (ADT) can be used to decrease the size of the prostate for brachytherapy, but it may not always be effective and there are additional risks for side effects with ADT [3]. Brachytherapy can be used as a definitive treatment for early-stage disease (very low, low, or favorable intermediate risk) or as a boost for higher-risk cancers to improve the overall effect of radiation treatment [3]. Brachytherapy can be used as a boost for patients with high-risk disease who are also receiving ADT [3]. Brachytherapy has been shown to increase overall control, but with more evidence of toxicity [3]. It is a common practice to give ADT for 2–3 years in patients with high-risk disease receiving a combination of external beam radiation therapy and brachytherapy, but the advantages of the addition of ADT are unclear in the data available [3]. Brachytherapy salvage treatment could be considered in men with biochemical recurrence who have had external beam radiation therapy in the past and can be considered in carefully selected patients who have had prior brachytherapy to the prostate [3].

There are some advantages and disadvantages to brachytherapy for prostate cancers. Patients are usually treated in 1 or 2 days, which decreases time away from work and regular daily activities. If patients have not previously had a TURP, the risk for urinary incontinence is low [3]. Erectile function has also been seen to be preserved in the short term after radiation therapy [24]. Disadvantages of brachytherapy include the need for general anesthesia and the risk for acute urinary retention after treatment. Some of the voiding symptoms may last up to 1 year after therapy [3].

High-dose-rate brachytherapy, or HDR brachytherapy, involves temporary insertion of a radioactive source into the prostate for a prescribed amount of time followed by removal [3]. This is considered a newer method of prostate brachytherapy. HDR brachytherapy sources are often introduced via catheters placed through the rectum and into the prostate tissue via ultrasound guidance.

Low-dose-rate brachytherapy, or LDR brachytherapy, often involves the placement of permanent seeds into the prostate that emit radiation and provide therapy over time. Radiation from the seeds is of a short range, so toxicity to the bladder and rectum is decreased [3]. After the use of low-dose-rate brachytherapy, dosimetry should be performed to assess the quality of the implant [3]. LDR brachytherapy should be avoided in patients with local disease and a prior transurethral resection of the prostate or with significant lower urinary tract symptoms not related to the cancer [4]. IMRT has been found to cause less genitourinary side effects in the short and long terms than with brachytherapy seed implants [25]. Because LDR brachytherapy with radioactive seeds remains in the prostate to emit radiation and provide therapy over time, internal radiation precautions are taken.

Because HDR brachytherapy involves the temporary placement of radioactive sources in the prostate gland, patients are not considered radioactive after therapy. Patients treated with low-dose radiotherapy have implanted seeds that, while uncommon, can migrate from the prostate. There is some evidence for decreased urinary symptoms and rectal discomfort with HDR brachytherapy compared to LDR brachytherapy [26]. HDR brachytherapy may also have a decreased risk for erectile dysfunction after treatment compared to LDR brachytherapy [26].

Radiopharmaceuticals, or radioactive compounds used to treat prostate cancer, are discussed in a later chapter.

## Radiation Therapy Based on Prostate Cancer Staging

Prostate cancer is categorized into low-risk, favorable intermediate-risk, unfavorable intermediate-risk, and high-risk disease based on staging at diagnosis, taking into account the physical exam, Gleason score, and prostate-specific antigen (PSA). For patients with early-stage disease, external beam radiation therapy is considered to be similar to radical prostatectomy in terms of progression-free survival when patients are classified according to staging [3]. Radiation may be a better option for patients with comorbidities that make the surgical intervention more risky or for patients who are not interested in surgery. Radiation therapy for prostate cancer should not be considered in patients with prior pelvic radiation therapy, active inflammatory disease of the pelvis, or permanent urinary catheters [3]. Caution should be used in patients with low bladder capacity, chronic diarrhea, bladder outlet obstruction requiring a suprapubic tube, and inactive ulcerative colitis [3].

Patients with very-low-risk prostate cancer are generally advised to enroll in active surveillance instead of treatment. No imaging studies are recommended at the time of diagnosis if patients are asymptomatic [4]. Patients with very-low-risk prostate cancer and a life expectancy of less than or equal to 5 years should be encouraged to pursue active surveillance [4].

Patients with low-risk prostate cancer are also often advised to undergo active surveillance. If radiation therapy is considered for patients with low-risk prostate cancer, the use of highly conformal radiation therapy is recommended. Pelvic nodal radiation is not recommended, nor is concurrent ADT [3]. Patients with low-risk disease can be offered either EBRT or brachytherapy for definitive treatment [4].

In patients with favorable intermediate-risk disease, radiation therapy and radical prostatectomy should be offered [4]. Generally, pelvic nodal radiation therapy and ADT are not used, though they may be added if there are signs of increased risk for the individual [3]. Patients can be offered either EBRT or brachytherapy as a single modality or in combination for intermediate-risk disease [4].

Men with unfavorable intermediate-risk prostate cancer should have staging imaging with a CT scan or MRI and a bone scan prior to the start of definitive treatment to assess for evidence of metastatic disease [4]. Nodal radiation can be considered depending on the clinical scenario and imaging studies. ADT is recommended for most patients, unless there are comorbidities that preclude the use or other factors that indicate the disease may be less aggressive [3].

High-risk prostate cancer patients should have staging imaging with a CT scan or MRI and a bone scan at diagnosis to assess for evidence of metastatic disease [4]. Nodal radiation can be considered and ADT is given unless contraindicated [3]. Men with high-risk prostate cancer can be offered EBRT alone or in combination with brachytherapy, but this should be given with ADT [4]. The various hypofractionation schedules should be discussed with patients if nodal radiation therapy is not going to be given [4].

Very-high-risk prostate cancer patients should have pretreatment imaging with a CT or MRI and a bone scan to assess for metastatic disease [5]. Nodal radiation should be considered and ADT is used unless medically contraindicated [3].

For men with locally advanced disease with evidence of metastatic nodal involvement who are receiving radiation therapy, nodal radiation should be used and the involved nodes should receive the maximum dose within usual tissue constraints [3]. ADT is used unless contraindicated and the use of abiraterone, an antiandrogen, plus prednisone can be considered [3].

## Fractionation Schedules and Dosing

Several radiation fractionation schedules have been shown to be effective with reasonable side effect profiles for prostate cancer. Dose escalation has been found to be most effective in patients with intermediate- or high-risk disease. For patients with low-risk cancers, radiation doses of 75.6–79.2 Gy are considered to be appropriate, while patients with intermediate- or high-risk disease should have doses of up to 81 Gy [3]. A common standard fractionation for prostate cancer is 78 Gy given over 39 fractions or 2 Gy per fraction.

### *Moderate Hypofractionation*

Hypofractionation is radiation therapy that is given in a smaller number of doses with each fraction being a higher dose than the standard fractionation. Image-guided radiation therapy (IGRT) is recommended when giving hypofractionated regimens for safety and accuracy [5]. IMRT is recommended over 3D conformal radiation therapy when treating with hypofractionated regimens [5]. Generally, moderate hypofractionation regimens, such as 60 Gy in 20 fractions or 70 Gy in 28 fractions, are supported when considering a moderate hypofractionation regimen for prostate cancer [5]. However, the best dose and fractionation has not been determined, and these regimens have not been compared directly in clinical trials [5]. Moderate hypofractionation should be offered to patients receiving EBRT with low risk, intermediate risk, and high risk where pelvic radiation therapy is not indicated due to similar side effect profiles compared to standard fractionation and improved convenience for patients [5]. Patients should be counseled on the slightly higher risk for acute gastrointestinal side effects and less data on long-term outcomes with moderate hypofractionation [5]. Genitourinary and chronic gastrointestinal side effects seem to be similar with standard fractionation [5].

### *Ultrahypofractionated Regimens*

Ultrahypofractionated regimens can be used in the treatment of prostate cancer and are usually administered as more than 5 Gy per fraction, often 36.25 Gy in five fractions [3]. However, the data available on these regimens are more limited than with moderate hypofractionation [5]. Therefore, a detailed discussion should be had with patients regarding risks, benefits, and available information. Patients with low-risk prostate cancer who elect EBRT may be offered ultrahypofractionated regimens [5]. Ultrahypofractionation is also recommended for intermediate-risk patients, but guidelines do recommend that patients with intermediate-risk disease be enrolled in a clinical trial or institutional registry, if possible, when treated with an ultrahypofractionated regimen [5]. Generally, ultrahypofractionated regimens are not recommended for patients with a high-risk disease [5].

### *Accuracy*

As discussed above, image-guided radiation therapy (IGRT) can be an integral method for ensuring the accuracy of fractionated radiation therapy for prostate cancer. Fiducial markers, often small gold seeds, can be placed into the prostate under ultrasound guidance from the rectum to better identify the prostate and treatment field when planning radiation therapy. Some method of ensuring accuracy should be used daily during radiation therapy in all patients, such as IGRT with CT, ultrasound, implanted fiducials, or electromagnetic targeting [3]. Endorectal balloons may be used for prostate immobilization [3].

## Palliative Radiation Therapy

Bony metastases tend to be common in prostate cancer patients with metastatic disease. Radiation therapy can be an effective means of controlling symptoms related to metastatic bone disease. Often, radiation doses of 8 Gy in a single fraction to a site of bone metastasis are effective for palliation of pain [3]. Palliative radiation therapy to the prostate can be used for patients with metastatic disease to prevent lower urinary symptoms related to the disease. Radiation therapy can include standard radiation doses and frequency or could use a common palliative fractionation, such as 30 Gy in 10 fractions or 37.5 Gy in 15 fractions [3].

## Use of Androgen Deprivation Therapy (ADT) with Radiotherapy

Androgen deprivation therapy (ADT) in combination with radiotherapy has been found to be effective in improving the outcomes in certain men with prostate cancer. Generally, men who have unfavorable intermediate-risk prostate cancer and high- or very-high-risk prostate cancer at diagnosis are considered for treatment with concurrent ADT and radiation therapy. ADT usually involves the administration of luteinizing hormone-releasing (LHRH) agonists, such as leuprolide and goserelin, and an antiandrogen, such as bicalutamide or flutamide.

### *Unfavorable Intermediate-Risk Disease*

In men with unfavorable intermediate-risk prostate cancer who are treated with radiation therapy, a short course of ADT, given for 4–6 months, is often used. With shorter courses of radiation therapy, such as brachytherapy or SBRT, the duration of ADT may be shortened to 4 months [3]. ADT is usually started 2–3 months prior to the initiation of radiation therapy and continued through the duration of the radiation treatments.

Several trials have shown an improvement in cancer-free survival and overall survival in patients treated with radiotherapy plus short-course ADT in intermediate-risk disease [3]. The EORTC 22991 trial randomized 819 patients with localized prostate cancer, of which approximately 75% had an intermediate-risk disease and 25% had a high-risk disease, to either radiation therapy alone or radiation therapy plus 6 months of ADT [27]. The addition of 6 months of ADT to radiotherapy significantly improved biochemical disease-free survival than for patients receiving radiation therapy alone (HR, 0.52; 95% CI, 0.41–0.66; $P < 0.001$) and clinical progression-free survival (HR, 0.63; 95% CI, 0.48–0.84; $P = 0.001$) at a median follow-up of 7.2 years [27]. In another trial, 818 patients with T2b, T2c, T3, and T4 N0 M0 prostate cancer were randomized to radiation monotherapy, 3 months of ADT with radiotherapy, or 6 months of ADT with radiotherapy [29]. ADT was started 2 months prior to radiation therapy in the 3-month arm and 5 months prior to radiation therapy in the 6-month arm [29]. After a median follow-up of 10.6 years, the 3 and 6 months of ADT plus radiotherapy groups showed a decrease in PSA progression and local progression compared to radiotherapy alone. In addition, 6 months of ADT significantly decreased distant progression (HR 0.49, CI 0.31–0.76; $P = 0.001$) and prostate cancer mortality (HR 0.49, CI 0.32–0.74;

$p = 0.0008$) compared to radiation monotherapy [29]. Finally, RTOG 9910 was a phase 3 randomized trial of 1579 intermediate-risk prostate cancer patients who were assigned to either ADT 8 weeks prior to radiation therapy and during radiotherapy (16 weeks in total) or ADT 28 weeks prior to and then during radiation therapy (36 weeks in total) [30]. Follow-up at 10 years showed no significant difference between the two groups in disease-specific survival, overall survival, local progression, distant metastases, or prostate-specific antigen recurrence, thereby showing little benefit of ADT beyond 4 months [30].

## *High-Risk and Very-High-Risk Disease*

For patients with high-risk disease, ADT is generally given for a total of 2–3 years along with radiation therapy. Studies have shown an improvement in overall survival and disease-free survival in patients treated with a combination of radiation therapy and ADT for a high-risk disease [3]. ADT is usually started 2–3 months prior to radiation therapy and then continued for the duration of the 2–3 year period for high-risk disease.

Clinical trials have shown benefits with ADT added to radiotherapy for high-risk prostate cancer with improvement in overall survival over radiotherapy alone [3]. EORTC 22863 was a randomized phase 3 clinical trial of 415 patients with localized prostate cancer with a high risk for metastasis (T1-2 with WHO histologic grade 3 disease or T3-4 with any histologic grade) in which patients were randomized to radiotherapy alone or radiotherapy plus 3 years of ADT [31]. Patients in the radiotherapy plus ADT arm were found to have significant improvement in disease-free survival and overall survival compared to the radiotherapy-alone group [31]. After a median follow-up of 9.1 years, disease-free survival was 22.7% in the radiotherapy-alone group versus 47.7% in the radiotherapy plus ADT group (HR 0.42, 95% CI 0.33–0.55, $p < 0.0001$) and overall survival was 39.8% in the radiotherapy-alone group versus 58.1% in the radiotherapy plus ADT group (HR 0.60, 95% CI 0.45–0.80, $p = 0.0004$) [31]. RTOG 85-31 was a phase 3 randomized trial in which 977 patients with prostate cancer at a high risk of relapse and poor outcomes, either clinical T3 disease or with regional lymph node involvement were randomized to either radiotherapy plus adjuvant ADT or radiotherapy followed by observation and ADT at relapse [32]. In patients in the radiotherapy plus ADT arm, the ADT was started at the end of radiation therapy and continued until there was evidence of progression of disease [32]. Patients who previously had a prostatectomy were included if they had evidence of extracapsular extension or seminal vesicle involvement on pathology [32]. At the 10-year follow-up, the absolute survival, local recurrence, and distant recurrence were all lower for the radiotherapy plus ADT arm [32]. Absolute survival was significantly better, with 49% of patients alive in the radiotherapy plus ADT arm versus 39% in the radiotherapy plus observation arm ($p = 0.002$) [32]. Local recurrence in the radiotherapy plus ADT was 23% versus 38% in the radiotherapy plus observation arm ($p < 0.0001$) and development of distant metastases was 24% in the radiotherapy plus ADT arm versus 39% in the radiotherapy plus observation arm ($p < 0.0001$) [32]. RTOG 9202 was a randomized trial which enrolled 1521 patients with T2c-T4 prostate cancers with a PSA of less than 150 ng/mL and no nodal disease outside of the pelvis [33]. All patients received radiation therapy plus ADT with flutamide and goserelin 2 months prior to radiation therapy start and until the completion of radiation therapy [33]. Patients were then randomized to receive no additional ADT or an additional 2 years of ADT with monthly goserelin [33]. After 10 years of follow-up, the patients who received additional long-term ADT had a significant improvement in disease-free survival of 13.2% for the short-term ADT arm versus 22.5% in the additional long-term ADT arm ($P < 0.0001$), local progression (22.2% versus 12.3%, $P < 0.0001$), and distant metastasis (22.8% versus 14.8%, $P < 0.0001$) [33]. Overall survival, however, was not found to be statistically significant, with 51.6% survival in the short-term ADT arm versus 53.9% in the additional long-term ADT arm ($P = 0.36$), although a subgroup analysis showed that patients with Gleason scores of 8–10 had an increased overall survival in the additional long-term ADT arm (31.9% versus 45.1%, $P = 0.0061$) [33].

### *Possible Side Effects*

The addition of ADT to a treatment regimen for prostate cancer does introduce possible additional side effects. Side effects of ADT include, but are not limited to, sexual dysfunction, hot flushes, fatigue, decreased muscle strength, breast enlargement, weight gain, risk for cardiac disease, memory changes, emotional liability, and bone loss [34]. Men treated with ADT tend to have more sexual side effects and fatigue related to treatment [35]. Patients with coexisting cardiac disease should be evaluated closely, as there has been some evidence that cardiac-related events are increased with ADT [35].

## Unique Toxicities: Recognition, Treatment, and Management

### *Fatigue*

Fatigue during radiation therapy is common, especially later in the course of radiation therapy and for the first several weeks afterward. Fatigue and systemic side effects related to radiation therapy are due to the release of cytokines by the tissues that are exposed [1]. Most patients notice an improvement in fatigue within a month after treatment, though others can have some mild fatigue for 2–3 months after the completion of therapy. One study that evaluated 681 patients undergoing radiation therapy for prostate cancer found that age younger than 60, depressive symptoms, and concurrent ADT may be factors linked to increased fatigue during radiotherapy [9].

There is some evidence that regular exercise can help to manage fatigue during radiation therapy [10, 11]. Patients should be instructed regarding adequate sleep and pacing activity to conserve energy. Regular, moderate exercise can often help with overall energy as well as with improving sleep at night. Patients should be encouraged to adhere to a healthy diet and regular meals with adequate hydration.

## *Urinary Toxicities*

As many as 50% of patients have some acute bladder or bowel toxicity during and shortly after radiation therapy [3]. Acute urinary symptoms during or immediately after radiation therapy often include frequency, urgency, dysuria, hematuria, enuresis, and nocturia [36]. The symptoms are likely related to acute radiation cystitis or inflammation of the bladder after radiation therapy [36]. Urinary symptoms often start later during the course of radiation therapy for those receiving standard fractionation or moderately hypofractionated regimens. For those receiving ultrafractionated regimens, urinary symptoms may not develop until the completion of therapy. Urinary tract infections should be ruled out in the setting of urinary frequency, urgency, or dysuria during radiation therapy. If infection is ruled out, medications, such as phenazopyridine or ibuprofen, can be used to treat dysuria due to radiation therapy. Patients should be encouraged to drink adequate fluids. Patients who are on anticoagulant medications should be monitored closely for hematuria during or after radiation therapy. Acute urinary symptoms often resolve within 4–6 weeks after the completion of radiotherapy but can persist in some patients for up to 2–3 months.

Men should be informed that chronic urinary symptoms are possible in some patients who receive radiation therapy for prostate cancer [4]. However, it is also thought that some patients can have a decrease in obstructive urinary symptoms after radiation therapy, which may be related to shrinking of the prostate after treatment [7]. In one study in which a prostate cancer database was reviewed for urethral stricture after prostate cancer treatment, radical prostatectomy had the highest incidence of stricture (8.4%) followed by prostate brachytherapy plus EBRT (5.2%) [21]. Most patients were treated with urethral dilation [21]. A clinical trial of patients treated with radiation therapy after radical prostatectomy did find that urethral stricture, incontinence, and proctitis were more common in patients treated with radiation therapy than without [6]. Radiation therapy can also worsen urinary incontinence after radical prostatectomy [4]. The incidence of urinary incontinence after radiation therapy alone is likely close to 1% [7].

Chronic radiation cystitis is a possible long-term side effect of radiation therapy. The incidence of chronic radiation cystitis is low, likely around 5%, especially if the dose of radiation to the bladder is limited to lower than 75 Gy [38]. In one study of 309 prostate cancer patients treated with IMRT, 78 Gy in 39 fractions, and followed for a median of 104 months, the most common GU toxicity grade 2 or higher was hematuria (11.2%), with radiation cystitis observed endoscopically in most patients [37]. In addition, hematuria and incontinence increased in incidence after 60 months while other symptoms decreased in the initial 60 months of follow-up [37]. Because of the late onset of toxicity seen in this study, the researchers recommended a follow-up of greater than 5 years for men treated with radiation therapy to monitor for delayed GU toxicities [37].

Men with delayed urinary symptoms after radiation therapy for prostate cancer should first be evaluated for another cause of the symptoms. Differential diagnosis for men with new-onset urinary lower urinary tract symptoms or hematuria includes urinary tract infection, urolithiasis, bladder cancer, or other malignancies invading the urinary tract. Men with dysuria should have a urinalysis and urine culture obtained to rule out infection. In addition, those with hematuria should be seen by a urologist with a hematuria workup, including urine for cytology, cystoscopy, and upper urinary tract imaging, such as a CT urogram [36].

If men are found to have radiation-related hemorrhagic cystitis, treatment is generally based on the severity and grade. For patients with grade 1 hemorrhagic cystitis, treatment generally includes supportive measures and hydration with close monitoring. Anticholinergic medications can help with bladder spasms in the setting of cystitis [36]. Those with grade 2 or 3 hemorrhagic cystitis may require continuous bladder irrigation or cystoscopy assessment, and astringents, such as silver nitrate, can be used to treat areas of bleeding [36]. If grade 3 or 4 toxicities develop, patients may require blood transfusions and other interventions, such as formalin instillation or electrocautery to the bladder [36]. There is some evidence that lasers may be helpful in controlling bleeding [36]. Temporary urinary diversion and cystectomy may be considered in the most severe cases [36]. Hyperbaric oxygen therapy may be an effective treatment for certain patients, as well.

The International Prostate Symptom Score, or I-PSS, was initially developed as a tool to assess urinary symptoms related to benign prostatic hyperplasia, but can be an effective tool for monitoring urinary symptoms during and after radiation therapy. The tool asks patients to rank the severity of urinary symptoms over the past month, including frequency, urgency, weak stream, intermittency, incomplete emptying, straining, and nocturia from 0 (not at all) to 5 (almost always) [22]. It then asks the patient about overall quality of life, from delighted to terrible [22]. If completed regularly, the tool can be helpful in assessing urinary symptoms compared to pretreatment levels and as the patient progresses after radiation therapy.

## *Gastrointestinal Toxicities*

Acute radiation proctitis during and immediately after radiation therapy for prostate cancer is caused by radiation exposure and damage to the rectal mucosa. Gastrointestinal side effects after radiation therapy can manifest as abdominal pain or cramping, loose or more frequent stools, urgency with bowel movements, or blood per rectum. There have not been any large studies to evaluate the optimal treatment of radiation proctitis. Symptoms can often be managed with antidiarrheal medications and a low residue diet. There has also been some evidence that short-chain fatty acids can have benefit in acute radiation proctitis. A small double-blind placebo-controlled cross-over study of 20 patients treated with pelvic radiation therapy who developed acute radiation proctitis found that those treated with a short-chain fatty acid enema, sodium butyrate, had an improvement in symptoms compared to the placebo group [17]. Acute gastrointestinal side effects resolve within a month for most men, but may take up to 2–3 months to fully resolve for some.

Chronic gastrointestinal symptoms after radiation therapy usually include radiation proctitis. Chronic radiation proctitis is defined by RTOG as rectal discomfort or urgency with bowel movements along with mucus or blood in the bowel movements. It may also include loose or frequent stools [28]. The incidence of radiation proctitis ranges from 5% to 30% depending on the treatment volume and dose of radiation [7]. Chronic radiation proctitis often occurs between 9 and 14 months after completion of radiation therapy but can occur up to 30 years after treatment [8]. Radiation proctitis is generally caused by fibrosis and chronic changes to the rectal mucosa that ultimately cause some ischemia from prior radiation therapy.

Patients with a change in bowel movements or new rectal bleeding need to be evaluated for radiation proctitis as well as other causes. Stool samples looking for an infectious cause may be indicated for patients with loose or watery stools. A complete blood count should be obtained in men who are experiencing bleeding with bowel movements. Patients should be referred for a colonoscopy or sigmoidoscopy to evaluate for other causes of symptoms, such as a new malignancy or possibly inflammatory bowel disease. Barium enema or cross-sectional imaging should be considered in patients with severe symptoms to rule out fistula or small perforation [19].

No large, placebo-controlled studies have been done to evaluate the best treatment for chronic radiation proctitis. Treatment options for chronic radiation proctitis often initially include sucralfate enemas or glucocorticoid enemas or suppositories. If patients do not improve within a few weeks, endoscopic intervention with colonoscopy or sigmoidoscopy is indicated. Most commonly used to treat symptoms or chronic radiation proctitis is argon plasma coagulation (APC). APC has been shown to be effective in reducing bleeding in chronic radiation proctitis but available studies involved a small number of patients [20]. Due to the lack of randomized controlled trials, it is difficult to assess the overall efficacy of APC, and additional research is needed [18]. Formalin application to the rectum has been used to decrease recurrent bleeding related to radiation proctitis and has been evaluated in small studies [18]. Formalin causes coagulation of the rectal tissue when applied. Evidence for the regular use of formalin for the treatment of bleeding from chronic radiation proctitis is insufficient due to lack of high-level evidence [18]. Laser therapies, cryoablation, radiofrequency ablation, and electrocoagulation have also been used but data are lacking in their overall efficacy, as well [18]. Hyperbaric oxygen may be an effective treatment option for chronic radiation proctitis but the cost and time requirements make it more difficult to complete a treatment course compared to some other options [18]. Other therapies that have been investigated in small studies include Vitamin A, 5-aminosalicylic acid (5-ASA) enemas, and mesalamine plus betamethasone enemas with the addition of oral metronidazole [18]. Surgical interventions for chronic radiation proctitis should only be used in patients with severe symptoms or complications, such as uncontrolled bleeding, rectal stricture, or fistula. Tissue changes after radiation therapy can make surgical intervention difficult.

## *Sexual Dysfunction*

Sexual dysfunction is a common side effect after radiation therapy for prostate cancer. Radiation techniques may affect sexual function after treatment, while IMRT and more precise techniques potentially may cause less sexual dysfunction. Generally, sexual dysfunction seems to decline after radiation therapy [7]. Patients treated with both ADT and radiation therapy are more likely to have difficulty with sexual function after treatment [24].

The International Index of Erectile Function, or IIEF, is a questionnaire that can be given to patients to assess their sexual function [39]. Often, it is helpful to get an IIEF prior to any treatment for prostate cancer and then continue to follow the scores over time. The tool, which includes questions about sexual function and desire, can be helpful in identifying patients who are having a decline in sexual function over time or as a way to open discussions with patients about their sexual function and quality of life.

A model has been developed to attempt to predict which patients will be at risk for developing sexual dysfunction after prostate cancer treatment and those who are less likely to develop dysfunction [13]. Certain factors, including lower PSA and lower risk category, better pretreatment sexual function scoring, lower AUA symptom assessment, younger age, and absence of androgen deprivation therapy use have been associated with a higher likelihood of adequate sexual function 2 years after EBRT [13].

In one series in which patients were sent questionnaires regarding their side effects and quality of life over a 2-year period after radiation therapy for prostate cancer, sexual dysfunction seemed to be an issue for more patients compared to urinary or bowel side effects [14]. In addition, sexual dysfunction quality of life seemed to worsen over time with the number of men reporting increased issues with sexual dysfunction between baseline and 24 months [14].

Treatments usually start with phosphodiesterase-5 inhibitors, such as sildenafil or tadalafil. Several studies have been done to show that phosphodiesterase-5 inhibitors can be effective in treating erectile dysfunction in men after radiation therapy [15, 16]. Patients should be assessed for possible contraindications and drug interactions prior to therapy, as well as educated regarding how to use the medications and possible side effects. The use of nitrates is contraindicated with phosphodiesterase-5 inhibitors. Testosterone replacement should not be used in patients with a history of prostate cancer. Other options for treatment of erectile dysfunction include vacuum devices, urethral alprostadil, and penile injections with alprostadil and papaverine can also be helpful for erectile dysfunction. Penile implants are sometimes used if patients do not have good outcomes with nonsurgical methods. Often, men who have mild sexual dysfunction after treatment for prostate cancer may need oral medications alone. For those who do not respond to oral medications or have contraindications to some erectile dysfunction treatments, referral to a urologist with specialization in erectile dysfunction can be helpful. In addition, social work and psychotherapy can be helpful for men who are struggling with sexual dysfunction after prostate cancer treatment. Sexual health counselors or relationship counselors can also play an important role for men and their partners.

## *Stress Fractures*

Stress fractures or insufficiency fractures are an uncommon but possible complication of radiation therapy to the pelvis. In one series, the charts of 134 patients were reviewed to assess the incidence and timing of insufficiency fractures after whole pelvic radiation therapy for prostate cancer. After a median follow-up period of 68 months, eight patients were found to have had insufficiency fractures after treatment [12]. The 5-year incidence of insufficiency fracture was 6.8% with a median time to development of a fracture of 20 months from the time of completion of treatment [12]. Most patients presented with back pain, so it is important to differentiate an insufficiency fracture from evidence of metastatic disease [12]. In this review, there were no clear risk factors identified for patients who developed insufficiency fractures after radiation therapy [12]. Most patients are treated with conservative measures.

## *Methods of Minimizing Adverse Effects*

Perirectal spacers, usually made of a hydrogel material, can be used for patients in which the targeted therapy may be inadequate to spare the surrounding structures or to reduce side effects to the patient based on anatomy [3]. In clinical trials, the spacer arm showed a decrease in rectal toxicities, grade greater than or equal to 1, by 75% at 3 years, and there were no reported grade 2 or greater toxicities noted in the spacer arm [29]. Perirectal spacers should not be used in patients who have evidence of rectal invasion or T3 disease with posterior extension. In addition, many clinicians will have patients undergo treatment with a full bladder in order to raise the bladder further out of the radiation field to decrease the dose to the bladder.

## Survivorship after Radiotherapy

### Urinary Recovery

Acute urinary symptoms after radiation therapy usually improve within 4–6 weeks after treatment. Patients should be followed closely after radiation therapy to ensure that the symptoms improve. Patients who develop new dysuria after radiation therapy should have an evaluation to rule out an underlying urinary tract infection. Patients should be monitored for evidence of chronic radiation cystitis and referred to a urologist promptly for further evaluation, especially in the setting of hematuria.

### Sexual Recovery

As above, patients are often treated with oral medications for sexual dysfunction first as long as they are not contraindicated. Patients treated with ADT are likely to have more prolonged sexual dysfunction than those treated with radiation alone. If men do not have a good response to oral medications, referral to urology to discuss additional medications and surgical interventions should be discussed. Patients who are experiencing sexual dysfunction should be offered counseling, along with their partners, as part of management. As discussed above, sexual function should be addressed at each postradiation therapy follow-up visit and patients offered intervention, if warranted.

### Bowel Toxicity

Patients should be monitored closely for evidence of chronic effects of radiation therapy on the GI system. Patients should be encouraged to have regular colon cancer screenings. Referral to a gastroenterologist experienced in treating patients with chronic radiation proctitis can also be helpful if symptoms develop. Diet can have a significant role in bowel management after radiation therapy, so dietary education and referral to a registered dietician should be considered.

### Secondary Malignancies

While uncommon, secondary malignancies are possible after radiation therapy for prostate cancer. There is usually an approximately 1% risk of malignancy for every year after the second decade after radiation therapy [1]. The risk of bladder and rectal cancer doubles starting 10 years after radiation therapy, though the overall incidence is still low [2]. Therefore, the patient's age at the time of radiation therapy can be important when considering the risk for secondary cancers in the future. Patients should be encouraged to remain up to date with regular cancer screenings.

### *Other Survivorship Considerations*

Men who have received ADT should be monitored for evidence of bone density loss depending on the duration, and adequate calcium and vitamin D intake should be encouraged throughout ADT treatment. Weight management and regular exercise, according to physical abilities, should be encouraged. Lymphedema to the groin or lower extremities is uncommon in men who have radiation to the prostate alone but can occur at higher rates if the pelvic lymph nodes are radiated or in men who have surgery plus radiation [38]. Men who are treated for prostate cancer should be regularly assessed for depression and anxiety related to diagnosis and treatment.

### *Assessing for Recurrence*

Regular monitoring of the prostate-specific antigen (PSA) after definitive radiation therapy is critical in evaluating the overall success of treatment. Patients should be instructed about the importance of checking the PSA as well as the planned schedule for surveillance. Generally, the PSA is checked every 3–6 months for the first 3 years after treatment and then annually thereafter. The PSA can continue to fall for several months to years after radiation therapy [40]. The PSA nadir is the lowest recorded level after radiation therapy. A PSA that is rising after definitive radiation therapy is concerning for recurrent disease. The Phoenix criteria were developed in 2005 as a joint consensus among specialists who reviewed available data on rising PSAs after definitive radiation therapy. The Phoenix criteria state that a PSA rise of 2 ng/mL or greater above the nadir is the definition of biochemical failure after EBRT with or without ADT [41]. Any patient who meets the criteria for biochemical recurrence by PSA should have an evaluation for evidence of metastatic disease or local recurrence. Repeat prostate biopsy can be considered, though the biopsy can be difficult to interpret after radiotherapy.

## Conclusion

Radiation therapy for prostate cancer has been a standard treatment approach for many years, and radiation techniques have been evolving to reduce side effects while improving overall outcomes. Additional studies are currently underway to assess various optimal fractionation schedules for patients that can limit side effects and duration of therapy while ensuring adequate control of the disease. Studies have also been evaluating medications in combination with radiation therapy to improve patient outcomes.

Patients should always be fully informed about the options for prostate cancer treatment based on their staging as well as possible acute and chronic side effects of radiation therapy prior to treatment. More evidence is needed to determine the best methods for managing patients after some side effects of radiation therapy, such as radiation proctitis.

Advanced practice providers (APPs) can play an important role in patients undergoing radiation therapy for prostate cancer. APPs can have a key role in patient education and reinforcing teaching regarding what patients will experience during and after radiation therapy. APPs can have an important role in managing side effects after radiation therapy and monitoring for evidence of recurrent disease.

**Clinical Pearls**

- Highly targeted radiation therapy techniques should be used to treat localized prostate cancer in order to minimize radiation doses to adjacent structures, including the bladder, rectum, pelvic bones, and femoral heads.
- Hypofractionated regimens should be used by departments with required experience and training when clinically appropriate for the patient.
- Brachytherapy can be used as a definitive treatment for patients with localized disease or as part of a boost dose in patients with high-risk disease, but specialty training is required.
- Photon and proton beam therapies are considered to be similar in efficacy.
- Radiation therapy can be an effective alternative to radical prostatectomy in patients who may have comorbidities that preclude surgery.
- Patients should be educated about possible side effects, both acute and late, of radiation therapy prior to treatment.
- Radiation-related side effects can be adequately managed in the majority of patients, but more research is needed to determine the best practice of managing some side effects.
- Radiation therapy for prostate cancer should not be considered in patients with prior pelvic radiation therapy, active inflammatory disease of the pelvis, or permanent urinary catheters. Caution should be used in patients with low bladder capacity, chronic diarrhea, bladder outlet obstruction requiring suprapubic tube, and inactive ulcerative colitis.

# References

1. Jameson JL, Fauci AS, Kasper DL, Hauser SL, Longo DL, Loscalzo J. Principles of cancer treatment. In: Harrison's principles of internal medicine. 20th ed. New York: McGraw-Hill; 2018. Available from http://accessmedicine.mhmedical.com/content.aspx?bookid=2129&sectionid=192014984.
2. Bhojani N, Capitanio U, Saurdi N, Jeldres C, Isbam H, Shariat SF, et al. The rate of secondary malignancies after radical prostatectomy versus external beam radiation therapy for localized prostate cancer: a population-based study on 17,845 patients [internet]. Int J Radiat Oncol Biol Phys. 2010;76(2):342–8; [cited 27 Oct 2018]. Available from: https://www.ncbi.nlm.nih.gov/pubmed/20117287. https://doi.org/10.1016/j.ijrobp.2009.02.011.
3. National Comprehensive Cancer Network (NCCN). NCCN guidelines version 4.2018 prostate cancer. 2018. Available from https://www.nccn.org/professionals/physician_gls/pdf/prostate.pdf. Accessed 8 Nov 2018.
4. American Urological Association (AUA). Clinically localized prostate cancer: AUA/ASTRO/SUO guideline [internet]. 2017. Available from https://www.auanet.org/guidelines/prostate-cancer-clinically-localized-guideline.
5. Morgan SC, Hoffman K, Loblaw DA, Buyyounouski MK, Patton C, Barocas D, et al. Hypofractionated radiation therapy for localized prostate cancer: an ASTRO, ASCO, and AUA evidence-based guideline. J Urol. [internet] 2018 (cited 13 Jan 2019). Available from https://www.jurology.com/doi/abs/10.1016/j.juro.2018.10.001. https://doi.org/10.1016/j.juro.2018.10.001.
6. Swanson GP, Thompson IM, Tangen C, Paradelo J, Canby-Hagino E, Crawford ED, et al. Update of SWOG 8794: adjuvant radiotherapy for pT3 prostate cancer improves metastasis free survival [internet]. Int J Radiat Oncol Biol Phys. 2008;72(1 suppl):S31; [cited 13 Jan 2019]. Available from https://www.redjournal.org/article/S0360-3016(08)01051-1/fulltext. https://doi.org/10.1016/j.ijrobp.2008.06.835.
7. DiBiase SJ, Roach M. External beam radiation therapy for localized prostate cancer. 2019 January 8 [cited 3 Feb 2019]. In UptoDate [internet]. UptoDate, Inc. Available from https://www.uptodate.com/contents/external-beam-radiation-therapy-for-localized-prostate-cancer?source=history_widget#H20.
8. Friedman LS. Clinical manifestations, diagnosis, and treatment of radiation proctitis. 2018 May 22 [cited 3 Feb 2019]. In UptoDate [internet]. UptoDate, Inc. Available from https://www.uptodate.com/contents/clinical-manifestations-diagnosis-and-treatment-of-radiation-proctitis?topicRef=6946&source=see_link#H520853351.
9. Chao HH, Doucette A, Raizen D, Vapiwala N. Factors associated with fatigue in prostate cancer (PC) patients undergoing external beam radiation therapy (EBRT) [internet]. Pract Radiat Oncol. 2018;8(3):e139–48; [cited 31 Jan 2019]. Available from https://www.sciencedirect.com/science/article/pii/S187985001730259X?via%3Dihub. https://doi.org/10.1016/j.prro.2017.09.002.
10. Windsor PM, Nicol K, Potter J. A randomized, controlled trial of aerobic exercise for treatment-related fatigue in men receiving radical external beam radiotherapy for localized prostate carcinoma [internet]. Cancer. 2004;101(3):550–7; [cited 31 Jan 2019]. Available from https://onlinelibrary.wiley.com/doi/full/10.1002/cncr.20378. https://doi.org/10.1002/cncr.20378.
11. Segal RJ, Reid RD, Courney KS, Sigal RJ, Kenny GP, Prud'Homme DG, et al. Randomized controlled trial of resistance or aerobic exercise in med receiving radiation therapy for prostate cancer [internet]. J Clin Oncol. 2009;27(3):344–51; [cited 31 Jan 2019]. Available from http://ascopubs.org/doi/full/10.1200/JCO.2007.15.4963?url_ver=Z39.88-2003&rfr_id=ori:rid:crossref.org&rfr_dat=cr_pub%3dpubmed63.
12. Igdem S, Alco G, Ercan T, Barlan M, Ganiyusufoclu K, Unalan B, et al. Insufficiency fractures after pelvic radiotherapy in patients with prostate cancer [internet]. Int J Radiat Oncol Biol Phys. 2010;77(3):818–23; [cited 2 Feb 2019]. Available from https://www.sciencedi-

rect.com/science/article/pii/S0360301609009067?via%3Dihub. https://doi.org/10.1016/j/ijrobp.2009.05.059.
13. Alemozaffar M, Regan MM, Cooperberg MR, Wei JT, Michalski JM, Sandler HM, et al. Prediction of erectile function following treatment for prostate cancer [internet]. JAMA. 2011;306(11):1205–14; [cited 2 Feb 2019]. Available from https://jamanetwork.com/journals/jama/fullarticle/1104401. https://doi.org/10.1001/jama.2011.1333.
14. Hamilton AS, Stanford JL, Filliland FD, Albertsen PC, Stephenson RA, Hoffman RM, et al. Health outcomes after external-beam radiation therapy for clinically localized prostate cancer: results from the prostate center outcomes study [internet]. J Clin Oncol. 2001;19(9):2517–26; [cited 2 Feb 2019]. Available from http://ascopubs.org/doi/pdf/10.1200/JCO.2001.19.9.2517. https://doi.org/10.1200/JCO.2001.19.9.2517.
15. Incrocci L, Koper PCM, Hop WCJ, Slob AK. Sildenafil citrate (Viagra) and erectile dysfunction following external beam radiotherapy for prostate cancer: a randomized, double-blind, placebo-controlled, cross-over study [internet]. Int J Radiat Oncol Biol Phys. 2001;51(5):1190–5; [cited 3 Feb 2019]. Available from https://www.sciencedirect.com/science/article/pii/S0360301601017679?via%3Dihub. https://doi.org/10.1016/S0360-3016(01)01767-9.
16. Incrocci L, Slagter C, Slob AK, WCJ H. A randomized, double-blind, placebo-controlled, cross-over study to assess the efficacy of tadalafil (Cialis) in the treatment of erectile dysfunction following three-dimensional conformal external-beam radiotherapy for prostatic carcinoma [internet]. Int J Radiat Oncol Biol Phys. 2006;66(2):439–44; [cited 3 Feb 2019]. Available from https://www.sciencedirect.com/science/article/pii/S0360301606009448?via%3Dihub. https://doi.org/10.1016/j.ijrobp.2006.04.047.
17. Vernia P, Fracasso PL, Casale V, Villotti G, Marcheggiano A, Stigliano V, et al. Topical butyrate for acute radiation proctitis: randomized crossover trial [internet]. Lancet. 2000;356(9237):1232–5; [cited 3 Feb 2019]. Available from https://www.sciencedirect.com/science/article/pii/S0140673600027872?via%3Dihub. https://doi.org/10.1016/S0140-6736(00)02787-2.
18. Hanson B, MacDonald R, Shaukat A. Endoscopic and medical therapy for chronic radiation proctopathy: a systematic review [internet]. Dis Colon Rectum. 2012;55(10):1081–95; [cited 3 Feb 2019]. Available from https://insights.ovid.com/pubmed?pmid=22965408. https://doi.org/10.1097/DCR.0b013e3182587aef.
19. Kennedy GD, Heise CP. Radiation colitis and proctitis [internet]. Clin Colon Rectal Surg. 2007;20(1):64–72; [cited 3 Feb 2019]. Available from https://www.ncbi.nlm.nih.gov/pmc/articles/PMC2780150/#r20064-54. https://doi.org/10.1055/s-2007-970202.
20. Do NL, Nagle D, Poylin VY. Radiation proctitis: current strategies in management [internet]. Gastroenterol Res Pract. 2011; [cited 3 Feb 2019]. Published online 17 Nov 2011. Available from https://www.ncbi.nlm.nih.gov/pmc/articles/PMC3226317/#B31; https://doi.org/10.1155/2011/917941.
21. Elliott SP, Meng MV, Elkin EP, McAninch JW, Duchane J, Carroll PR. Incidence of urethral stricture after primary treatment for prostate cancer: data from CaPSURE [internet]. J Urol. 2007;178(2):529–34; [cited 3 Feb 2019]. Available from https://www.sciencedirect.com/science/article/pii/S0022534707007744#bib5. https://doi.org/10.1016/j.juro.2007.03.126.
22. Halpern JA, Sedrakyan A, Hsu WC, Mao J, Daskivich TJ, Nguyen PL, et al. Utilization, complications, and costs of stereotactic body radiation therapy (SBRT) for localized prostate cancer [internet]. Cancer. 2016;122(16):2496–504; [cited 3 Feb 2019]. Available from https://www.ncbi.nlm.nih.gov/pmc/articles/PMC4974119/. https://doi.org/10.1002/cncr.30101.
23. American Society for Radiation Oncology. ASTRO model policies: proton beam therapy (PRT) [internet]. Arlington. [2017 June; cited 3 Feb 2019]. Available from https://www.astro.org/uploadedFiles/_MAIN_SITE/Daily_Practice/Reimbursement/Model_Policies/Content_Pieces/ASTROPBTModelPolicy.pdf.
24. Sanda MG, Dunn RL, Michalski J, Sandler HM, Northouse L, Hembroff L, et al. Quality of life and satisfaction with outcome among prostate-cancer survivors [internet]. N Engl J Med. 2008;358:1250–61; [cited 3 Feb 2019]. Available from https://www.nejm.org/doi/10.1056/

NEJMoa074311?url_ver=Z39.88-2003&rfr_id=ori%3Arid%3Acrossref.org&rfr_dat=cr_pub%3Dwww.ncbi.nlm.nih.gov. https://doi.org/10.1056/NEJMoa074311.
25. Eade TN, Horwitz EM, Ruth K, Buyyounouski MK, D'Ambrosio DJ, Feigenberg SJ, et al. A comparison of acute and chronic toxicity for men with low-risk prostate cancer treated with intensity-modulated radiation therapy or $^{125}$I permanent implant [internet]. Int J Radiat Oncol Biol Phys. 2008;71(2):338–45; [cited 3 Feb 2019].
26. Grills IS, Martinez AA, Hollander M, Huang R, Goldman K, Chen PY, et al. High dose rate brachytherapy as prostate monotherapy reduces toxicity compared to low dose rate palladium seed [internet]. J Urol. 2004;171(3):1098–104; [cited 3 Feb 2019]. Available from https://www.sciencedirect.com/science/article/pii/S0022534705624226?via%3Dihub. https://doi.org/10.1097/01.ju.0000113299.34404.22.
27. Bolla M, Maingon P, Carrie C, Villa S, Kistios P, Phillip MP, et al. Short acting androgen suppression and radiation dose escalation for intermediate and high risk localized prostate cancer: results of EORTC trial 2291 [internet]. J Clin Oncol. 2016;34(15):1748–56; [cited 3 Feb 2019]. Available from http://ascopubs.org/doi/full/10.1200/JCO.2015.64.8055?url_ver=Z39.88-2003&rfr_id=ori%3Arid%3Acrossref.org&rfr_dat=cr_pub%3Dpubmed&. https://doi.org/10.1200/JCO.2015.64.8055.
28. Radiation Therapy Oncology Group. RTOG/EORTC late radiation morbidity scoring schema. 2019. Available from https://www.rtog.org/researchassociates/adverseeventreporting/rtogeortclateradiationmorbidityscoringschema.aspx.
29. Denham JW, Steigler A, Lamb DS, Joseph D, Turner S, Matthews J, et al. Short-term neoadjuvant androgen deprivation and radiotherapy for locally advanced prostate cancer: 10-year data from the TROG 96.01 randomised trial [internet]. Lancet. 2011;12(5):451–9; [cited 17 Feb 2019]. Available from https://www.sciencedirect.com/science/article/pii/S1470204511700638?via%3Dihub. https://doi.org/10.1016/S1470-2045(11)70063-8.
30. Pisansky TM, Hung D, Gomella L, Amin MB, Balogh AG, Chinn DM, et al. Duration of androgen suppression before radiotherapy for localized prostate cancer: Radiation Therapy Oncology Group randomized clinical trial 9910 [internet]. J Clin Oncol. 2015;33(4):332–9. Available from http://ascopubs.org/doi/pdf/10.1200/JCO.2014.58.0662. https://doi.org/10.1200/JCO.2014.58.0662.
31. Bolla M, Van Tienhoven G, Warde P, Dubois JB, Mirimanoff RO, Storme G, et al. External irradiation with or without long-term androgen suppression for prostate cancer with high metastatic risk: 10-year results of an EORTC randomised study [internet]. Lancet Oncol. 2010;11(11):1066–73; [cited 17 Feb 2019]. Available from https://www.sciencedirect.com/science/article/pii/S1470204510702230?via%3Dihub. https://doi.org/10.1016/S1470-2045(10)70223-0.
32. Pilepich MV, Winter K, Lawton CA, Krisch RE, Wolkov HB, Movsas B, et al. Androgen suppression adjuvant to definitive radiotherapy in prostate carcinoma – long term results of phase III RTOG 85-31 [internet]. Int J Radiat Oncol Biol Phys. 2005;61(5):1285–90; [cited 17 Feb 2019]. Available from https://www.sciencedirect.com/science/article/pii/S036030160402468X?via%3Dihub. https://doi.org/10.1016/j.irobp.2004.08.047.
33. Horwitz EM, Bae K, Hanks GE, Porter A, Grignon DJ, Brereton HD, et al. Ten-year follow-up of radiation therapy oncology group protocol 92-02: a phase III trial of the duration of elective androgen deprivation in locally advanced prostate cancer [internet]. J Clin Oncol. 2008;26(15):2497–504; [cited 17 Feb 2019]. Available from: http://ascopubs.org/doi/pdf/10.1200/JCO.2007.14.9021. https://doi.org/10.1200/JCO.2007.14.9021.
34. Smith MR. Side effects of androgen deprivation therapy. 2018 February 13 [cited 2019 February 17]. In UptoDate [internet]. UptoDate, Inc. Available from https://www.uptodate.com/contents/side-effects-of-androgen-deprivation-therapy?search=adt%20and%20radiation%20therapy%20prostate%20cancer&topicRef=6947&source=see_link#H22.
35. Ward JF, Vogelzang N, Davis BJ. Initial management of regionally localized intermediate-, high-, and very high – risk prostate cancer and those with clinical lymph node involvement. 2019 February 11 [cited 17 Feb 2019]. In UptoDate [internet]. UptoDate, Inc. Available from

https://www.uptodate.com/contents/initial-management-of-regionally-localized-intermediate-high-and-very-high-risk-prostate-cancer-and-those-with-clinical-lymph-node-involvement?search=adt%20and%20radiation%20therapy%20prostate%20cancer&source=search_result&selectedTitle=1~150&usage_type=default&display_rank=1#H2956464.
36. Moy B, Linder BJ, Chao NJ, Gounder MM. Hemorrhagic cystitis in cancer patients. 2018 [cited 4 Mar 2019]. In UptoDate [internet]. UptoDate, Inc. Available from https://www.uptodate.com/contents/hemorrhagic-cystitis-in-cancer-patients?source=history_widget#H1760164724.
37. Inokuchi H, Mizowaki T, Norihisa Y, Takayama K, Ikeda I, Nakamura K, et al. Correlation between urinary dose and delayed radiation cystitis after 78 Gy intensity-modulated radiotherapy for high-risk prostate cancer: a 10-year follow-up study of genitourinary toxicity in clinical practice [internet]. Clin Transl Radiat Oncol. 2017 6:31–36; [cited 3 Mar 2019]. Available from https://www.ncbi.nlm.nih.gov/pmc/articles/PMC5862643/. https://doi.org/10.1016/j.ctro.2017.09.005.
38. Chapter 29 – Prostate. In: Radiation oncology: management decisions. Philadelphia: Lippincott Williams & Wilkins; 2019. Available from http://ovidsp.tx.ovid.com/sp-3.32.2a/ovidweb.cgi?QS2=434f4e1a73d37e8c4c7d6b65ba1a76f10a5f0eeeb99837e07ca68deaddb0a4b0cd2925ebbbcf384b7dca20bf0c0be6a2c11e50864caec7a3a6905907355151f83559bac33189355c15f613aa0c5c4bc695b0712cb5be03f6e75da3efa37e15de05ef9ff00ff8edfdaad11b48e66bb81abe196e04da6dbc37a27d3371db5421f95f3a65aaff7455c7ce0a8aac7eef55c9455ae740464cbfd95c597c4515565370da52469f485779d6a22988d6d5688441aa384cdca6d673fba30369ecd1a6f62e2dc66094e535b427a2569c021d2837af9161979d31ef93174b74895b892efb6f.
39. Rosen RC, Riley A, Wagner G, Osterloh IH, Kirkpatrick J, Mishra A. The international index of erectile function (IIEF): a multidimensional scale for assessment of erectile dysfunction [internet]. Urology. 1997;49(6):822–30; [cited 2019 March 12]. Available from https://www.sciencedirect.com/science/article/pii/S0090429597002380?via%3Dihub. https://doi.org/10.1016/S0090-4295(97)00238-0.
40. Moul JW, Lee WR. Rising serum PSA following local therapy for prostate cancer: definition, natural history, and risk stratification. 2019 [cited 12 Mar 2019]. In UptoDate [internet]. UptoDate, Inc. Available from https://www.uptodate.com/contents/rising-serum-psa-following-local-therapy-for-prostate-cancer-definition-natural-history-and-risk-stratification#H6.
41. Roach M, Hanks G, Thames H Jr, Schellhammer P, Shipley WU, Sokol GH, et al. Defining biochemical failure following radiotherapy with or without hormonal therapy in men with clinically localized prostate cancer: recommendations of the RTOG-ASTRO Phoenix Consensus Conference [internet]. Int J Radiat Oncol Bio Phys. 2006;65(4):965–74; [cited 11 Mar 2019]. Available from https://www.sciencedirect.com/science/article/pii/S0360301606006638?via%3Dihub. https://doi.org/10.1016/j.ijrobp.2006.04.029.

# Chapter 7
# Androgen Deprivation Therapy

**Charlene Reyes, Carla Groshel, and Robert Given**

## Introduction

Androgen deprivation therapy (ADT) has been the standard of care for treating advanced prostate cancer for many decades. Prostate cancer proliferation is, in part, attributed to male androgens. Androgen deprivation therapy is utilized in the suppression of testosterone production. Castrate levels of testosterone are defined as less than 50 ng/dl testosterone. The American Urologic Association is constantly revising its standards. Currently, 25 ng/ml of testosterone is being considered for a new castrate level. The first-line treatment methods of achieving castration target 90–95% of testosterone production in the testes. Many forms of hormone manipulation are used to achieve castrate levels of testosterone. These methods include surgical castration, luteinizing hormone-releasing hormone agonists, and gonadotropin-releasing hormone antagonists. Earlier use of synthetic estrogens, such as diethylstilbestrol (DES), was abandoned due to increased risk of mortality from cardiac causes [1].

There is a small amount of testosterone produced by the adrenal glands. The first-line agents do not suppress this production. This small amount of testosterone production is blocked by using steroidal and nonsteroidal antiandrogens. Complete testosterone blockade requires a multimodal approach.

C. Reyes
Department of Oncology, Urology of Virginia, Virginia Beach, VA, USA
e-mail: charlenereyes@urologyofva.net

C. Groshel (✉)
Urology of Virginia, Schellhammer Cancer Center, Virginia Beach, VA, USA
e-mail: CarlaGroshel@Urologyofva.net

R. Given
Urology of Virginia, LLC, Virginia Beach, VA, USA
e-mail: robertgiven@urologyofva.net



E. J. Trabulsi et al. (eds.), *Chemotherapy and Immunotherapy in Urologic Oncology*, https://doi.org/10.1007/978-3-030-52021-2_7

As discussed in Chap. 5, it is the standard of care to offer adjuvant ADT to radiation as a primary treatment to patients with unfavorable intermediate-risk and high-risk, or very high-risk group [40]. Studies show that patients with higher risk disease undergoing radiation treatment have been shown to prolong survival with neoadjuvant and adjuvant ADT [2, 3]. Short-term ADT (4–6 months) is recommended in patients with intermediate disease. Long-term ADT (18–36 months) should be offered for high-risk and very high-risk patients [40]. One study compared the use of short-term ADT ( 4 months) versus long-term ADT (24 months) in men with locally advanced cancers (cT2c-T4N0-1M0 and Gleason scores 8–10). Men receiving long-term ADT to had an improved overall survival and disease specific. Short-term ADT consists of 2 months of neoadjuvant ADT and 2 months of adjuvant ADT [2]. Another study compared men with localized higher risk prostate cancer (PSA equal to or greater than 10 ng/mL and/or Gleason grade 7 or higher, cT3) receiving radiation monotherapy or combined radiation with 6 months of ADT. The study revealed that the overall and disease-specific survival rates were better in the men who received ADT [3].

ADT may be used as a sole or primary treatment. It is utilized in men with prostate cancer who are of advanced age, have significant comorbidities, and for those who decline curative therapy. One large study compared cancer-specific survival and overall survival in men with localized prostate cancer who received primary ADT versus men on surveillance. The study concluded that primary ADT did not provide a survival benefit in the majority of men compared to those on observation [4].

ADT has significant side effects such as hot flashes, decreased libido, osteoporosis, decline in sexual function and drive, and metabolic and cardiac effects. Most are mild to moderate and a good quality of life can be achieved with its use.

In this chapter, we review the general mechanism of action of ADT, side effect management, patient counseling, health lifestyle, and second-line hormonal manipulations.

## Mechanism of Action

### *Regulation of Androgen Production*

In order to understand the mechanism of action of ADT, it is important to review the testosterone production pathways. Testosterone is regulated by two mechanisms in the body. The hypothalamic–pituitary–gonadal (HPG) axis, see Fig. 7.1, is responsible for the production and regulation of testosterone by the testicles. The hypothalamic–pituitary–adrenal (HPA) axis, see Fig. 7.2, is responsible for a very small amount of testosterone released from the adrenal glands. Gonadotropin-releasing hormone (GnRH) and corticotrophin-releasing factor (CRF) are neurohormones produced in the hypothalamus. GnRH simulates in pulses the secretion of two

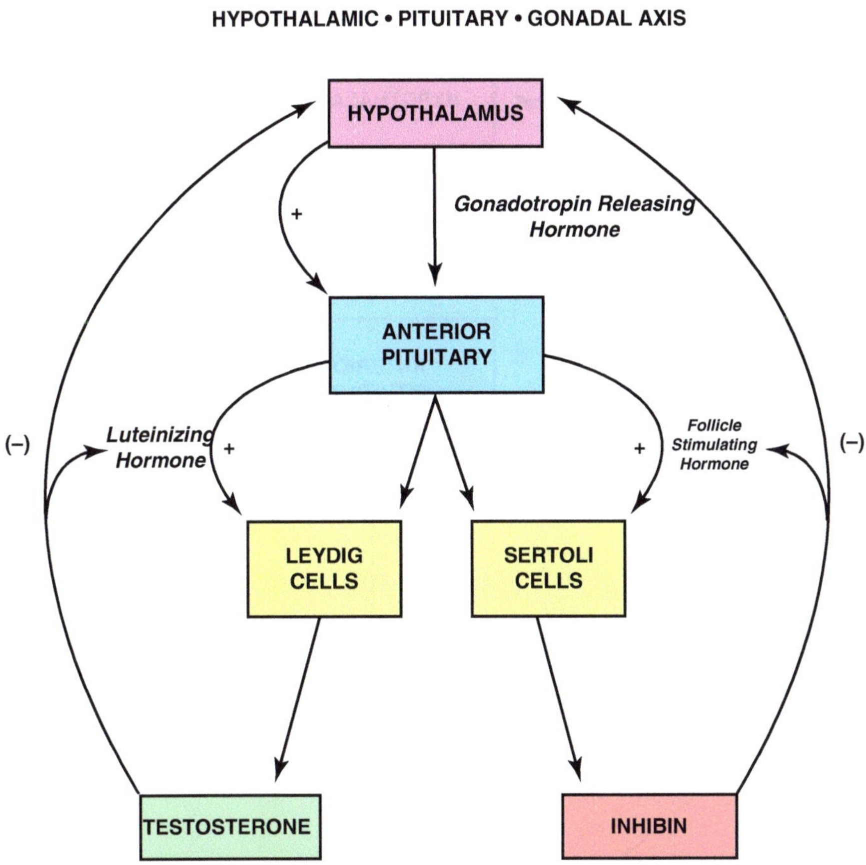


**Fig. 7.1** Hypothalamic–pituitary–gonadal axis

gonadotropins, luteinizing hormone (LH) and follicle-stimulating hormone (FSH) from the anterior pituitary gland. CRF stimulates the release of adrenocorticotropic hormone (ACTH) also from the anterior pituitary gland. LH is responsible for 95% of circulating testosterone production through receptors on the surface of Leydig cells in the testes. ACTH acts on the adrenal glands to produce androstenedione and dehydroepiandrosterone. These intermediate metabolites become androgens that are more active in prostate tissue [5].

Testosterone levels are maintained within a narrow range by a negative feedback mechanism. When testosterone is decreased, GnRH and LH secretion are increased. When testosterone is elevated, GnRH and LH secretion are decreased. Continuous stimulation of the pituitary gland leads to an increase in the secretion of GnRH resulting in a decrease in secretion of LH and consequently a decrease in testosterone production.

Similarly, cortisol regulation is maintained by stimulation and inhibition of CRF and ACTH on the hypothalamus and pituitary gland [6, 7].

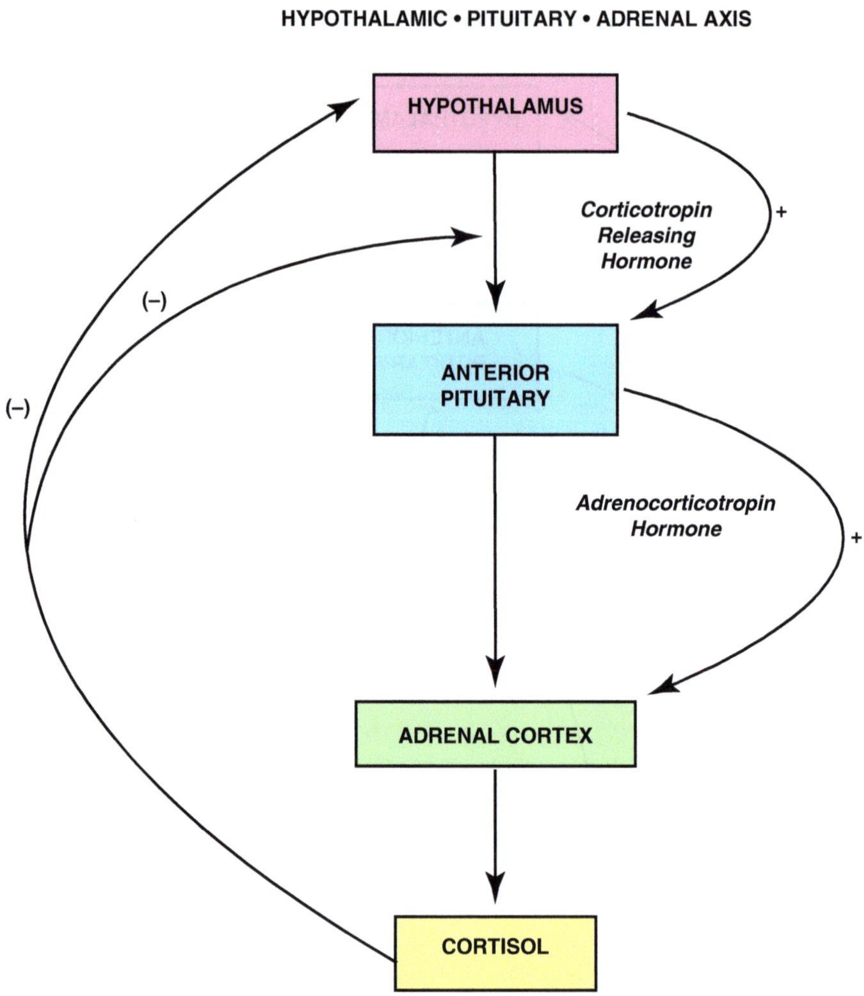


**Fig. 7.2** Hypothalamic–pituitary–adrenal axis

## Agents of Treatment

Prostate cancer cells are generally androgen-dependent, and most patients with advanced disease will respond to ADT in some form or another [8]. There are four methods to block androgen: (1) removal of sources of androgens, (2) use of LHRH agonists/GnRH antagonists, (3) use of antiandrogens, and (4) inhibition of androgen synthesis.

## *Removal of Sources of Androgens*

Bilateral orchiectomy historically was considered the gold standard for the treatment of advanced prostate cancer. Removal of the testes results in the inhibition of testosterone and dihydrotestosterone (DHT) and an increase in luteinizing hormone and follicle-stimulating hormone (FSH). This method results in a 95% reduction in testosterone hormone levels. One study revealed that greater than 90% of testosterone levels were reduced within 24 hours of castration [9]. Although more cost-effective, the major disadvantage of orchiectomy is its irreversibility. Treatment by orchiectomy should only be considered in men with advanced prostate cancer who require indefinite ADT.

## *Use of LHRH Agonists and GnRH Antagonists*

An alternative to orchiectomy is pharmacologic androgen suppression using LHRH receptor agonists and GnRH antagonists. LHRH receptor agonists function to suppress androgens produced at the level of the testes, not the adrenal glands. Initially, agonist action causes a rise in LH, FSH, testosterone, and DHT. This elevation in hormone levels produces what is known as "testosterone surge" and may contribute to the exacerbation of clinical symptoms in men with bone metastases. LH increases up to ten-fold during the flare and may last as long as 10–20 days [10]. Testosterone flare is blocked by prior administration with an antiandrogen, which will be discussed later in this chapter.

The goal of androgen suppression is attaining a testosterone level less than 50 ng/dl within 3 weeks of administration. Chronic stimulation of the pituitary gland results in desensitizing and suppressing the LHRH receptors, which ultimately causes a decrease in hormone levels, see Fig. 7.3. FSH is only partially suppressed as compared to LH. FSH levels begin to rise after a few weeks to baseline concentration, which is known as the "FSH escape." FSH receptors located on the surface of prostate cancer cells and blood vessels within tumors may promote progression of prostate cancer [11].

Examples of LHRH agonists, routes of administration, doses, and interval of administration are listed in Table 7.1. The most common agonist used is leuprolide acetate. It can be administered subcutaneously or intramuscularly.

GNRH receptor antagonists are the most recently introduced class of hormonal treatments. GnRH receptor antagonists rapidly and competitively bind to GnRH receptors in the pituitary, blocking the release of gonadotropins, causing a decrease in LH, FSH, and testosterone. See Fig. 7.4. Testosterone suppression occurs rapidly with the use of GnRH receptor antagonists and does not produce the testosterone flare associated with the receptor agonists; therefore, antiandrogens are not coadministered with the antagonists. GnRH antagonists are preferred for an initial treatment therapy for men with bone metastases. A recent study comparing the ability of

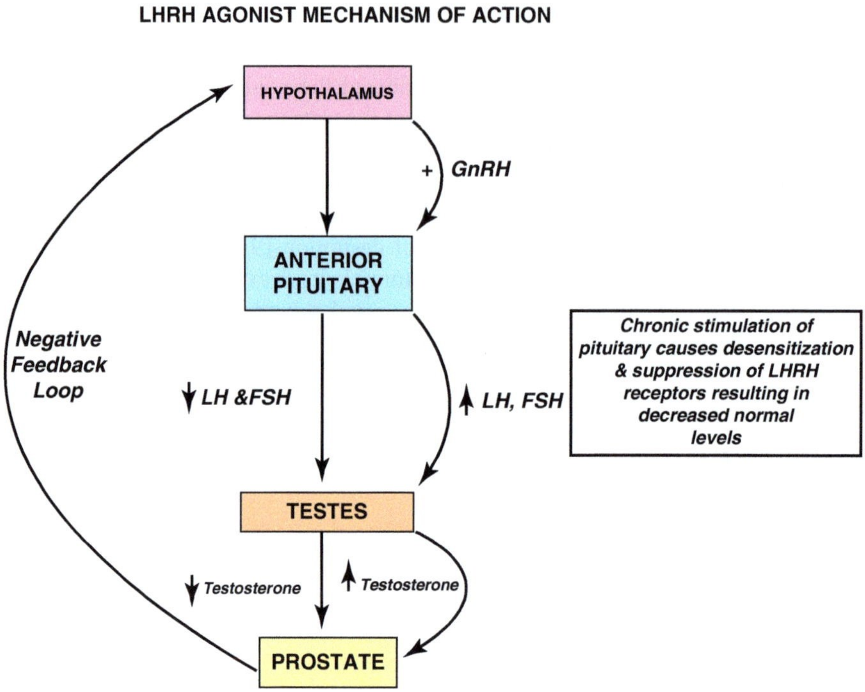


**Fig. 7.3** Mechanism of action of LHRH agonist

**Table 7.1** Examples of luteinizing hormone-releasing hormone

| Generic name | Brand name | Route | Dose (mg) | Dose interval |
|---|---|---|---|---|
| Leuprolide acetate injection | Eligard® | Subcutaneous | 7.5<br>22.5<br>30<br>45 | 1 month<br>3 months<br>4 months<br>6 months |
| Leuprolide acetate depot | Lupron® | Intramuscular | 7.5<br>22.5<br>30<br>45 | 1 month<br>3 months<br>4 months<br>6 months |
| Triptorelin pamoate injection | Trelstar® | Intramuscular | 3.75<br>11.25<br>22.5 | 1 month<br>3 months<br>6 months |
| Goserelin acetate implant | Zoladex® | Subcutaneous | 3.6<br>10.8 | 1 month<br>3 months |
| Histrelin acetate implant | Vantas® | Subcutaneous | 50 | 1 year |

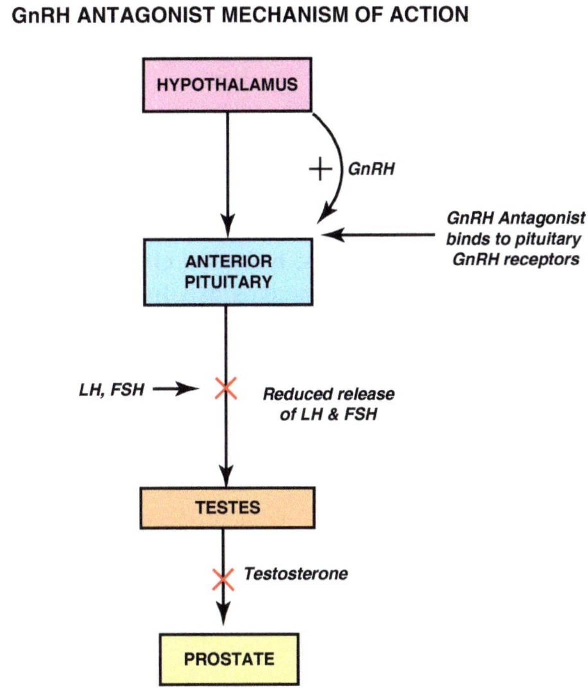


**Fig. 7.4** Mechanism of action of GNRH antagonist

GNRH antagonists and agonists to suppress FSH revealed that GNRH antagonists were superior at suppressing and maintaining lower FSH levels than the agonists, which could account for better prostate cancer control [12].

Firmagon® (degarelix) is the only GnRH receptor antagonist administered by subcutaneous injection monthly. The initial loading dose is 240 mg, given as two 120 mg injections administered simultaneously. The monthly maintenance dose is 80 mg, which is currently the only dose available.

The primary advantage of GnRH receptor antagonists is their ability to lower testosterone rapidly. In one clinical trial, the efficacy of degarelix compared to leuprolide in lowering testosterone to castrate levels was measured. During a period of 28 days, 620 patients were randomized to degarelix or leuprolide. Degarelix lowered testosterone to castrate levels in 52% of men after 1 day and 96% after 3 days. Leuprolide lowered testosterone to castrate levels in 18% of men after 14 days and 100% after 28 days [13].

## *Antiandrogens: Nonsteroidal and Steroidal Antiandrogens*

There are two categories of antiandrogens: steroidal and nonsteroidal antiandrogens. Nonsteroidal antiandrogens, also called androgen receptor antagonists, bind to and inhibit the androgen receptor, thereby inhibiting activation of the receptor

**Table 7.2** Nonsteroidal antiandrogens

| Generic name | Brand name | Route | Dose | Dosing interval |
|---|---|---|---|---|
| Flutamide | Eulexin® | Oral | 250 mg | 3 times daily |
| Nilutamide | Nilandron® | Oral | 300 mg (1st month) | Daily |
| | | | 150 mg | Daily |
| Bicalutamide | Casodex® | Oral | 50 mg | Daily |

and limiting the androgens' biological effects. Nonsteroidal antiandrogens do not inhibit the hypothalamic-pituitary axis from producing testosterone. Testosterone levels will not lower with the use of nonsteroidal antiandrogens. They are not recommended as a monotherapy for advanced prostate cancer.

First-generation nonsteroidal antiandrogens are often used as an adjuvant therapy with LHRH agonists to provide maximum androgen blockade. They are prescribed 2–3 weeks prior to LHRH receptor agonists to prevent the potential clinical effects of the testosterone flare in men with metastatic prostate cancer. Examples of nonsteroidal antiandrogens include bicalutamide, flutamide, and nilutamide. These are listed in Table 7.2 with their dosing information [14]. Enzalutamide and apalutamide, potent antiandrogens, will be discussed in another chapter.

Flutamide was the first nonsteroidal antiandrogen produced for the treatment of prostate cancer. Flutamide was prescribed in 250 mg doses three times daily due to its short half-life of 6 hours. Eliminated through renal excretion, flutamide is not recommended for patients with renal impairment. Flutamide is rarely used since the introduction of longer acting antiandrogens.

Another nonsteroidal antiandrogen, nilutamide, has a longer half-life of 56 hours. It is prescribed for once-daily dosing, which allows for better compliance. The initial dose is 300 mg for the first month, followed by 150 mg daily maintenance dose. Nilutamide should be taken with food. It is eliminated through hepatic clearance [15].

Bicalutamide is the most recently developed nonsteroidal antiandrogen. Bicalutamide is prescribed as a 50-mg dose for once a day. It has a half-life of 6 days. It may be taken with or without food. Metabolism occurs via the liver; however, patients with mild to moderate hepatic impairment are not excluded from taking bicalutamide [15]. Periodic liver function tests should be performed in patients with moderate hepatic impairment, who remain on chronic bicalutamide therapy. Bicalutamide is well tolerated with very few side effects. It is a more potent nonsteroidal antiandrogen than its predecessors, with a much greater binding affinity for the androgen receptor [16].

Steroidal antiandrogens inhibit the binding of dihydrotestosterone to prostate cancer cells. Unlike nonsteroidal antiandrogens, steroidal antiandrogens, such as cyproterone acetate (CPA), are involved in the negative feedback mechanism exerted on the hypothalamic–pituitary axis, which leads to decrease in LH and subsequently lowers testosterone. CPA is less effective at controlling prostate cancer than LHRH agonists and GnRH antagonists, and CPA has a higher side-effect profile including significant cardiovascular complications in up to 10% of men [17]. CPA is not available in the United States.

## Antiandrogen Withdrawal

When a person has used combined androgen blockade using LHRH agonists and antiandrogens, a withdrawal effect can occur when the antiandrogen is removed from the combination. This withdrawal effect results in a decrease in the PSA. In this setting, a possible mutation in the androgen receptor allows the antiandrogen activity to shift from an antagonist to an agonistic exertion on prostate cancer cells [18]. This withdrawal phenomenon has been shown in flutamide, nilutamide, and bicalutamide antiandrogens. PSA decrease after flutamide withdrawal has been seen within 4 weeks, whereas nilutamide and bicalutamide withdrawal yielded a PSA decrease within 6 weeks [19]. Two studies revealed that antiandrogen withdrawal effect on PSA occurred in 15–30% of patients with a more than a 50% decrease in PSA level over an average of 3.5–5 months [20, 21].

## Side Effects Management

Androgen deprivation therapy (ADT) has side effects for most men. The common side effects vary in intensity, frequency, and duration but most side effects reported in clinical trials were mild to moderate [13, 24]. Common side effects in order of their frequency include hot flashes, injection site pain, fatigue, weight gain, muscle loss, weakness, decrease of libido, sexual dysfunction, depression, osteoporosis, heart disease, and uncontrolled blood sugar [25]. The side effects in this discussion are not an exhaustive list. There are other side effects such as cognitive loss, gynecomastia, or anemia to name a few. They are not discussed in this chapter, as their rate of occurrence is very low and generally not a significant deterrent to treatment.

The most common side effects in the use of ADT are hot flashes. These are a vasomotor symptom of decreased testosterone. They are described as a short burst of heat generally originating in the head with or without perspiration [26]. They range in intensity, duration, and frequency, but the vast majority fall in the mild to moderate category. The rate of reported hot flashes varies depending on the drug given to start with and the study reviewed. Reports of the rate of hot flashes range from 20% to 88% of men depending on the drug and the study being reviewed [24, 26]. It is safe to assume that more than 30% of patients using ADT will experience hot flashes.

Patients report more hot flashes within the first 3 months with degarelix than leuprolide. This is due to the antagonistic effect of degarelix and the speed with which it reduces testosterone compared to slower acting leuprolide. After 3 months, it is unlikely for a patient to start experiencing hot flashes.

The main risk factor for developing hot flashes appears to be with men who have a higher BMI or slower heart rate. The exact reason for these predictors is speculative. Having a higher BMI is associated with lower testosterone levels at baseline and may hasten the suppression. For heart rate, it is thought that hypothyroid conditions may play a role in contributing to hot flashes [26].

There are several ways to manage hot flashes. The method of management should be commensurate with the severity, i.e., the more severe the hot flashes, the more invasive the treatment.

Studies in Europe have shown that cyproterone acetate, an antiandrogen/progestin, has a 95% success rate in resolving hot flashes. Cyproterone acetate is not used as a first line regardless of its efficacy in reducing hot flashes because it can interfere with the ADT therapy [25, 27].

Medroxyprogestrone acetate is 83% effective in resolving hot flashes and is considered the first-line treatment for hot flashes [25, 27]. Since depomedroxyprogesterone acetate (Depo-provera®) is readily available in 150 mg IM doses in the United States, it is most often dosed at 300IM q6mos as needed for hot flashes. Be aware that depomedroxyprogesterone has the potential for serious side effects. Thromboembolism, breast cancer, depression, seizures, bone density loss, and hepatic impairment are just a few [39].

Venlafaxine ER 75 mg daily is about 47% effective at reducing and/or eliminating hot flashes [27]. Venlafaxine has serious side effects of its own such as suicidal ideation and worsening depression, serotonin syndrome, seizures, and arrhythmias to name a few. Initially, close follow-up after starting this medication is recommended. This medicine must not be stopped abruptly, so refills need to be maintained on time and the patient needs to be compliant and reliable [28].

Alternative or complementary treatments such as soy, black cohosh, or Mexican yam have some anecdotal effect. However, this may be a placebo effect. In a very small study of 33 men undergoing ADT, soy protein did not show improvement in vasomotor symptoms. Acupuncture was tested and found to be effective with 95% improvement, but none of the acupuncture studies was randomized or placebo-controlled [25].

Injection site pain occurs more often with degarelix (35%) as opposed to leuprolide (1%). When experienced it is mostly mild to moderate and is usually in the first injection only. The first injection of degarelix is two180 mg doses vs. one 80 mg dose for maintenance. This medication forms a disc or nodule under the skin and is more viscous than a traditional vaccine. The best management is patient education. Tylenol is sufficient to help with residual pain. Over-the-counter hydrocortisone cream can also help with redness.

Fatigue is a noticeable side effect of ADT that can affect the quality of life. Fatigue, as a symptom of hypogonadism, is so recognizable that it is used as a marketable tool for men's health clinics. Fatigue is reported about 3–11% depending on the study referencing [13, 24]. The only evidence-based management for ADT-induced fatigue is exercise. In a systematic review of all peer-reviewed articles published between 1980 and 2013 focusing on exercise and the treatment-related adverse effects of prostate cancer, none of the outcomes reported worsening fatigue with exercise. All studies reviewed showed improvement or equivocal results. The studies that showed improvement varied from as little as 30 min 3 days a week to 60 min 3–5 days a week. The one commonality the positive studies had was some form of resistance training to improve muscle mass/definition [29, 31].

After only 9 months of ADT, about 80% of men will have a decrease in bone mineral density (BMD) [32]. A decrease in BMD leads to osteopenia, osteoporosis, and increased risk for fractures. The risk for fractures increases with longer duration of use. The National Comprehensive Cancer Network (NCCN) guidelines recommend men have a serum 25-hydroxy vitamin D and a DEXA bone scan for baseline information [33]. The National Osteoporosis Foundation recommends men older than 50 years of age, have a daily intake of 1200 mg calcium, and 800–1000 IU vitamin D [25]. It is reasonable to recommend patients start a calcium and vitamin D supplement such as Caltrate® or Citracal®. The upper limit of safe vitamin D3 supplement in a 50-year-old or older with normal vitamin D levels is 4000 IU daily. If vitamin D levels drop below normal (<20 ng/ml), the patient should be replenished [33]. In high-risk patients, such as ADT-treated patients, vitamin D is often replaced when levels drop below 30 ng/ml. vitamin D3 is sold in stores in 2000 IU and 4000 IU doses. The common practice is to recommend 2000 IU of vitamin D3 in addition to the calcium and vitamin D supplement. If a severe deficiency occurs <10 ng/ml, 50,000 IU of vitamin D2 once a week should be prescribed. Repeat 25-hydroxy levels 3 months after treatment, is recommended to ensure they have returned to normal. If vitamin D levels fail to increase with over-the-counter D3 supplementation, 50,000 IU of vitamin D2 weekly should be prescribed. Patients who have 25-hydroxy serum levels <10 ng/ml at the baseline evaluation are at risk for osteomalacia, referral to their primary care for further evaluation is recommended [33].

There is no evidence-based guideline set by the AUA or NCCN on how often vitamin D should be monitored. The NCCN suggests yearly screening at a minimum. Conservative management practices choose to monitor every 6 months.

The NCCN guidelines recommend denosumab (60 mg subcutaneously every 6 months), for men who have a 10-year risk of fracture ≥3%, based on the Fracture Risk Assessment Tool (FRAX) algorithm, or if the baseline DEXA scan shows osteopenia. The FRAX algorithm can be accessed at https://www.sheffield.ac.uk/FRAX/. When using the FRAX algorithm, select yes for "secondary osteoporosis" due to ADT [25, 34].

A cascade of side effects occurs with the increase in fat mass, loss of lean muscle mass, and increase in waist circumference. Men are at risk of having metabolic syndrome, which is a significant risk factor for diabetes and heart disease [35]. Studies have shown that as little as 12 weeks of ADT can result in a decrease in insulin sensitivity and an increase in plasma insulin. In multiple studies, greater than 1 year of ADT, 28–44% of the men had fasting glucose in the diabetic range [25]. No definitive prevention or guidelines have been set to address the risk of diabetes. Some preliminary studies have shown positive outcomes with metformin usage [25, 30]. Prescribing this is not the standard of care to date, and managing diabetes or prediabetes is not in the purview of urology.

Regular monitoring of blood glucose level every 6 months is a sound clinical decision. Also working in concert with a patient's primary care provider will help ensure patient health while on ADT.

The FDA has required the drug manufacturers of leuprolide to list an association with increased risk in cardiac harm. The studies regarding this have mixed results. There are multiple studies to show an association between ADT use and increased incidents of coronary artery disease (CAD), myocardial infarction (MI), and congestive heart failure (CHF). The cause for this is unknown. Lack of testosterone alone may not be the culprit. Men who have undergone orchiectomies do not show an increased risk for CAD. This would suggest the problem lies with the pharmacology of the medication or a secondary problem arising from the metabolic effects of weight gain, decreased lean muscle mass, increase in central obesity, and increase in serum lipids. All of which have known cardiovascular risk factors. The use of ADT does not increase the overall morbidity due to CAD unless the patient had CAD, CHF, or a history of MI prior to start of ADT [25, 30, 36]. Careful patient selection and monitoring are key to the prevention of CAD complications.

The use of ADT can significantly affect the quality of life with decreased libido and erectile dysfunction. This can lead to loss of feeling of masculinity and depression [37].

Decrease in testosterone results in a loss of libido. Over time, it can increase venous leakage, decrease arterial flow, and impair nitric oxide leading to sexual dysfunction. There is also significant atrophy of the penis and testes [25]. This can lead to feelings of loss of masculinity, particularly in men who are younger and define masculinity with sexual function. Men who have erectile dysfunction prior to treatment due to age, medication, or comorbid conditions are less bothered by this. Loss of sexual function can be particularly stressful in men who are single or not in long-term relationships. Navigating a new relationship can be tricky when one partner cannot perform sexually and may lead men to avoid social situations or dating. Men in relationships, also worry about their partner leaving them if they cannot satisfy them [37].

This loss of masculinity and self-identity can lead to depression. Men should be screened for depression and thoughts of suicide. If patients are willing to admit to thoughts of depression, sadness, or loss of self-worth, referral to their primary care providers for antidepressants is recommended. Three studies have shown that moderate to high-intensity exercise can improve sexual function in men. This translates to $\geq$3000 kcal/week or 450 kcal/day [30]. The average man would need to walk briskly for an hour a day to achieve this. That is a lot of exercise, and most Americans do not have the self-discipline or physical health to accomplish this.

## Healthy Lifestyle

It is important that patients adopt a healthy lifestyle while receiving ADT. Exercise, both aerobic and strength training, is important in mitigating side effects such as fatigue, erectile dysfunction, and hot flashes. Weight-bearing exercises are important for bone density. Consistent aerobic exercise is a known benefit for cardiovascular health. Diet, as a solution for the side effects of ADT, is under continual study.

Challenges arise when studying diet, mainly in compliance and reporting. There are to date no known foods that will reverse hot flashes or improve ED [29]. We know that patients who have a waist circumference of greater than 40 inches are at higher risk for metabolic syndrome and CAD. A heart-healthy diet low in refined carbohydrates and sugars can help reduce waist circumference. We have discussed that patients with a BMI greater than 30 and regular alcohol consumption are more prone to hot flashes. Adopting a healthy lifestyle with exercise and diet are the keys to reducing the risks of side effects of ADT, but there is no proof that these will eliminate them all together [25, 30]. At the end of the day, eating healthy and exercising regularly will improve a patient's outlook and mood. That may be the best way to ensure good quality of life despite the side effects.

## Patient Counseling

Many large urology groups have dedicated Advance Prostate Cancer Clinics (APCC) where an MD or an APC spends 30–40 minutes educating patients when they start an ADT medication. It is important to manage patient expectations when starting this medication. Patients should be aware of all of the side effect potentials with this treatment.

By educating the patients about the risks that ADT presents, they can keep open dialogue with all their providers.

Knowing the cardiac and metabolic effects can help patients understand the role this treatment will play in managing their existing cardiac or diabetic conditions. Feelings of depression or loss of quality of life can be discussed without shame when patients know the medicine is causing their problems. Patients need to know there are potential solutions before the symptoms arise to prevent frustration and noncompliance with treatment.

Discussing sexual function and depression are sensitive intimate discussions. Taking time to review this treatment helps the provider and patient build a relationship that fosters open communication. This will lead to more "shared decision-making" (SDM). SDM leads to higher patient satisfaction scores, and patients report better quality of life if they feel they have chosen their treatments. When patients feel that they have control of their healthcare, they will be more likely to be compliant with treatment regimens [38].

## Second-Line Hormone Manipulation

### *Ketoconazole*

Historically, second-line therapies such as ketoconazole have been used off-label in men with castrate-resistant prostate cancer before and after chemotherapy. One example of a second-line hormonal therapy is ketoconazole, which is a nonselective steroid 17α-hydroxylase/17, 20 lyase (CYP17A1) inhibitor that blocks the synthesis of adrenal testosterone. It is prescribed at 200 mg or 400 mg three times daily along with prednisone due to adrenal suppression. Testosterone suppression to castrate levels is immediate. One study noted that castrate levels of testosterone occurred within 4 hours [22]. Currently, ketoconazole is utilized as palliative therapy for patients with advanced prostate cancer with symptomatic spinal cord compression and in a setting with limited access to GnRH receptor antagonists [23]. More recent second-line therapies (abiraterone, enzalutamide, and apalutamide) have superseded the need for ketoconazole beyond the urgent need for castration in the symptomatic spinal cord compression patient and will be discussed in another chapter.

**Clinical Pearls**

- Start ADT treatment with a GNRH antagonist or a nonsteroidal antiandrogen if the patient is metastatic to avoid “surge.”
- Choose ADT recipients carefully. Men with uncontrolled diabetes or heart disease may not be good candidates.
- Monitor bone health with DEXA scans and serum vitamin D.
- Side effects can be improved with exercise and heart-healthy diet.

## References


1. Nelson JB. Hormone therapy for prostate cancer. In: Campbell-Walsh urology, vol. 3. 10th ed. Amsterdam: Elsevier Inc; 2012. p. 2935.
2. Hanks GE, Pajak TF, Porter A, Grignon D, Brereton H, Venkatesan V, Horwitz EM, Lawton C, Rosenthal SA, Sandler HM, Shipley WU, Radiation Therapy Oncology Group. Phase III trial of long-term adjuvant androgen deprivation after neoadjuvant hormonal cytoreduction and radiotherapy in locally advanced carcinoma of the prostate: the Radiation Therapy Oncology Group Protocol 92-02. J Clin Oncol. 2003;21(21):3972–8.
3. D’Amico AV, Manola J, Loffredo M, Renshaw AA, DellaCroce A, Kantoff PW. 6-month androgen suppression plus radiation therapy vs radiation therapy alone for patients with clinically localized prostate cancer: a randomized controlled trial. JAMA. 2004;292(7):821–7.
4. Lu-Yao GL, Albertsen PC, Moore DF, Shih W, Lin Y, DiPaola RS, Yao SL. Survival following primary androgen deprivation therapy among men with localized prostate cancer. JAMA. 2008;300(2):173–81. https://doi.org/10.1001/jama.300.2.173.
5. Denmeade SR, Isaacs JT. Overview of regulation of systemic androgen levels. In: Holland-Frei cancer medicine. 6th ed. Hamilton: BC Decker Inc; 2003.
6. Up To Date. Physiology of gonadotropin-releasing hormone. http://www.uptodate.com. Accessed 29 Dec 2018.
7. Up To Date. Adrenal steroid biosynthesis. http://uptodate.com. Accessed 29 Dec 2018.
8. Tanagho EA, McAninch JW. Smith’s general urology. 17th ed. New York: McGraw-Hill Companies, Inc; 2008. p. 367.
9. Maatman TJ, Gupta MK, Montie JE. Effectiveness of castration versus intravenous estrogen therapy in producing rapid endocrine control of metastatic cancer of the prostate. J Urol. 1985;133(4):620–1.
10. Weckermann D, Harzmann R. Hormone therapy in prostate cancer: LHRH antagonists versus LHRH analogues. Eur Urol. 2004;46(3):279–83.

11. Lepor H, Shore ND. LHRH agonists for the treatment of prostate cancer: 2012. Rev Urol. 2012;14(1–2):1–12.
12. Crawford ED, Tombal B, Boccardo F, Miller K, Shore N, Moul JW, Damber JE, Collette L, Persson BE. FSH suppression and tumour control in patients with prostate cancer during androgen deprivation with a GnRH agonist or antagonist. Scand J Urol. 2019;9:1–9. https://doi.org/10.1080/21681805.1522372.
13. Klotz L, Boccon-Gibod L, Shore ND, Andreou C, Persson BE, Cantor P, Jensen JK, Olesen TK, Schroder FH. The efficacy and safety of degarelix: a 12-month, comparative, randomized, open-label, parallel-group phase III study in patients with prostate cancer. BJU Int. 2008;102(11):1531–8. https://doi.org/10.1111/j.1464-410X.2008.08183.x.
14. Up To Date. ADT plus first-generation antiandrogens. Http://www.uptodate.com. Accessed 16 Jan 2019.
15. Mahler C, Verhelst J, Denis L. Clinical pharmacokinetics of the antiandrogens and their efficacy in prostate cancer. Clin Pharmacokinet. 1998;34(5):405–17.
16. Mukherjee A, Kirkovsky L, Yao XT, Yates RC, Miller DD, Dalton JT. Enantioselective binding of Casodex to the androgen receptor. Xenobiotica. 1996;26(2):117–22.
17. de Voogt HJ, Smith PH, Pavone-Macaluso M, DePauw M, Suciu S. Cardiovascular side effects of diethylstilbestrol, cyproterone acetate, medroxyprogesterone acetate and estramustine phosphate used for the treatment of advanced prostate cancer: results from European Organization for Research on Treatment of Cancer trials 30761 and 30762. J Urol. 1986;135(2):303–7.
18. Taplin ME, Bubley GJ, Shuster TD, Frantz ME, Spooner AE. Mutation of the androgen-receptor gene in metastatic androgen-independent prostate cancer. N Engl J Med. 1995;332(21):1393–8.
19. Nieh PT. Withdrawal phenomenon with the antiandrogen casodex. J Urol. 1995;153(3 Pt 2):1070–2.
20. Kelly WK, Scher HI. Prostate specific antigen decline after antiandrogen withdrawal: the flutamide withdrawal syndrome. J Urol. 1993;149(3):607–9.
21. Small EJ, Srinivas S. The antiandrogen withdrawal syndrome. Experience in a large cohort of unselected patients with advanced prostate cancer. Cancer. 1995;76(8):1428–34.
22. Trachtenberg J, Halpern N, Pont A. Ketoconazole: a novel and rapid treatment for advanced prostate cancer. J Urol. 1983;130(1):152–3.
23. Patel V, Liaw B, Oh W. The role of ketoconazole in current prostate cancer care. Natl Rev Urol. 2018;15(10):643–51. https://doi.org/10.1038/s41585-018-0077-y.
24. Spitz A, Young JM, Larsen L, Mattia-Goldberg C, Donnelly J, Chwalisz K. Efficacy and safety of leuprolide acetate 6-month depot for suppression of testosterone in patients with prostate cancer. Prostate Cancer Prostatic Dis. 2012;15(1):93–9. https://doi.org/10.1038/pcan.2011.50. Epub 25 Oct 2011. PubMed PMID: 22025196; PubMed Central PMCID: PMC3278745.
25. Nguyen PL, Alibhai SM, Basaria S, D'Amico AV, Kantoff PW, Keating NL, Penson DF, Rosario DJ, Tombal B, Smith MR. Adverse effects of androgen deprivation therapy and strategies to mitigate them. Eur Urol. 2015;67(5):825–36. Epub 2 Aug 2014. Review. PubMed PMID: 25097095. https://doi.org/10.1016/j.eururo.2014.07.010.
26. Iversen P, Karup C, van der Meulen E, Tankó LB, Huhtaniemi I. Hot flushes in prostatic cancer patients during androgen-deprivation therapy with monthly dose of degarelix or leuprolide. Prostate Cancer Prostatic Dis. 2011;14(2):184–90. Epub 29 Mar 2011. PubMed PMID: 21445092. https://doi.org/10.1038/pcan.2011.11.
27. Irani J, Salomon L, Oba R, Bouchard P, Mottet N. Efficacy of venlafaxine, medroxyprogesterone acetate, and cyproterone acetate for the treatment of vasomotor hot flushes in men taking gonadotropin-releasing hormone analogues for prostate cancer: a double-blind, randomised trial. Lancet Oncol. 2010;11(2):147–54. Epub 4 Dec 2009. PubMed PMID: 19963436. https://doi.org/10.1016/S1470-2045(09)70338-9.
28. Up To Date. Venlafaxine drug information Lexicomp. 1978-2018. http://www.uptodate.com. Accessed 12 Dec 2018.
29. Moyad MA, Newton RU, Tunn UW, Gruca D. Integrating diet and exercise into care of prostate cancer patients on androgen deprivation therapy. Res Rep Urol. 2016;8:133–43. eCol-

lection 2016. Review. PubMed PMID: 27574584; PubMed Central PMCID: PMC4993404. https://doi.org/10.2147/RRU.S107852.
30. Gardner JR, Livingston PM, Fraser SF. Effects of exercise on treatment-related adverse effects for patients with prostate cancer receiving androgen-deprivation therapy: a systematic review. J Clin Oncol. 2014;32(4):335–46. Epub 16 Dec 2013. Review. PubMed PMID: 24344218. https://doi.org/10.1200/JCO.2013.49.5523.
31. Yu EY, Kuo KF, Gulati R, Chen S, Gambol TE, Hall SP, Jiang PY, Pitzel P, Higano CS. Long-term dynamics of bone mineral density during intermittent androgen deprivation for men with nonmetastatic, hormone-sensitive prostate cancer. J Clin Oncol. 2012;30(15):1864–70. Epub 9 Apr 2012. PubMed PMID: 22493411; PubMed Central PMCID: PMC3383183. https://doi.org/10.1200/JCO.2011.38.3745.
32. Up To Date. Vitamin D deficiency. http://www.uptodate.com. Accessed 12 Dec 2018.
33. Principals of androgen deprivation therapy. NCCN guidelines version 3.2016, Prostate cancer. 2016. Http://NCCN.org. Accessed 12 Dec 2018.
34. Ziehr DR, Chen MH, Zhang D, Braccioforte MH, Moran BJ, Mahal BA, Hyatt AS, Basaria SS, Beard CJ, Beckman JA, Choueiri TK, D'Amico AV, Hoffman KE, Hu JC, Martin NE, Sweeney CJ, Trinh QD, Nguyen PL. Association of androgen-deprivation therapy with excess cardiac-specific mortality in men with prostate cancer. BJU Int. 2015;116(3):358–65. Epub 29 Oct 2014. PubMed PMID: 25124891. https://doi.org/10.1111/bju.12905.
35. Nguyen PL, Jarolim P, Basaria S, Zuflacht JP, Milian J, Kadivar S, Graham PL, Hyatt A, Kantoff PW, Beckman JA. Androgen deprivation therapy reversibly increases endothelium-dependent vasodilation in men with prostate cancer. J Am Heart Assoc. 2015;4(4):e001914. PubMed PMID: 25896892; PubMed Central PMCID: PMC4579953. https://doi.org/10.1161/JAHA.115.001914.
36. Jones JM, Kohli M, Loprinzi CL. Androgen deprivation therapy-associated vasomotor symptoms. Asian J Androl. 2012;14(2):193–7. Epub 30 Jan 2012. Review. PubMed PMID: 22286861; PubMed Central PMCID: PMC3338189. https://doi.org/10.1161/JAHA.115.001914.
37. Chambers SK, Chung E, Wittert G, Hyde MK. Erectile dysfunction, masculinity, and psychosocial outcomes: a review of the experiences of men after prostate cancer treatment. Transl Androl Urol. 2017;6(1):60–8. Review. PubMed PMID: 28217451; PubMed Central PMCID: PMC5313306. https://doi.org/10.21037/tau.2016.08.12.
38. Martinez LS, Schwartz JS, Freres D, Fraze T, Hornik RC. Patient-clinician information engagement increases treatment decision satisfaction among cancer patients through feeling of being informed. Patient Educ Couns. 2009;77:384.
39. Pfizer.com, Depo Provera injection. http://labeling.pfizer.com/ShowLabeling.aspx?id=522. Accessed 2 Nov 2019.
40. NCCN Guidelines version 4.2018, prostate cancer, risk stratification and staging work up, p 11–17. https://www.nccn.org/professionals/physician_gls/pdf/prostate.pdf. Accessed 2 Dec 2019.

# Chapter 8
# Second-Generation Androgen-Targeted Agents

**Laura P. Gurten and Jamison S. Jaffe**

## Second-Generation Androgen-Targeted Agents

Prostate cancer is the most commonly diagnosed solid organ cancer and the second leading cause of cancer death among men in the United States [1]. The National Cancer Institute (NCI) estimated approximately 161,360 men were diagnosed with the disease in 2017, with 26,730 estimated deaths as a result [2]. That number rose to approximately 165,000 diagnoses and close to 30,000 deaths in 2018 [1]. Despite early detection, as well as advances in surgical and radiation techniques, the disease can recur.

Studies suggest that 15–40% of men with prostate cancer will go on to develop recurrent, biochemical recurrence (BCR), and/or metastatic disease within 10 years of initial treatment [3]. The median time to BCR is typically 2–3 years, which has been strongly associated with PSA doubling time (PSADT) [3]. Moreover, research provides evidential support that the risk of metastases increases as PSADT decreases [3]. The American Urologic Association (AUA) defines biochemical recurrence as a PSA > 0.2 ng/ml measured greater than or equal to 6 weeks post radical prostatectomy with a confirmatory check of a PSA persistently >0.2 ng/ml [3]. Additionally, in 1996, the American Society for Therapeutic Radiology and Oncology (ASTRO) established a definition of biochemical failure after external beam radiotherapy [4]. The ASTRO definition defined biochemical failure as occurring after three consecutive PSA rises after a nadir with the date of failure as the point halfway between the nadir date and the first rise or any rise great enough to provoke initiation of therapy [4].

It was discovered in 1941, by Huggins and Hodges, that prostate cancer is an androgen-dependent disease [5]. Further research revealed that, although patients with metastatic prostate cancer experienced significant tumor regression and

L. P. Gurten (✉) · J. S. Jaffe
Department of Urology, St. Mary Medical Center, Langhorne, PA, USA



E. J. Trabulsi et al. (eds.), *Chemotherapy and Immunotherapy in Urologic Oncology*, https://doi.org/10.1007/978-3-030-52021-2_8

palliation of symptoms after medical or surgical castration, endocrine therapy alone often failed to control the disease long term leading to a castrate-resistant state [5]. Castration-resistant prostate cancer (CRPC) is defined by disease progression despite androgen-deprivation therapy (ADT) and may present as a continuous rise in serum levels of PSA, progression of preexisting disease, and/or appearance of new metastases [6]. Patients inevitably progress to a castrate-resistant state, despite initial response to ADT, and the cancer continues to progress even with low levels of serum testosterone [5]. For decades, patients with CRPC were thought to have hormone-refractory tumors with the assumption that additional hormonal manipulations would be ineffective due to the fact that patients were already experiencing clinical progression in the setting of low levels of serum testosterone [5].

The exact process of transitioning from castration-sensitive to castration-resistant prostate cancer is unknown [1]. We do know the androgen receptor remains active and continues to drive prostate cancer progression, despite castrate levels of androgens [1]. Continued dependence of androgen receptor signaling is clearly evident through rising levels of PSA, an androgen receptor target gene, which occurs in virtually all patients with progressive disease [5]. There are multiple mechanisms that contribute to continued androgen receptor signaling including genomic amplification and overexpression of androgen receptors, alterations in androgen transport, increased synthesis of extragonadal androgens and many more [5]. Developing agents that completely block androgen receptor signaling has posed a challenge to many researchers.

Until recently, the options for medical management for patients with CRPC were extremely limited. Prior to 2004, treatments were administered for the sole purpose of palliation once patients failed primary androgen deprivation [1]. As our knowledge base grows regarding the understanding of tumor biology, the treatment of CRPC has dramatically changed over the last decade. The mainstay of treatment, for patients with newly diagnosed advanced disease, remains suppression of gonadal androgens using a gonadotropin-releasing hormone (GnRH) analog alone or in combination with an anti-androgen agent [5].

Historically, conventional, first-generation anti-androgen agents such as bicalutamide, flutamide, and nilutamide have been used in combination with a GnRH agonists and antagonists. In recent years, research regarding the limitations of first-generation anti-androgens, their agonist potential and weak affinity for androgen receptors, has resulted in an apparent need to develop novel, potent, and pure second-generation androgen receptor antagonists that directly target the androgen-receptor-binding domain and impair nuclear translocation [5].

A multitude of clinical trials have been performed as a result of the need for, better, more potent medications. More specifically, trials such as SPARTAN, PROSPER, PREVAIL, LATITUDE, and STAMPEDE have resulted in the Food and Drug Administration (FDA) approval of agents designed specifically to affect the androgen axis. Since 2010, the FDA has approved five new drugs for the treatment of metastatic castration-resistant prostate cancer (mCRPC); however, progress has been slower in the treatment of nonmetastatic castration-resistant prostate cancer (nmCRPC) [7]. With such a significant increase in the number of therapeutic agents available for the treatment of CRPC, clinical decision-making has become more complex as providers are presented with many treatment options and various sequencing of these agents [1]. In the wake of such advancements, the AUA issued an amendment to their CRPC guideline statement in April 2018. The new guideline, which profiles six index patients, was created to help providers in their daily clinical decision-making.

## Usage, Indications, and Side Effects of Abiraterone, Enzalutamide, Apalutamide, and Darolutamide

### *Abiraterone (ZYTIGA™, YONSA™)*

Abiraterone, in combination with prednisone, is indicated for the treatment of patients with metastatic castration-resistant prostate cancer (mCRPC) [8]. The medication was initially FDA approved in 2011 for this use; however, it has recently received attention for its approval and indication in men with metastatic castration-sensitive prostate cancer (mCSPC). Brand names of the medication include Zytiga™ and Yonsa™.

The STAMPEDE trial, which included 1917 patients, was a randomized multi-arm study performed from November 2011 to January 2014 on men with locally advanced or metastatic prostate cancer [9]. This trial concluded that ADT plus abiraterone and prednisolone was associated with significantly higher overall survival rates, as well as higher rates of progression-free survival [9]. Additionally, the LATITUDE trial, which followed 1199 men with mCSPC, proved that the addition of abiraterone and prednisone to ADT significantly increased overall survival and radiographic progression-free survival in men with newly diagnosed mCSPC [10].

The mechanism of action of abiraterone is its ability to inhibit CYP17 [8]. The enzyme CYP17 is required for androgen biosynthesis and can be found in testicular, adrenal, and prostatic tissues [8]. The inhibition of CYP17 can also result in increased mineralocorticoid production by the adrenal glands [8].

The potential for adverse reactions must be taken into consideration when prescribing. Serious side effects can include hypertension, hypokalemia, arrhythmias, cardiac failure, adrenal insufficiency, hepatotoxicity, fulminant hepatitis, and acute hepatic failure [8]. More common side effects can include nausea, hypertriglyceridemia, hypercholesterolemia, elevated LFTs, hyperglycemia, fatigue, URI, lymphopenia, UTI, arthralgia, headache, hypokalemia, dyspnea, edema, contusion, hypophosphatemia, cough, anemia, hot flashes, diarrhea, vomiting, hypernatremia, constipation, diarrhea, hematuria, insomnia, and dyspepsia [8, 9]. There have been post-marketing reports of noninfectious pneumonitis, myopathy including rhabdomyolysis, and acute hepatic failure resulting in death [8].

Abiraterone should be used with caution in patients with a history of cardiovascular disease. Safety has not been established for those with LVEF <50% or those patients considered to be NYHA Class III or IV heart failure [8]. Hypertension, hypokalemia, and fluid retention can occur as a result of increased mineralocorticoid production due to CYP17 inhibition [8]. Adrenocortical insufficiency can occur following interruption of daily steroids and/or in situations of concurrent infection or stress [8]. Caution must be used when administering abiraterone to patients with hepatic impairment, Child-Pugh Class B [8]. Men with female partners, of reproductive potential, should be advised to use some form of contraceptive during treatment and for 3 weeks after their final dose [8]. Male patients should be advised that the use of abiraterone may impair fertility [8]. Also, women who are pregnant or may become pregnant should not handle abiraterone uncoated tablets or other tablets if broken, crushed, or damaged without protection such as gloves [8].

Prior to initiating therapy, baseline LFTs should be performed [8]. Subsequent follow-up includes monitoring LFTs every 2 weeks for 3 months, then monthly [8]. If Child-Pugh Class B, then LFTs should be monitored weekly for 4 weeks, every 2 weeks for 8 weeks, then monthly [8]. Blood pressure and potassium should be performed at baseline, then monitored monthly thereafter [8]. Signs and symptoms of edema should be monitored monthly [8]. Adrenal function should be monitored throughout the duration of therapy [8].

The recommended dosage of Zytiga™, for the use of mCRPC, is 1000 mg (two 500 mg tablets or four 250 mg tablets) to be taken orally once daily with 5 mg of prednisone every 12 hours [8]. The recommended dosage of Yonsa™, for the use of mCRPC, is 500 mg (four 125 mg tablets) to be taken orally once daily with 4 mg of methylprednisolone twice daily [8]. The recommended dosage of Zytiga™, for the use of metastatic high-risk castration-sensitive prostate cancer, is 1000 mg (two 500 mg tablets or four 250 mg tablets) to be taken orally once daily with 5 mg of prednisone every 12 hours [8]. Patients receiving abiraterone should also receive a GnRH analog, such as leuprolide, concurrently or should have had bilateral orchiectomy [8].

Drug-to-drug interactions should always be taken into consideration. Notably, the concomitant use of abiraterone with drugs that are strong CYP3A4 inducers should be avoided, as this may decrease the systemic exposure of abiraterone [8]. Examples of strong CYP3A4 inducers include carbamazepine, phenytoin, dexamethasone, and St. John's Wart. If the combination must be used, it is recommended to increase the abiraterone dosing to twice daily [8]. Concomitant use of medications primarily metabolized by CYP2D6 and CYP2C8 should also be avoided, as abiraterone may increase the therapeutic effect of these medications [8]. One common example is amiodarone.

## *Enzalutamide (XTANDI™)*

Enzalutamide, brand name Xtandi™, is indicated for the treatment of castration-resistant prostate cancer, both metastatic and nonmetastatic, as well as metastatic castration-sensitive prostate cancer [11]. Until recently, there were no FDA-approved medications available to treat all three groups, making this a pivotal transition in the way we treat prostate cancer. Enzalutamide was first FDA approved in 2012 for the treatment of men with mCRPC [12]. The hallmark approval of the medication, for the treatment of men with nmCRPC, came on July 13, 2018 [12]. Finally, the medication was approved for the treatment of men with mCSPC on December 16, 2019 [13]. With this final approval, Enzalutamide became the first and only oral medication used in the treatment of these three distinct groups of advanced prostate cancer.

Extensive research was performed to ensure the efficacy of this medication to all three groups. The PROSPER trial, a phase 3 double-blind trial, studied 1401 patients with nmCRPC and had a primary endpoint of metastasis-free survival [14]. From the PROSPER trial, it was concluded that among men with nmCRPC and a rapidly rising PSA, treatment with enzalutamide led to a significant 71% lower risk of metastasis or death than placebo alone [14].

Additionally, a double-blind phase 3 trial was performed on 1717 patients with mCRPC [15]. The PREVAIL trial had co-primary endpoints of radiographic progression-free survival, as well as overall survival [15]. Conclusions from this trial revealed that enzalutamide did significantly decrease the risk of radiographic progression, death, and delayed the initiation of chemotherapy in men with mCRPC [15].

The most recent research regarding enzalutamide comes from the ARCHES trial, a double-blind phase 3 trial, involving 1150 men with mHSPC (metastatic hormone-sensitive prostate cancer) and a primary endpoint of radiographic progression-free survival [16]. Results from the ARCHES trial revealed a significant reduction of radiographic progression or death with the use of enzalutamide plus ADT versus placebo plus ADT, in men with mHSPC [16]. This included those men with low volume disease and/or prior treatment with docetaxel. In addition, it was concluded that enzalutamide plus ADT significantly reduced the risk of PSA progression, first symptomatic skeletal event, initiation of new antineoplastic therapy, pain progression, and castration resistance [16].

Enzalutamide functions as an androgen receptor inhibitor [11]. It works by competitively inhibiting the act of androgen binding to androgen receptors [11]. Enzalutamide also inhibits androgen receptor nuclear translocation and interaction with DNA resulting in decreased proliferation and induced cell death [11]. This is an extremely important mechanism that first-generation anti-androgen agents lack.

Despite the efficacy of the medication, adverse reactions can still occur. During clinical trials, serious adverse reactions were noted and included seizures, posterior reversible encephalopathy syndrome (PRES), neutropenia, severe infection, hypersensitivity reaction, ischemic heart disease, fractures, and falls [11, 14]. More common adverse reactions included asthenia, fatigue, back pain, constipation, arthralgia, diarrhea, hot flashes, decreased appetite, musculoskeletal pain, neutropenia, peripheral edema, weight loss, headache, respiratory infection, dyspnea, dizziness, vertigo, hypertension, nausea, falls, fractures, muscle weakness, insomnia, hematuria, dysgeusia, paresthesia, anxiety, thrombocytopenia, mental impairment, pollakiuria, hypesthesia, pruritus, xeroderma, gynecomastia, epistaxis, hyperbilirubinemia, and musculoskeletal stiffness [11, 14]. There have been post-marketing reports of vomiting, rash, and edema of the face, tongue, lip, or pharynx [11].

Enzalutamide should be used with caution in patients who have a history of seizure or suffer from seizure disorder [11]. The medication must be permanently discontinued in any patient that develops a seizure during treatment [11]. Caution should be used in patients with a history of cardiovascular disease, especially ischemic heart disease [11, 14]. Enzalutamide must be discontinued for any grade 3–4 ischemic cardiac reaction [11]. Cardiovascular risk factors such as hypertension, diabetes, or dyslipidemia should be optimized prior to treatment [11]. Caution should be used in those patients more at risk for falls and fractures, and the use of bone-targeted agents should be considered [11]. The medication must be discontinued in any patient who develops PRES, which must be confirmed by brain imaging such as MRI [11]. Men with female partners, of reproductive potential, should be advised to use some form of contraceptive during treatment and for 3 months after their final dose [11]. Male patients should also be advised that the use of enzalutamide may impair fertility [11].

There are no routine tests or monitoring recommended during treatment [11]. Pharmacokinetic data pulled from multiple clinical trials showed no significant difference in enzalutamide clearance for those with preexisting mild to moderate renal impairment as compared to patients with normal renal function [11]. No initial dose adjustment is necessary for patients with mild to moderate renal impairment [11]. The use of enzalutamide in patients with severe to end-stage renal disease has not been assessed [11]. Dedicated hepatic trials revealed patients receiving enzalutamide with baseline mild, moderate, or severe hepatic impairment had similar systemic exposure as those patients with normal hepatic function [11]. No initial dose adjustment is necessary for patients with hepatic impairment [11].

The recommended dose of enzalutamide is 160 mg (four 40 mg capsules) to be taken orally once daily [11]. The medication can be taken with or without food. The medication should not be crushed, chewed, dissolved, or the capsules opened. Patients receiving enzalutamide should also receive a GnRH analog concurrently or should have had bilateral orchiectomy [11].

There are multiple drug-to-drug interactions that must be taken into consideration. It is recommended that concomitant use of enzalutamide and strong CYP2C8 inhibitors be avoided [11]. The combination can decrease the efficacy of medications such as warfarin. If unable to avoid the combination, the enzalutamide dose should be reduced to 80 mg once daily [11]. Avoidance of coadministration of enzalutamide and strong CYP3A4 inducers is recommended, as this combination can reduce the efficacy of enzalutamide [11]. If unable to avoid the combination, the enzalutamide dose should be increased from 160 to 240 mg once daily [11]. Concomitant use of medications primarily metabolized by CYP3A4 substrate, CYP2C9 substrate, and CYP2C19 should also be avoided, as enzalutamide may decrease the efficacy of these medications [11].

## *Apalutamide (ERLEADA™)*

Apalutamide, brand name Erleada™, is indicated for the treatment of patients with nonmetastatic castration-resistant prostate cancer [17]. In February 2018, apalutamide became the first FDA-approved drug of its kind for the treatment of men with nmCRPC [2].

The SPARTAN trial, a double-blind phase 3 study, was designed to prove that the use of apalutamide in men with nmCRPC would lead to a longer period of metastasis-free survival [18]. The study followed 1207 men with nmCRPC and a PSDAT of 10 months or less [18]. Results of the study showed a significantly longer metastasis-free survival for those in the apalutamide group, as opposed to the placebo group [18]. The median time to metastasis-free survival was 40.5 months in the apalutamide group, compared to 16.2 months in the placebo group [18]. A secondary endpoint of progression-free survival and an exploratory endpoint of PSA response were also evaluated, revealing positive results for the apalutamide group in both categories [18]. Median progression-free survival was 40.5 months for the apalutamide group, compared to 14.7 for the placebo group [18]. Moreover, 89.7% of patients in the apalutamide group experienced a PSA response, as opposed to 2.2% in the placebo group [18].

Like enzalutamide, apalutamide is an androgen receptor inhibitor that binds directly to the ligand-binding domain of the androgen receptor [17]. Apalutamide inhibits the nuclear translocation of the androgen receptor, inhibits DNA binding, and impedes androgen receptor transcription causing decreased tumor cell proliferation and increased apoptosis leading to decreased tumor volume [17].

Serious reactions of the medication can include fractures, seizures, HTN, cardiac ischemia, heart failure, and hyperkalemia [17]. During clinical trials, more specifically the SPARTAN trial, eight patients (1%) treated with Erleada™ died from serious adverse reactions [17, 18]. The cause of death among these patients included infection, myocardial infarction, and cerebral hemorrhage [17, 18]. More common adverse reactions can include hypercholesterolemia, anemia, hyperglycemia, hypertriglyceridemia, leukopenia, lymphopenia, fatigue, rash, diarrhea, nausea, arthralgia, falls, weight loss, hot flashes, decreased appetite, peripheral edema, hypothyroidism, pruritus, and CHF [17].

Apalutamide should be used with caution in patients who have a history of seizure or suffer from seizure disorder [17]. Apalutamide must be permanently discontinued in any patient that develops a seizure during treatment [17]. It is unknown whether or not antiepileptic medications will prevent seizures during treatment [17]. Caution should be used in those patients more at risk for falls and fractures and use of bone-targeted agents should be considered [17]. Men with female partners, of reproductive potential, should be advised to use some form of contraceptive during treatment and for 3 months after their final dose [17]. Male patients should be advised that the use of apalutamide may impair fertility, and they should not donate sperm for 3 months following their last dose of apalutamide [17].

Due to the risk of hypothyroidism during treatment, it has been recommended that TSH be monitored every 4 months [19]. It is advisable to perform a baseline TSH prior to therapy. There were no clinically significant differences in the pharmacokinetics of apalutamide observed in patients with mild to moderate renal impairment or mild to moderate hepatic impairment [17]. The effect on those with severe renal impairment or severe hepatic impairment is unknown [17].

The recommended dose of apalutamide is 240 mg (four 60 mg tablets) administered orally once daily [17]. The tablet should be swallowed whole and can be taken with or without food [17]. Patients receiving apalutamide should also receive a GnRH analog concurrently or should have had bilateral orchiectomy [17].

Multiple drug-to-drug interactions have been observed and must be taken into consideration when prescribing apalutamide. Concomitant use with medications that are sensitive substrates of CYP3A4, CYP2C19, CYP2C9, UGT, P-gp, breast cancer resistance protein (BCRP), or OATP1B1 may result in loss of activity of these medications [17]. Strong CYP2C8 inhibitors and strong CYP3A4 inhibitors have been shown to increase the steady state of apalutamide [17]. Additionally, CYP3A4/CYP2C8 inducers have been shown to decrease the steady state of apalutamide [17]. Acid lowering agents, such as proton pump inhibitors and H2 receptor antagonist, are not expected to affect the bioavailability or solubility of apalutamide [17].

## *Darolutamide (NUBEQA™)*

Darolutamide, brand name Nubeqa™, is indicated for the treatment of patients with nonmetastatic castration-resistant prostate cancer [20]. In July 2019, darolutamide became the newest drug on the market for the treatment of nmCRPC [21]. What is more significant, darolutamide offers the potential for fewer and less severe toxic effects than apalutamide and enzalutamide because of its distinct structure [22].

The ARAMIS trial, which set out to prove the efficacy of this medication, was a randomized double-blind, phase 3, placebo-controlled study that included 1509 patients with nmCRPC and a PSADT of 10 months or less [22]. The study's primary endpoint was metastasis-free survival, with the presence of metastasis determined by radiographic imaging every 16 weeks [22]. From the ARAMIS trial, it was concluded that, among men with nmCRPC, metastasis-free survival time was significantly longer with darolutamide than with placebo alone [22]. The median metastasis-free survival time was 40.4 months for those individuals treated with darolutamide, as opposed to 18.4 months in the placebo group [22]. Secondary endpoints including overall survival, time to symptomatic skeletal event, time to cytotoxic chemotherapy, and time to pain progression were also studied with all positive outcomes noted [22].

Like apalutamide and enzalutamide, darolutamide is an androgen receptor inhibitor [20]. Darolutamide inhibits androgen receptor binding, androgen receptor nuclear translocation, and androgen-receptor-mediated translocation resulting in decreased prostate cancer cell proliferation and tumor volume [20]. As stated previously, due to its distinct structure, darolutamide has low penetration of the blood–brain barrier and low binding affinity for γ-aminobutyric acid type A receptors resulting in fewer and less severe toxic effects than other drugs on the market today [22].

With any medication, the potential for serious adverse reactions must be taken into consideration when prescribing darolutamide. During clinical trials, serious adverse reactions were noted and included cardiac failure, cardiac arrest, general physical health deterioration, pulmonary embolism, urinary retention, pneumonia, neutropenia, hematuria, and death [20]. More common adverse reactions included increased bilirubin, increased aspartate aminotransferase, fatigue, rash, neutropenia, and extremity pain [20].

Darolutamide should be used with caution in patients who have moderate hepatic impairment, Child-Pugh Class B [20]. Caution should also be used in patients with severe renal impairment or eGFR 15–29 mL/min/1.73 $m^2$, who are not receiving hemodialysis [20]. Overall, there were no differences in the safety or efficacy of the medication observed between the geriatric population and younger patients [20]. Male patients should be advised that the use of darolutamide may impair fertility [20]. The safety and efficacy of darolutamide have not been established in female patients; however, due to the mechanism of action, it has been noted that the medication has the potential to cause fetal harm and/or loss of pregnancy [20]. Males with female partners, of reproductive potential, should be advised to use some form of contraceptive during the entirety of treatment and 1 week after the last dose of darolutamide is administered [20].

There are no routine tests or monitoring recommended during treatment [20]. It is advisable that baseline hepatic and renal function be assessed prior to initiating treatment. Dosing should be held or reduced if the patient experiences a greater than or equal to Grade 3 toxicity or an intolerable adverse reaction [20]. Normal dosing may be resumed once the patient's symptoms have improved [20].

The recommended dose of darolutamide is 600 mg (two 300 mg film-coated tablets) taken orally twice daily [20]. The medication should be taken with food [20]. When administered with food, the bioavailability of darolutamide increases 2.0 to 2.5-fold [20]. The medication should not be crushed, chewed, or dissolved. Patients receiving darolutamide should also receive a GnRH analog concurrently or should have had bilateral orchiectomy [20]. Patients with moderate hepatic impairment have a higher exposure to darolutamide, and dosage reduction is recommended [20]. The recommended dose for this patient population is 300 mg twice daily [20]. No dose reduction is needed for patients with mild hepatic impairment [20]. The effect of severe hepatic impairment (Child-Pugh C) with the use of darolutamide is unknown [20]. Patients with severe renal impairment also have a higher exposure to darolutamide, and dosage reduction is recommend [20]. The recommended dose for this patient population is 300 mg twice daily [20]. No dose reduction is needed for patients with mild to moderate renal impairment (eGFR 30–89 mL/min/1.73 $m^2$) [20]. The effect of end-stage renal disease (eGFR $\leq$15 mL/min/1.73 $m^2$) with the use of darolutamide is unknown [20]. Dose reduction below 300 mg twice daily is not recommended [20].

Drug-to-drug interactions must be taken into consideration when prescribing this medication. Darolutamide is a P-gp and CYP3A4 substrate, BCRP transporter inhibitor, and OATP1B1 and OATP1B3 inhibitor [20]. Coadministration of darolutamide and combined P-gp and/or moderate to strong CYP3A4 inducers should be avoided [20]. When given in combination with these medications, the activity of darolutamide may be decreased [20]. Coadministration of darolutamide along with combined P-gp and strong CYP3A4 inhibitors increases the exposure of darolutamide, which may increase the risk of adverse reactions associated with darolutamide [20]. If these medications must be administered concomitantly, increased monitoring of adverse reactions or dosage adjustment is warranted [20]. Lastly, concomitant use of darolutamide with BCRP substrates should be avoided if possible [20]. This combination may increase the risk of BCRP substrate-related toxicities [20]. If these medications must be administered together, more frequent monitoring of adverse reactions and reduction in dosage of the BRCP substrate drug must be considered [20].

## Conclusion

Metastatic-castration-resistant prostate cancer remains incurable. Despite this, men suffering from this disease are living substantially longer due to advances in research and the rate at which new medications are becoming available. Second-generation androgen-targeted agents have dramatically changed the way we treat prostate cancer. The uses of these medications continue to grow as well. Consequentially, more research is warranted. With an aging population and increased frequency at which advanced prostate cancer is being diagnosed, caring for men with prostate cancer has become a major global healthcare challenge [23]. In the wake of studies exploring disease molecular stratification, as well as correlation to disease predictive biomarkers, there may be a new generation of medications to look forward to and new exciting uses of the second-generation androgen targeting agents we currently use today.

**Clinical Pearls**

- The diagnosis of incurable cancer can be a difficult conversation to have with patients and it is important to ensure they have an appropriate support system set in place. If a support system such as family and/or friends is unavailable to the patient, a nurse navigator should be considered to help guide them and answer any questions they may have.
- Quality of life and the patient's expectations should always be discussed prior to initiating any treatment.
- A multidisciplinary approach to patient care should be considered and can often lead to better outcomes.
- A patient's overall health status should be known and optimized prior to initiating any treatment.

## References


1. American Urologic Association. Castration-resistant prostate cancer: 2018 guideline amendment. American Urological Association; 2018.
2. Food and Drug Administration [news release]. FDA approves new treatment for a certain type of prostate cancer using novel clinical trial endpoint. U.S. Food and Drug Administration; 2018.
3. Morgans AK. M0 CRPC: emerging treatment options: Powerpoint Presentation. Northwestern University; 2018.
4. Roach M, Hanks G, Thames H Jr, Schellhammer P, Shipley WU, Sokol GH, Sandler H. Defining biochemical failure following radiotherapy with or without hormonal therapy in men with clinically localized prostate cancer: recommendations of the RTOG-ASTRO Phoenix Consensus Conference. Int J Radiat Oncol Biol Phys. 2006;65(4):965–74.
5. Rathkopf D, Scher HI. Androgen receptor antagonists in castration-resistant prostate cancer. Cancer J. 2013;19(1):43–9.
6. Hotte SJ, Saad F. Current management of castrate-resistant prostate cancer. Curr Oncol. 2010;17(Suppl 2):S72–9.
7. Smith MR. Progress in nonmetastatic prostate cancer. N Engl J Med. 2018;378:2531–2.
8. Zytiga (Abiraterone) [prescribing information]. Horsham: Janssen Pharmaceutical Companies; 2018.
9. James ND, de Bono JS, Spears MR, Clarke NW, Mason MD, Dearnaley DP, et al. Abiraterone for prostate cancer not previously treated with hormone therapy. N Engl J Med. 2017;377:338–51.
10. Fizazi K, Tran NP, Fein L, Rodriguez-Antolin A, Alekseev BY, Ozguroglu M, Ye D, Feyerabend S, Protheroe A, De Porre P, Kheoh T, et al. Abiraterone plus prednisone in metastatic, castration-sensitive prostate cancer. N Engl J Med. 2017;377:352–60.
11. Xtandi (Enzalutamide) [prescribing information]. Northbrook: Astellas Pharma US, Inc.; 2018.
12. Astellas [news release]. U.S. FDA approves XTANDI® (enzalutamide) for the treatment of men with non-metastatic castration-resistant prostate cancer (CRPC). Astellas; 2018.
13. Food and Drug Administration [news release]. FDA approves enzalutamide for metastatic castration sensitive prostate cancer. U.S. Food and Drug Administration; 2019.
14. Hussain M, Fizazi K, Saad F, Rathenborg P, Shore N, Ferreira U, Ivashchenko P, et al. Enzalutamide in men with nonmetastatic, castration-resistant prostate cancer. N Engl J Med. 2018;378:2465–74.
15. Beer TM, Armstrong AJ, Rathkopf DE, Loriot Y, Sternberg CN, Higano CS, et al. Enzalutamide in metastatic prostate cancer before chemotherapy. N Engl J Med. 2014;371:424–33.
16. Armstrong AJ, Szmulewitz R, Petrylak D, Holzbeierlein J, Villers A, Azad A, et al. ARCHES: a randomized, phase III study of androgen deprivation therapy with enzalutamide or placebo in men with metastatic hormone-sensitive prostate cancer. J Clin Oncol. 2019;37:2974–86.
17. Erleada (Apalutamide) [prescribing information]. Janssen Pharmaceutical Companies: Horsham; 2018.
18. Smith MR, Saad F, Chowdhury S, Oudard S, Hadaschik BA, Graff J, et al. Apalutamide treatment and metastasis-free survival in prostate cancer. N Engl J Med. 2018;378:1408–18.
19. UpToDate. Aplalutamide: drug information. Wolters Kluwer UpToDate, Inc.; 1978–2019.
20. Nubeqa (Darolutamide) [prescribing information]. Whippany: Bayer HealthCare Pharmaceuticals Inc; 2019.
21. Food and Drug Administration [news release]. FDA approves darolutamide for non-metastatic castration-resistant prostate cancer. U.S. Food and Drug Administration; 2019.
22. Fizazi K, Shore N, Tammela T, Ulys A, Vjaters E, Polyakov S, et al. Darolutamide in nonmetastatic, castration-resistant prostate cancer. N Engl J Med. 2019;380:1235–46.
23. Sartor O, de Bono JS. Metastatic prostate cancer. N Engl J Med. 2018;378:645–57.

# Chapter 9
# Chemotherapy and Prostate Cancer

**Miranda L. Tsang**

## Introduction

While many options of first-line chemotherapy are available for other cancer types, it is not the case for prostate cancer (PC). Based on the most recent National Comprehensive Cancer Network (NCCN) guideline [1], clinicians will consider using chemotherapy when a patient has (i) metastatic hormone-sensitive prostate cancer (mHSPC) with high-risk feature; or (ii) metastatic castration-resistant prostate cancer (mCRPC), with or without visceral metastases. The most common use of cytotoxic chemotherapy is a taxane derivative. Docetaxel is used as first-line chemotherapy with mHSPC and mCRPC patients. Cabazitaxel is used as second-line chemotherapy when patients do not tolerate docetaxel during treatment or progressed after completion of docetaxel. The taxane derivatives have shown to improve overall survival in men with mCRPC. Other chemotherapy may also be used during the cause of treatment due to the progression of disease or mCRPC with a small-cell feature. We are going to discuss the treatment options for both mHSPC and mCRPC patients, chemotherapies dosage, mechanism of action, administration and monitoring, common side effects, and management.

## Metastatic Hormone-Sensitive Prostate Cancer (mHSPC)

Prior to 2016, the option of chemotherapy was reserved for patients with mCRPC only. Hormone-sensitive prostate cancer (HSPC) means that the prostate cancer cells still respond to the withdrawal of androgen deprivation therapy (ADT). It is

M. L. Tsang (✉)
Sidney Kimmel Cancer Center – Jefferson Health, Thomas Jefferson University Hospital, Philadelphia, PA, USA
e-mail: miranda.tsang@jefferson.edu



E. J. Trabulsi et al. (eds.), *Chemotherapy and Immunotherapy in Urologic Oncology*, https://doi.org/10.1007/978-3-030-52021-2_9

**Table 9.1** Comparison of CHAARTED [2] and STAMPEDE [5]

| | CHAARTED [2] ($n = 790$) | STAMPEDE [5] ($n = 2962$) |
|---|---|---|
| Publication year | 2015 | 2016 |
| Treatment arm | ADT + docetaxel ($n = 397$) | ADT + docetaxel ($n = 592$) |
| Other arm(s) | ADT | ADT |
| | | ADT + zoledronic acid |
| | | ADT + zoledronic acid + docetaxel |
| Median age | 63 | 65 |
| Media overall survival (months) | 57.6 | 81 |
| | (ADT alone: 44.0) | (ADT alone: 71) |
| *P* | <0.001 | <0.001 |

also known as "castration-naive" [1]. Men with evidence of metastatic disease with HSPC are the candidate for chemotherapy treatment. This group of men will receive docetaxel and ADT upfront. CHAARTED [2] study was published in 2016 and provided evidence of improved overall survival in men with mHSPC using docetaxel with ADT upfront compared to ADT alone. STAMPEDE [3] study also supports these findings in the next year. Both CHAARTED [2] and STAMPEDE [3] studies improved overall survival in this group of patients compared to treatment with ADT alone. Comparison of these two clinical trials is listed in Table 9.1. Abiraterone acetate (AA) with ADT can also be used in men with mHSPC, which demonstrated increased overall survival and radiographic progression-free survival from the LATITUDE study [4]. In addition, another STAMPEDE [5] study compared docetaxel with ADT and AA with ADT, which shows no evidence of a difference in overall or prostate cancer-specific survival. Moreover, the cost of docetaxel and AA were also compared in a recent study. Docetaxel with ADT is more cost-effective than AA with ADT [6]. Additional ongoing clinical trials are also providing evidence of benefit with docetaxel as first-line therapy in HSPC population.

## Metastatic Castration-Resistant Prostate Cancer (mCRPC)

Castration-resistant prostate cancer (CRPC) is defined as cancer that progresses clinically, radiographically, or biochemically, despite castrate levels of serum testosterone (<50 ng/dL; 1.7 nmol/L) [1]. Once a metastatic disease is confirmed by radiographic imaging, additional treatment should be considered in addition to ADT [1].

Before the investigation of taxanes, the only FDA-approved chemotherapy for symptomatic mCRPC patients was mitoxantrone plus prednisone (1996). While mitoxantrone provided a palliative benefit, there was no improvement in overall survival when compared to prednisone alone. In the pivotal studies (1996 and 1999), it demonstrated pain improvement in one-third of the symptomatic CRPC patients. Therefore, it was used as a palliative care approach [7, 8].

The first chemotherapy that presented with a survival benefit for mCRPC came out in 2004. In the TAX 327 study [9], docetaxel plus daily prednisone was compared to mitoxantrone plus prednisone. Docetaxel every 3 weeks with prednisone showed improved overall survival; better pain control and quality of life; and higher proportion of patients with declines in serum PSA level. In 2013, the SWOG S0421 trial [10] compared docetaxel with atrasentan, an endothelin receptor antagonist, in the effectiveness of treating mCRPC patients with bone metastases. There have been multiple trials looking at docetaxel combinations; however, none have improved overall outcomes compared to docetaxel plus prednisone alone. Single-agent docetaxel remains a standard of care for mCRPC patients. A comparison of TAX 327 [9] and SWOG S0421 [10] is listed in Table 9.2.

In 2010, a second-generation taxane, cabazitaxel, was approved by FDA for mCRPC patients who progressed on docetaxel in the first-line setting. In the TROPIC study [11], cabazitaxel plus prednisone was compared to mitoxantrone plus prednisone in men with mCRPC who had progressed after docetaxel-based chemotherapy. The study showed cabazitaxel plus prednisone improves overall survival in men that have progressed during or after docetaxel-based therapy. In 2017, PROSELICA study [12] compared low-dose cabazitaxel (20 mg/m$^2$) to standard-dose cabazitaxel (25 mg/m$^2$), which showed that low-dose cabazitaxel has similar clinical benefit to standard-dose cabazitaxel with fewer side effects. The evolution and development of chemotherapy for prostate cancer are illustrated in Fig. 9.1.

**Table 9.2** Comparison of TAX 327 [9] and SWIG S0421 [10]

| | TAX 327 [9] (*n* = 1006) | SWOG S0421 [10] (*n* = 996) |
|---|---|---|
| Publication year | 2004 | 2013 |
| Treatment arm | Docetaxel + prednisone every 3 weeks (*n* = 335) | Docetaxel + astasentan (*n* = 500) |
| Other arm(s) | Mitoxantrone + prednisone every 3 weeks | Docetaxel + placebo |
| | Docetaxel + prednisone weekly | |
| Median age | 68 | 69 |
| Media overall survival (months) | 18.9 | 17.8 |
| | (Mitoxantrone: 16.5) | (Placebo: 17.6) |
| | (Docetaxel weekly: 17.4) | |

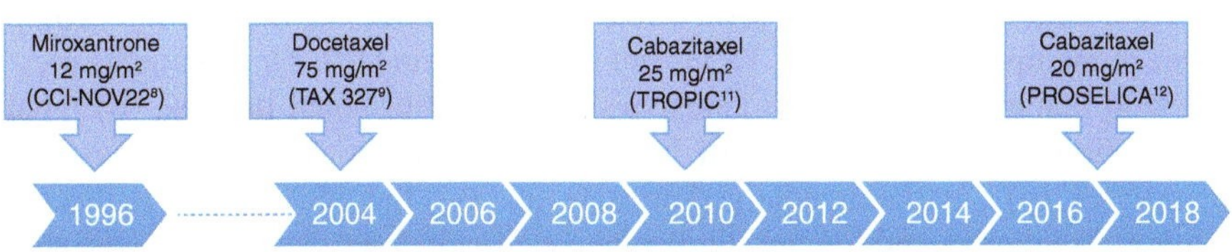


**Fig. 9.1** Evolution of chemotherapy for prostate cancer [8, 9, 11, 12]

First-line treatment options for mCPRC include oral therapy (i.e., abiraterone with prednisone [13], enzalutamide [14]), and chemotherapy (i.e., docetaxel). Determination between oral therapy and chemotherapy depends on the patient's current symptoms of PC, performance status, ability to maintain medication adherence, previous exposure to the above medications, and drug–drug interaction with patient's current medications. For symptomatic mCRPC patients with good performance status, docetaxel with concurrent steroid may be considered. Patients who previously received docetaxel in castration-naive setting may also have benefits from receiving docetaxel again [1].

If the progression of disease occurs after docetaxel in the castration-resistant setting, cabazitaxel will be a second-line treatment option of chemotherapy. Patients who are not able to tolerate docetaxel should be considered for cabazitaxel [1].

Clinicians should also consider dose reduction and/or delay treatment if the patient presents with pronounced toxicities during the administration of these chemotherapies. The result of a meta-analysis revealed that cabazitaxel is associated with lower rates of peripheral neuropathy than docetaxel, but there is no evidence of superior efficacy of cabazitaxel over docetaxel. At this time, there are no data suggesting that other chemotherapy regimens will improve the overall survival rate or quality of life after cabazitaxel [1, 15].

## Metastatic Neuroendocrine Carcinoma

For patients with visceral metastases, clinicians should consider biopsy to the area. If the biopsy result shows adenocarcinoma, treatment decision is made as those without visceral metastases. In a rare case, it may present with a small-cell feature (neuroendocrine carcinoma). Neuroendocrine prostate cancer (NEPC) is one of the rarest and most aggressive malignancies of the prostate cancer. This occurs more frequently with patients who have disease progression while on abiraterone, enzalutamide, or perhaps docetaxel or cabazitaxel. NEPC is an area where clinicians have minimal understanding due to lack of research. This is defined in various ways. "In normal cells, the neuroendocrine phenotype may play a role in regulating growth and differentiation of epithelia. However, the neuroendocrine phenotype in prostate cancer presented as a more aggressive pathological feature, indicating poor clinical outcomes relative to primary neuroendocrine cancer from other organ systems" [16]. Some scientists think that these tumors might relate to manipulation of RB1, TP53, and PTEN protein [17]. These patients present with features including (i) unresponsiveness to hormonal therapy, (ii) rapid progression, (iii) increased risk of lytic bone lesions, (iv) presence of visceral metastases, (v) a markedly enlarged prostate, and (vi) low PSA relative to disease burden. Treatment options are similar to small-cell lung cancer. Patients with NEPC are mostly responsive to chemotherapy (i.e., platinum-based therapy [18]) and radiation therapy. However, due to the rareness, aggressiveness, and short-term overall survival for this population, clinical trials supporting evidence are lacking in proving the effectiveness of these treatments [1, 16, 19, 20]. Examples of NCCN-recommended chemotherapy regimens for NEPC are listed in Table 9.3.

# Chemotherapy

## *Docetaxel*

*Docetaxel* is the first-line chemotherapy that is used for treatment with mHSPC and mCRPC. This is a taxane derivative. *Mechanism of action:* Taxanes are an antineoplastic agent, which also considered as a microtubule inhibitor. Cancer cells grow by mitosis. Taxanes interrupt the microtubular network in cells that is essential for mitotic and interphase cellular functions. It binds to free tubulin and promotes its assembly into microtubules while simultaneously inhibiting disassembly. This leads to the stabilization of microtubules, which results in the inhibition of mitosis [21, 22]. *Dosage and administration:* This is to be given 75 mg/m$^2$ every 3 weeks IV in combination with concurrent steroid premedication. Intravenous (IV) infusion is given over 1 hour, via peripheral IV or Infusaport. Docetaxel is an irritant with the vesicant-like feature; therefore, extravasation should be avoided during administration. The duration of chemotherapy should be determined by the patient's overall benefit and toxicities [1]. Given the survival benefit, patients can receive up to 10 cycles of treatment if no progression and no severe toxicities noted during chemotherapy. Retreatment of docetaxel can also be considered in men who have not demonstrated definitive evidence of progression on prior docetaxel-based therapy [1, 21]. Side effects are listed in Table 9.4.

**Table 9.3** NCCN-recommended chemotherapy regimen commonly used for patients with NEPC [1]

| Chemotherapy for neuroendocrine prostate cancer (NEPC) [1] |
|---|
| Carboplatin + cisplatin |
| Cisplatin + etoposide |
| Docetaxel + carboplatin |

**Table 9.4** Common side effects of docetaxel [21]

| | |
|---|---|
| CNS | Peripheral neuropathy, fatigue, fever |
| Cardiac | Edema |
| Respiratory | Pulmonary disorder |
| Endocrine and metabolism | Fluid retention |
| Gastrointestinal | Stomatitis, diarrhea, nausea, vomiting, increased serum transaminases |
| Genitourinary | – |
| Hematology | Neutropenia, leukopenia, anemia, thrombocytopenia, febrile neutropenia |
| Musculoskeletal | Asthenia, myalgia, neuromuscular reaction |
| Dermatological | Alopecia, rash, nail changes |

**Table 9.5** Common side effects of cabazitaxel [23]

| | |
|---|---|
| CNS | Fatigue, peripheral neuropathy, fever |
| Cardiac | – |
| Respiratory | – |
| Endocrine and metabolism | – |
| Gastrointestinal | Diarrhea, nausea, vomiting, constipation, decreased appetite, abdominal pain, anorexia, dysgeusia |
| Genitourinary | Hematuria, urinary tract infection |
| Hematology | Anemia, leukopenia, neutropenia, thrombocytopenia |
| Musculoskeletal | Dyspnea, cough |
| Dermatological | – |

## *Cabazitaxel*

*Cabazitaxel* is a second-generation taxane derivative. It is used as second-line chemotherapy for mCRPC patient who has progression of disease during or after docetaxel-based therapy. *Mechanism of action* is the same as docetaxel. *Dosage and administration:* This is to be given 25 mg/m$^2$ or 20 mg/m$^2$ every 3 weeks IV in combination with prednisone. Administration instruction is the same as docetaxel. Premedications are recommended at least 30 minutes prior to administrating cabazitaxel. Those included antihistamine (dexchlorpheniramine 5 mg or diphenhydramine 25 mg, or equivalent antihistamine), corticosteroid (dexamethasone 8 mg, or equivalent), and $H_2$ antagonist (ranitidine 50 mg, or equivalent) [23]. Side effects are listed in Table 9.5.

## *Mitoxantrone*

*Mitoxantrone* is the very first chemotherapy that is being used to treat mCRPC patients. This is an antineoplastic agent, also known as anthracenedione. *Mechanism of action:* Anthracenedione intercalates into DNA, causing cross-links and strand breaks. This inhibits DNA and RNA synthesis and hence decreases the replication of cells. It is active throughout the entire cell cycle. *Dosage and administration:* Mitoxantrone is an IV-only infusion. Dosage is either (i) 12 mg/m$^2$ once every 3 weeks (in combination with prednisone or prednisolone) for up to 10 cycles or (ii) 12–14 mg/m$^2$ once every 3 weeks (in combination with prednisone) until disease progression or unacceptable toxicity, up to the maximum cumulative dose of 144 mg/m$^2$. Each dose of mitoxantrone should be infused over 5–15 minutes via a free-flow setting. This is an irritant with vesicant-like properties and extravasation should be avoided [24]. Side effects are listed in Table 9.6. Since TAX327 [9], TROPIC [11], and PROSELICA [12] studies all show the benefits of taxanes over mitoxantrone, this drug is being used as a palliative approach and used in only in

**Table 9.6** Common side effects of mitoxantrone [24]

| | |
|---|---|
| CNS | Pain, fatigue, headache, fever |
| Cardiac | Edema, cardiac diseases/arrhythmia, ECG changes |
| Respiratory | Upper respiratory tract infection, pharyngitis, dyspnea, cough |
| Endocrine and metabolism | Hyperglycemia, weight gain/loss, increased gamma-glutamyl transferase |
| Gastrointestinal | Nausea, vomiting, mucositis, stomatitis, anorexia, constipation, GI bleed, abdominal pain, dyspepsia, increased serum alkaline phosphatase/transaminases |
| Genitourinary | Urinary tract infection, hematuria, urine abnormality, increased BUN/creatinine |
| Hematology | Neutropenia, leukopenia, lymphocytopenia, anemia, thrombocytopenia, febrile neutropenia, petechia |
| Musculoskeletal | Weakness |
| Dermatological | Alopecia, nail bed changes |

**Table 9.7** Cytotoxic chemotherapy options and dosage for mCNPC or mCRPC patients [1, 21, 23, 24]

| Chemotherapy | Docetaxel [21] | Cabazitaxel [23] | Mitoxantrone [24] |
|---|---|---|---|
| Indication | mCNPC or mCRPC | mCRPC with progression after docetaxel | mCRPC |
| Dose | 75 mg/m$^2$ every 3 weeks with concurrent steroid | 25 or 20 mg/m$^2$ every 3 weeks with concurrent steroid | 12–14 mg/m$^2$ every 3 weeks with concurrent steroid |

rare occasions at this time. Thus, the remainder of the discussion will focus how to manage the toxicities of the more commonly used taxanes. Cytotoxic chemotherapy options and dosage for mCNPC or mCRPC patients are listed in Table 9.7.

## Management of Side Effects for Taxanes Derivatives

Both docetaxel and cabazitaxel share a very similar side effect profile, which included by not limited to fatigue, nausea, vomiting, taste change, mouth sores, nail changes, liver toxicity, alopecia, renal toxicity, neutropenia, anemia, thrombocytopenia, and fluid retention/edema [21, 23]. Side effects vary from patient to patient. It is a very personal experience for each patient.

Close monitoring of the laboratory values and side effects of chemotherapy during treatment is crucial to help prevent toxicities. Laboratory values that help manage toxicities prior to each cycle of treatment include the absolute neutrophil count (ANC), hemoglobin (hgb), platelet, renal function, and liver function. Dose reduction and/or delays in treatment should be considered if the patient has pronounced toxicities during the administration of chemotherapy. Utilization of Common Terminology Criteria for Adverse Event (CTCAE) from the National Cancer

Institute (NCI) is very helpful in grading toxicity and monitoring symptoms [25]. Examples of CTCAE grading related to common side effects of taxane derivatives are illustrated in Table 9.8.

***Neutropenia*** If ANC < 1500 cells/mm$^3$, consider holding treatment for 1 week for the blood counts to recover. Granulocyte-colony stimulating factor (G-CSF) (i.e., filgrastim or pegfilgrastim) and granulocyte-macrophage colony-stimulating factor

**Table 9.8** Examples of CTCAE grading related to common side effects of taxane derivatives [25]

| Examples of common terminology criteria for adverse event (CTCAE) [25] | | | | | |
|---|---|---|---|---|---|
| | Grade 1 | Grade 2 | Grade 3 | Grade 4 | Grade 5 |
| Anemia | Hgb < LLN – 10.0 g/dL | Hgb < 10.0 – 8.0 g/dL | Hgb < 8.0 g/dL | Life-threatening consequences; urgent intervention indicate | Death |
| Diarrhea | Increase of <4 stools per day over baseline; mild increase in ostomy output compared to baseline | Increase of 4–6 stools per day over baseline; moderate increase in ostomy output compared to baseline; limiting instrumental ADL | Increase of ≥7 stools per day over baseline; hospitalization indicated; severe increase in ostomy output compared to baseline; limiting self-care ADL | Life-threatening consequences; urgent intervention indicate | Death |
| Fatigue | Fatigue relieved by rest | Fatigue not relieved by rest; limiting instrumental ADL | Fatigue not relieved by rest; limiting self-care ADL | – | – |
| Febrile neutropenia | | | ANC <1000/mm$^3$ with a single temp of >38.3 °C (101 °F) or a sustained temperature of ≥38 °C (100.4 °F) for more than 1 hour | Life-threatening consequences; urgent intervention indicate | Death |
| Nail changes | Present | – | – | – | – |
| Nausea | Loss of appetite without alteration in eating habits | Oral intake decreased without significant weight loss, dehydration, or malnutrition | Inadequate oral caloric or fluid intake; tube feeding, TPN, or hospitalization indicated | – | – |

**Table 9.8** (continued)

| Examples of common terminology criteria for adverse event (CTCAE) [25] | | | | | |
|---|---|---|---|---|---|
| | Grade 1 | Grade 2 | Grade 3 | Grade 4 | Grade 5 |
| Oral mucositis | Asymptomatic or mild symptoms; intervention not indicated | Moderate pain or ulcer that does not interfere with oral intake; modified diet indicated | Severe pain; interfering with oral intake | Life-threatening consequences; urgent intervention indicate | Death |
| Peripheral sensory neuropathy | Asymptomatic | Moderate symptoms; limiting instrumental ADL | Severe symptoms; limiting self-care ADL | Life-threatening consequences, urgent intervention indicate | – |

(GM-CSF) (i.e., sargramostim) can be given after each cycle of chemotherapy as secondary prophylaxis. These drugs stimulate the production, maturation, and activation of neutrophils to prevent neutropenia, neutropenic fever, and infection related to neutropenia. Pegfilgrastim has a prolonged duration of effect compared to filgrastim and reduced renal clearance. Sargramostim is limited to use following induction therapy for some hematological malignancy settings. If a patient presented with fever (≥38.3 °C or 101 °F) and/or neutropenia (ANC < 1000/mm$^3$), a complete workup including history and physical (H&P), epidemiologically relevant exposures, laboratory/radiology assessment (complete blood count with differentials, comprehensive metabolic panel, electrolytes, urine analysis, and chest X-ray), and microbiologic elevation (blood cultures, urine culture, site-specific culture, and viral diagnostics) is required. An empiric broad-spectrum antibiotic should also be utilized. Typical IV mono-antibiotic therapies are cefepime, imipenem/cilastatin, meropenem, piperacillin/tazobactam, or ceftazidime. IV combination therapy should also be considered if the patient has a known history or is suspicious for antimicrobial resistance [21, 23, 26–28].

***Hepatic Toxicity*** Taxanes are metabolized through the liver; therefore, an abnormal liver function test is common, which needs to be closely monitored. The US box warning of docetaxel suggests: *"Should not be given if bilirubin > ULN, or if AST and/or ALT > 1.5 × ULN concomitant with alkaline phosphatase (ALK) > 2.5 × ULN. LFT elevations increase risks of severe or life-threatening complications. Obtain LFTs before each treatment cycle."* Also note that it is very common for patients with prostate cancer to have an isolated elevation of ALK that is related to bone disease, not the liver. In this case, docetaxel is safe to administer [21, 23].

***Fluid Retention*** One of the more common side effects of docetaxel is fluid retention. Premedication of oral corticosteroids is recommended to all patients prior to each chemotherapy administration to reduce the incidence and severity of fluid retention and allergic reactions. Severe fluid retention (poorly tolerated peripheral edema, generalized edema, pleural effusion requiring urgent drainage, dyspnea at rest, cardiac tamponade, or pronounced abdominal distention) occurred in 6.5% of patients despite the use of a 3-day dexamethasone premedication regimen. The use of diuretics can be used to eliminate extra fluid retention along with holding further taxane therapy if severe. Patient should also be encouraged to utilize compression stockings and elevate lower extremities when able to reduce lower extremities edema [21, 23, 28].

***Anemia*** Marrow suppression is common with taxane-based chemotherapy including the development of anemia. Blood transfusions are considered for the treatment of symptomatic anemia (tachycardia, tachypnea, postural hypotension, shortness of breath, increased fatigue, and skin paleness). Chemotherapy can still be given while the patient is anemic based on provider decision and patient presentation. Erythropoietin therapy, such as epoetin alfa and darbepoetin alfa, can also be considered during active chemotherapy. Anemia workup should also be performed to rule out underlying causes, such as iron deficiency anemia or vitamin B12 deficiency [21, 23, 28, 29].

***Nausea and Vomiting*** Nausea and/or vomiting are common but manageable with taxanes. Both docetaxel and cabazitaxel are considered low-emetic-risk chemotherapy. Premedication of dexamethasone 8–12 mg PO/IV, metoclopramide 10–20 mg PO/IV, prochlorperazine 10 mg PO/IV, or ondansetron 8–16 mg PO can be used 30 minutes prior of chemotherapy administration and repeat daily as needed. In a case where severe nausea and vomiting are uncontrolled by the above recommendation, lorazepam 0.5–2 mg PO/SL/IV can also be used. Clinicians may also consider IV hydration for patients with frequent episodes of nausea and vomiting and decreased oral intake [21, 23, 28, 30].

***Diarrhea*** Diarrhea can occur up to 47% of patients who are receiving taxanes. Closely monitor signs and symptoms of dehydration and electrolyte imbalance. Antidiarrheal medication (i.e., loperamide) and fluid and electrolyte replacement may be necessary. If diarrhea is greater than or equal to seven stools per day over baseline, hospitalization is indicated, or if there is severe increase in ostomy output compared to baseline, limiting self-care ADL (CTCEA grade 3 or higher), treatment delay, and dose reduction are required [21, 23, 28].

***Oral Stomatitis/Taste Change*** Oral ulceration can present with patients on active treatment of taxanes. Patients are often recommended prophylactic oral care during chemotherapy, which included dental check-up prior to chemotherapy initiation, self-monitor, and oral care daily. Patients can rinse mouth throughout the day with a mixture of warm water, baking soda, and salt (one-half teaspoon of salt and one teaspoon of baking soda in a quart of water). Topical and systemic analgesia can also be used with some pain relief; "magic mouthwash" is commonly used and prescribed. Magic mouthwash usually contains at least three of the following medication: antibiotic, antihistamine or local anesthetic, antifungal, corticosteroid, and antacid. Taste change may also occur for some patients. Most of them described as "metallic taste" and have no appetite due to taste change. This is reversible once treatment is completed. Patients are often reminded to maintain proper nutrition and hydration when having oral stomatitis and taste change. Nutritional supplement drinks are often helpful [21, 23, 28].

***Fatigue*** Patients often experience fatigue during chemotherapy. Encourage patients to maintain their daily routine as much as possible with a well-balanced diet. Short naps of less than 1 hour during the days should be considered. Taking short walks and getting light exercise may increase the patients' energy level [21, 23, 28, 31].

***Peripheral Sensory Neuropathy*** Patients will often describe numbness, tingling, or pins and needles feelings of the hands and feet. Patients should be educated to report signs and symptoms of peripheral neuropathy, which included but not limited to, change in sensation with cold or hot, inability to feel pain on palms or planters, unable to button shirts or pants, or unable to pick up small objects like coins. Treatment delay or dose reduction should be considered if grade 2 or higher neuropathy is reported. Also, note that neuropathy is a delayed effect, so stopping chemotherapy earlier is the key [21, 23, 28].

***Nail Changes*** The color of fingernails and/or toenails may change while receiving docetaxel. In rare cases, nails may fall off. Educate patients that nails will generally grow back after completion of treatment. Nails should be kept clean and cut short. Gloves should be worn while performing household duties (i.e., dishwashing, cleaning) [21, 23, 28].

***Thrombocytopenia*** If platelet <100, clinicians should consider holding treatment for at least 1 week. Platelet usually recovers without additional intervention. Educate patients to implement bleeding precautions at home by brushing teeth with a soft bristle brush, wearing proper footwear both inside and outside, avoid sharp objects, and report any unexpected bleeding or brushing. They should also avoid over-the-counter aspirin or ibuprofen. In rare case, platelet transfusion can be given platelet <15 or <50 with active bleeding [21, 23, 28].

***Alopecia*** Hair loss can occur during active treatment. Educate patients that alopecia will be reversed once treatment is completed. A wig can be used during the time of transition [21, 23, 28].

***Allergic Reactions*** Severe allergic reaction is common if patients do not have adequate steroid prophylaxis. These symptoms include but not limited to generalized rash, erythema, hypotension, bronchospasm, or anaphylaxis. Follow individual institutional protocol for emergency allergic reaction management [21, 23, 28].

## Conclusion

Chemotherapy treatment options for prostate cancer are very limited. Taxane derivatives (i.e., docetaxel and cabazitaxel) are a class of chemotherapy that is commonly used to treat mHSPC with high-risk feature, and mCRPC with or without visceral metastases. For mHSPC patients, first-line treatment is docetaxel and ADT upfront. For mCRPC patient, the first-line treatment options include oral therapy (i.e., abiraterone with prednisone, or enzalutamide) or chemotherapy (i.e., docetaxel). Decision of chemotherapy over oral therapy is based upon patient's symptoms and performance status. The second-line treatment option is cabazitaxel. Other chemotherapies such as cisplatin, carboplatin, and etoposide may also be considered when a patient presents with NEPC. NEPC is one of the rarest and most aggressive malignancies of the prostate cancer. This occurs more frequently with patients who have disease progression while on abiraterone, enzalutamide, or perhaps docetaxel or cabazitaxel. Lab results and side effects should be closely monitored and assessed prior to each chemotehrapy administration. If toxicities present during treatment, treatment delay and/or dose reduction may require. Due to the limitation of chemotherapy options for PC patients, ongoing clinical trials are needed to investigate and develop more treatment options for patients with PC.

**Clinical Pearls**

- Clinicians will consider using chemotherapy when the patient has (i) metastatic hormone-sensitive prostate cancer (mHSPC) with high-risk feature; or (ii) metastatic castration-resistant prostate cancer (mCRPC), with or without visceral metastases.
- The most common use of cytotoxic chemotherapy is a taxane derivative.
- Both CHAARTED and STAMPEDE studies improved overall survival in men with mHSPC using docetaxel with ADT upfront compared to ADT alone.
- In mCRPC, mitoxantrone provides a palliative benefit alone.
- Single-agent docetaxel remains a standard of care for mCRPC patients.
- Patients who previously received docetaxel in castration-naive setting may also have benefits from receiving docetaxel again.
- If progression of disease occurs after docetaxel in the castration-resistant setting, cabazitaxel will be a second-line treatment option of chemotherapy.
- Patients with neuroendocrine prostate cancer are mostly responsive to chemotherapy (i.e., platinum-based therapy) and radiation therapy.
- Taxanes (docetaxel and cabazitaxel) are microtubule inhibitors.
- Side effects of taxanes include fatigue, nausea, vomiting, taste change, mouth sores, nail changes, liver toxicity, alopecia, renal toxicity, neutropenia, anemia, thrombocytopenia, fluid retention/ edema.

- Laboratory values that help screen for taxane toxicities prior to each cycle of treatment include the absolute neutrophil count (ANC), hemoglobin (hgb), platelet, renal function, and liver function.
- Taxanes are metabolized through the liver; therefore, an abnormal liver function test is common, which needs to be closely monitored.
- One of the more common side effects of docetaxel is fluid retention. Premedication of oral corticosteroids is recommended to help mitigate this and other side effects.

## References

1. NCCN. Prostate cancer [Internet]. 2018 Apr [cited 2018 Oct]. Available from: https://www.nccn.org/professionals/physician_gls/pdf/prostate.pdf.
2. Sweeney CJ, Chen YH, Carducci M, et al. Chemohormonal therapy in metastatic hormone-sensitive prostate cancer. N Engl J Med. 2015;373:737–46.
3. James ND, Sydes MR, Clarke NW, et al. Additional docetaxel, zoledronic acid, or both to first-line long-term hormone therapy in prostate cancer (STAMPEDE): survival results from an adaptive, multiarm, multistage, platform randomised controlled trial. Lancet. 2016;387:1163–77.
4. Fizazi K, Tran N, Fein L, et al. Abiraterone plus prednisone in metastatic, castration-sensitive prostate cancer. N Engl J Med. 2017;377:352–60.
5. Sydes MR, Spears MR, Manson MD, et al. Adding abiraterone or docetaxel to long-term hormone therapy for prostate cancer: directly randomized data from the STAMPEDE multi-arm, multi-stage platform protocol. Ann Oncol. 2018;29(5):1235–48.
6. Ramamurthy C, Correa AF, Handorf EA, et al. Cost-effectiveness analysis of abiraterone acetate (AA) versus docetaxel (D) for the management of metastatic hormone naïve prostate cancer (mHNPC). J Clin Oncol. 2018;36:6514.
7. Kantoff PW, Halabi S, Conaway M, et al. Hydrocortisone with or without mitoxantrone in men with hormone-refractory prostate cancer: results of the cancer and leukemia group B 9182 study. J Clin Oncol. 1999;17(8):2506.
8. Tannock IF, Osoba D, Stockler MR, et al. Chemotherapy with mitoxantrone plus prednisone or prednisone alone for symptomatic hormone-resistant prostate cancer: a Canadian randomized trial with palliative end points. J Clin Oncol. 1996;14(6):1756–64.
9. Tannock IF, Wit RD, Berry WR, et al. Docetaxel plus prednisone or mitoxantrone plus prednisone for advanced prostate cancer. N Engl J Med. 2004;351(15):1502–12.
10. Quinn DI, Tangen CM, Hussain M, et al. Docetaxel and atrasentan versus docetaxel and placebo for men with advanced castration-resistant prostate cancer (SWOG S0421): a randomized phase 3 trial. Lancet. 2013;14(9):893–900.
11. de Bono JS, Oudard S, Ozguroglu M, et al. Prednisone plus cabazitaxel or mitoxantrone for metastatic castration-resistant prostate cancer progressing after docetaxel treatment: a randomised open-label trial. Lancet. 2010;376(9747):1147–54.
12. Eisenberger M, Hardy-Bessard AC, Kim CS, et al. Phase III study comparing a reduced dose of cabazitaxel (20 mg/m2) and the currently approved dose (25 mg/m2) in post docetaxel patients with metastatic castration-resistant prostate cancer-PROSELICA. J Clin Oncol. 2017;35(28):3198–206.
13. Fizazi K, Scher HI, Molina A, et al. Abiraterone acetate for treatment of metastatic castration-resistant prostate cancer: final overall survival analysis of the COU-AA-301 randomized, double-blind, placebo-controlled phase 3 study. Lancet. 2012;13(10):983–92.

14. Beer TM, Armstrong AJ, Rathkopf DE, et al. Enzalutamide in metastatic prostate cancer before chemotherapy. N Engl J Med. 2014;371:424–33.
15. Song P, Huang C, Wang Y. The efficacy and safety comparison of docetaxel, cabazitaxel, estramustine, and mitoxantrone for castration-resistant prostate cancer: a network meta-analysis. Int J Surg. 2018;56:133–40.
16. Dicken H, Hensley PJ, Kyprianou N. Prostate tumor neuroendocrine differentiation via EMT: the road less traveled. Asian J Urol. 2019;6:82–90.
17. Tan HL, Sood A, Rahimi HA, et al. Rb loss is characteristic of prostatic small cell neuroendocrine carcinoma. Clin Cancer Res. 2013;20(4):890–903.
18. Beltran H, Tomlins S, Aparicio A, et al. Aggressive variants of castration-resistant prostate cancer. Clin Cancer Res. 2014;20(11):2845–50.
19. Nadal R, Schweizer M, Kryvenko ON, et al. Small cell carcinoma of the prostate. Nat Rev Urol. 2014;11(4):213–9.
20. Parimi V, Goyal R, Poropatich K, et al. Neuroendocrine differentiation of prostate cancer: a review. Am J Clin Exp Urol. 2014;2(4):273–85.
21. Taxotere™ (docetaxel) [Package insert]. Bridgewater: Sanofi-Aventis U.S. LLC; 2010. Available from: https://www.accessdata.fda.gov/drugsatfda_docs/label/2010/020449s059lbl.pdf.
22. De Morrée ES, Vogelzang NJ, Petrylak DP, et al. Association of survival benefit with docetaxel in prostate cancer and total number of cycles administered. JAMA Oncol. 2017;3(1):68.
23. Jevtana™ (cabazitaxel) [Package insert]. Bridgewater: Sanofi-Aventis U.S. LLC; 2010. Available from: https://www.accessdata.fda.gov/drugsatfda_docs/label/2010/201023lbl.pdf.
24. Novantrone™ (mitoxantrone) [Package insert]. Rockland: EMD Serono, Inc.; 2008. Available from: https://www.accessdata.fda.gov/drugsatfda_docs/label/2009/019297s030s031lbl.pdf.
25. NCI. Common terminology criteria for adverse events (CTCAE) [Internet]. 2017 Nov 27 [cited 2019 Jan]. Available from: https://ctep.cancer.gov/protocoldevelopment/electronic_applications/docs/ctcae_v5_quick_reference_8.5x11.pdf.
26. NCCN. Prevention and treatment of cancer-related infection [Internet]. 2019 Jan [cited 2019 Jan]. Available from: https://www.nccn.org/professionals/physician_gls/pdf/infections.pdf.
27. NCCN. Hematopoietic growth factor [Internet]. 2019 Jan [cited 2019 Mar]. Available from: https://www.nccn.org/professionals/physician_gls/pdf/growthfactors.pdf.
28. NIH. Side effects of cancer treatment [Internet]. Updated 2018 Aug [cited 2019 Jan]. Available from: https://www.cancer.gov/about-cancer/treatment/side-effects.
29. NCCN. Cancer- and chemotherapy-induced anemia [Internet]. 2018 Mar [cited 2019 Jan]. Available from: https://www.nccn.org/professionals/physician_gls/pdf/anemia.pdf.
30. NCCN. Antiemesis [Internet]. 2018 Mar [cited 2019 Jan]. Available from: https://www.nccn.org/professionals/physician_gls/pdf/antiemesis.pdf.
31. NCCN. Cancer-related fatigue [Internet]. 2018 Feb [cited 2019 Jan]. Available from: https://www.nccn.org/professionals/physician_gls/pdf/fatigue.pdf.

# Chapter 10
# Radiopharmaceuticals for Prostate Cancer

**Ann E. Donnelly and Mark D. Hurwitz**

## General Considerations for Radiopharmaceuticals

Only physicians and facilities with experience and licensing to handle and use these medications should administer radiopharmaceuticals. The American College of Radiology has a practice standard for the administration of radiopharmaceuticals, but state and local regulations must be followed as well. Candidates for intervention with radiopharmaceuticals should be assessed directly by the physician who will be overseeing treatment. Informed consent should be obtained before patients undergo treatment with radiopharmaceuticals. Physicians should have detailed discussions with patients about the possible side effects, logistics, and alternative treatments.

## Strontium-89

Strontium-89 is a beta-emitting radioactive isotope with a half-life of 50.5 days. It was the first radiopharmaceutical approved by the FDA for the treatment of pain related to known bony metastatic disease [5].

A. E. Donnelly (✉) · M. D. Hurwitz
Department of Radiation Oncology, Thomas Jefferson University Hospital, Philadelphia, PA, USA
e-mail: ann.donnelly@jefferson.edu



E. J. Trabulsi et al. (eds.), *Chemotherapy and Immunotherapy in Urologic Oncology*, https://doi.org/10.1007/978-3-030-52021-2_10

## Mechanism of Action

Strontium-89 acts in a way similar to calcium in the body and is deposited in bone with increased uptake in blastic lesions [5]. Strontium-89 then delivers radiation to the tissue by emitting beta particles. The beta particles have a maximum range of emission of 8 mm with a maximum energy of 1.463 MeV, so the effect on normal tissue is minimized [5].

## Pharmacokinetics

After administration, strontium-89 is cleared from the bloodstream quickly and taken up by primarily bone tissue [5]. Since strontium-89 acts like calcium in the body, it is taken up in much higher amounts in blastic metastatic bone lesions where the rate of osteogenesis is higher [5]. Strontium-89 has a half-life of 50.5 days; therefore, there is more exposure of both diseased and normal bone to radiation over time compared to other isotopes [5]. Strontium-89 remains in metastatic lesions for longer time periods than normal bone and over half of the injected doses is deposited in the bones after treatment [5]. Excretion is two-thirds renal and one-third fecal, and the urinary excretion is highest in the first 2 days after treatment [5].

## Dosage and Administration

Strontium-89 is given over IV push infusion over 1–2 minutes at a dose of 148 MBq, 4 mCi, or 1.5–2.2 MBq/kg, 40–60 μCi/kg body weight [5]. Repeat infusion can be considered but should only be done depending on how the patient tolerates the first infusion [5]. Infusions should not be given less than 90 days apart. Though there is no clear recommended alternative dosing for patients with renal insufficiency, caution should be taken in patients with decreased renal function given the high percentage of renal excretion [9].

## Adverse Reactions and Warnings

White blood cells and platelets are most often affected by strontium-89, and bone marrow effects are often seen. The prolonged half-life relative to radium-223 or samarium-153 has been associated with an extended delay in count recovery and, in some patients, a lack of full recovery. A complete blood count should be checked prior to administration and then should be checked every 2 weeks after injection [5]. Per the manufacturer's prescribing guidelines, caution should be used in patients with a platelet count below 60,000 and a white blood cell count below 2400 [5]. However, more conservative baseline parameters such as platelet counts of at least 100,000 and WBC counts of at least 3000 at baseline should be considered. Many patients experience a 30% or greater decrease in platelet levels with strontium-89 [5]. Generally, the blood count nadir was found to be 12–16 weeks after infusion, and it may take up to 6 months for blood cell counts to recover after treatment [9]. Some patients have noticed an increase in bone pain within 36–72 hours after infusion, which usually resolves with analgesics [5]. Flushing has been seen in patients when there is a rapid administration of the drug [9]. Other reported adverse reactions that are less common include chills, fever, hot flashes, and septicemia [9]. Strontium-89, like all radiopharmaceuticals, may cause fetal harm and should not be given to pregnant women [5]. Patients should be advised to avoid pregnancy. There are no known contraindications, but caution should be used in any patients with underlying bone marrow suppression [5]. There are no known significant drug interactions.

## *Safety Precautions and Patient Education*

Strontium-89 should only be given in facilities and by physicians who are trained in using radiopharmaceuticals. The strontium-89 should be stored in its original lead container or have adequate radiation shielding during handling [9]. Given the renal excretion, patients who are incontinent of urine should be catheterized to avoid contamination and exposures [5]. Patients should be instructed to flush the toilet multiple times after use and practice good hand washing. Typical onset of pain relief is 7–20 days after infusion [5].

## *Background and Clinical Considerations*

Strontium-89 has been evaluated in several clinical trials. In a small placebo-controlled trial of patients with castrate-resistant metastatic prostate cancer with painful bone metastases, patients were randomly assigned to receive either strontium-89 or placebo. After 5 weeks, patients were reassessed and a second injection could be given if the patient was still having pain. The patients' pain was evaluated with a scoring system and categorized as deteriorated, no significant change, some improvement, substantial improvement, or dramatic improvement [2]. The final analysis showed that only patients in the strontium-89 arm had full pain relief, and strontium-89 significantly reduced pain scores in more patients than those treated with placebo ($p < 0.01$) [2]. Strontium-89 was also evaluated in a phase III, randomized, placebo-controlled clinical trial to associate its effect as an adjunct treatment in patients with metastatic prostate cancer treated with external beam radiation therapy. A total of 126 patients with castrate-resistant prostate cancer were treated with local radiation therapy plus strontium-89 or placebo as a single injection and then followed with tumor markers and pain assessments [19]. Patients in the strontium-89 arm had a greater decrease in the amount of pain medication they were taking, decreased new sites of pain (1.213 in the placebo arm vs 0.587 in the strontium-89 arm, $p < 0.002$), and improved quality-of-life indicators in the strontium-89 arm with decreased pain and improved physical activity found to be statistically significant ($p < 0.05$) [19].

Strontium-89 has been evaluated with chemotherapy in several trials, as well. In a small, randomized, phase II clinical trial, 103 patients with metastatic castrate-resistant prostate cancer and either increasing cancer-related symptoms or rising PSA were treated with induction chemotherapy with doxorubicin, ketoconazole, vinblastine, and estramustine [11]. Patients with stable or improved disease after two to three cycles of chemotherapy were then randomized to receive 6 weeks of doxorubicin with or without one dose of strontium-89 [11]. One limitation of the study however was the use of doxorubicin, which is now recognized as having limited efficacy in the treatment of prostate cancer. Patients who received strontium-89 along with chemotherapy were found to have an increased overall survival, with a mean survival of 27.7 months compared to 16.8 months in the chemotherapy alone arm [11]. The TRAPEZE trial involved 757 patients with castrate-resistant metastatic prostate cancer, who were randomized to receive treatment on one of four arms: docetaxel alone, docetaxel with zoledronic acid, docetaxel with strontium-89, or docetaxel with both zoledronic acid and strontium-89. Chemotherapy with strontium-89 had a mild effect on the time to clinical disease progression with an increase of approximately 1 month (HR, 0.85; 95% CI, 0.73–0.99; $P = 0.03$) but with no improvement in overall survival [20].

Strontium-89 can be a beneficial tool for the treatment of patients with painful bony metastatic disease. Patients should have imaging studies or biopsy confirming the presence of bone metastases before treatment. The high affinity for blastic metastatic bone lesions and low area of tissue penetration help to target areas of cancer while limiting the effect to healthy tissue. In addition, strontium-89 may also be helpful in managing patients who have had persistent pain despite other therapies. Patients should be alerted to the possibility of pain flare 36–72 hours after injection and a strategy to address pain flare, including adjustment in pain medication dose, put in place prior. Because most patients do not see an onset of pain relief until 7–20 days after administration, it may not be the ideal treatment for patients with a very short life expectancy. In addition, the cost of producing strontium-89 has made it one of the more expensive radiopharmaceuticals and may limit its overall use [15]. The prolonged half-life and associated less favorable hemodynamic side effect profile of strontium-89 as compared with samarium-153 EDTMP has led to a wider utilization of samarium-153 EDTMP in the management of diffuse, predominately osteoblastic metastatic bone pain.

## Samarium-153

Samarium-153 EDTMP is a radioactive isotope that emits medium-energy beta particles. The half-life of samarium-153 at 1.93 days is considerably shorter than both radium-223 and strontium-89. Samarium-153 EDTMP is indicated for patients with pain from metastatic osteoblastic bone lesions confirmed on nuclear bone scan imaging [6].

### *Mechanism of Action*

Samarium-153 EDTMP is taken up by bone metastases, and local radiation is delivered to the lesions. Alone, the samarium-153 does not have a high affinity for bone uptake, but when chelated to form a complex with EDTMP (ethylenediamine tetramethylene phosphonic acid), it becomes more targeted to bone [16]. The exact method by which the drug decreases pain from bone metastases is not clear [6]. Samarium-153 EDTMP decays much faster than other radiopharmaceuticals, such as strontium-89, so the radiation dose is delivered quickly over a shorter period of time.

### *Pharmacokinetics*

Samarium-153 EDTMP is cleared rapidly from the blood stream after injection [16]. The samarium-153 EDTMP complex has an affinity for bone and is taken up by osteoblastic lesions approximately five times more than normal bone [6]. More of the drug is taken up by patients with a higher number of osteoblastic skeletal lesions, and there is an unknown benefit to patients with osteolytic lesions [6]. The drug that is not taken up by bone is cleared quickly and excreted through the urine [16]. Samarium-153 EDTMP is excreted in urine as an intact complex with 34.5% (±15%) excreted within the first 6 hours after administration and urinary excretion of radioactive material takes place over approximately 12 hours after administration [6]. Beta particles of samarium-153 EDTMP travel a maximum of 3 mm in soft tissues and 1.7 mm in bone [6]. In clinical studies, the age of the patient, including advanced age, did not seem to affect the pharmacokinetics of samarium-153 EDTMP [6].

### *Dosage and Administration*

Dosage of samarium-153 EDTMP is 1 mCi/kg or 37 MBq/kg given by IV push over 1 minute through a secure catheter. The IV should be flushed with saline after administration. The patient should be given 500 mL of oral or IV hydration prior to

IV push to promote excretion. Caution should be used in calculating doses for patients that are very thin or very obese [6].

## Adverse Effects and Precautions

Bone marrow suppression is a significant but generally predictable potential side effect for patients treated with samarium-153 EDTMP. In clinical trials, up to 95% of patients had a decrease in white blood cell counts and platelets counts of up to 40–50% from the pretreatment levels, and nadir of the counts was found 3–5 weeks after administration [6]. Most patients had return of counts to baseline levels within 8 weeks of treatment [6]. Patients should have weekly blood work to assess for bone marrow function for at least 8 weeks after treatment. In clinical trials, there were deaths in patients with disseminated intravascular coagulation (DIC) when receiving beta-emitting particles, so patients should be monitored closely. Caution should be taken in any patients with evidence of bone marrow insufficiency prior to treatment. Patients should generally not receive concurrent chemotherapy or external beam radiation therapy while undergoing treatment with samarium-153 EDTMP due to the risk for significant myelosuppression unless the benefit outweighs the risk [6].

Hypocalcemia has been reported in patients undergoing treatment [7]. Other less common side effects include arrhythmias, hypertension, stroke, dizziness, ecchymosis, diarrhea, bone pain, spinal cord compression, hematuria, bronchitis, and epistaxis [7]. Samaraium-153 EDTMP can cause fetal harm, so women of childbearing age should have a negative pregnancy test prior to administration [6]. Patients should be advised to avoid pregnancy and use effective contraception after treatment. Samarium-153 EDTMP is contraindicated in any patients with a known hypersensitivity to the compound [6].

Increased hydration is recommended to promote urinary excretion of the compound, so caution should be used in patients with a history of congestive heart failure and renal insufficiency. There are no clear guidelines regarding dose adjustments for renal function, as adequate studies have not been performed [6]. Precautions should be taken to avoid contact with the urine of patients treated with samardium-153 EDTMP, as urinary excretion of radioactive material takes place over approximately 12 hours after administration. Patients should be encouraged to void frequently after treatment to decrease bladder exposure [6].

## Patient Education

Patients should be instructed to take precautions to avoid exposure to radioactivity in their urine for 12 hours after administration [6]. Toilets should be flushed several times after use. Any soiled linens should be cleaned separately. Alternatively, linens can be stored for 1–2 weeks to allow for decay of the radioactivity [7]. Patients can use analgesics for any temporary bone pain that can be seen after treatment. The onset of pain relief is usually in 1 week with a full effect of pain relief within 3–4 weeks [6].

## *Background and Clinical Considerations*

The efficacy of samarium-153 EDTMP was evaluated in several clinical trials. In a randomized, double-blind study of 118 patients with bone metastases causing pain, patients received 0.5 or 1.0 mCi/kg versus placebo. The study found that 62–72% of patients who received 1.0 mCi/kg had some pain relief within the first 4 weeks after injections, while 31% reported "marked" or "complete" pain relief on patient-reported scores at 4 weeks after treatment [17]. Approximately 43% of patients who received the 1.0 mCi/kg dose also reported pain improvement 16 weeks after completion of treatment [17]. There were no grade 4 bone marrow adverse effects reported [17]. In another study, 152 men with metastatic castrate-resistant prostate cancer with bone metastases causing pain were enrolled in a randomized, double-blind clinical trial where patients were given either radioactive or nonradioactive samarium-153 complexes. Patients reported less pain with the radioactive samarium-153 compared with placebo within 1–2 weeks after administration [18]. Bone marrow suppression was also seen, but no grade 4 myelosuppression was noted [18].

Samarium-153 EDTMP has a shorter half-life than some other radiopharmaceuticals. For the majority of the radiation dose to be administered, it takes approximately 1 week for samarium-153, versus approximately 25 weeks for strontium-89 [16]. Repeat doses of samarium-153 EDTMP have been used in some patients who have had good pain control with recurrent symptoms after treatment and who have adequate bone marrow function [16]. Overall, samarium-153 EDTMP can be an effective tool in the treatment of pain from metastatic bone disease when patients are selected appropriately and monitored closely after treatment.

## Radium-223

Radium-223 is predominantly an alpha-emitting particle with a half-life of 11.4 days [14]. The energy emitted from radium-223 is 95.3% alpha particles, 3.6% beta particles, and 1.1% emitted as gamma-radiation [4]. Radium-223 is indicated for the treatment of bone metastases causing symptoms in castrate-resistant patients with no known visceral disease [4]. A key distinction of radium-223 is a defined survival advantage in the treatment of castrate-resistant prostate cancer.

## Mechanism of Action

The alpha-particle-emitting isotope radium-223 mimics calcium in the body, forming complexes with areas of new bone growth [10]. Alpha-emitting particles cause high linear energy transfer that causes breaks in double-stranded DNA to cause cell destruction; however, the range from radium-223 is less than 100 μm, so there is limited effect to surrounding healthy tissue [4].

## Pharmacokinetics

Radium-223 is quickly distributed from the blood to bone or excreted into the intestines. After 15 minutes, only 20% of the drug remains in blood circulation decreasing to only 4% at 4 hours [4]. In clinical trials, there was no significant uptake in organs such as the heart, liver, kidneys, urinary bladder, and spleen 4 hours after administration [4]. The highest doses absorbed by body organs include bone by osteogenic cells, red bone marrow, and the upper and lower large intestinal wall [4]. Radium-223 decays rather than undergoes metabolism through the body [4]. Approximately 63% of the radium-223 was excreted from the body within 7 days of infusion, which is mainly by fecal and urinary excretion [4]. Therefore, patients with slower gastrointestinal motility rates will experience higher radiation exposure to the intestines, but it is unclear if this causes an increase in gastrointestinal toxicities [4].

## Dosing and Administration

The dose of radium-223 is calculated based on the patient's body weight, dosage level, radioactivity concentration of the product, and decay correction factor to correct for physical decay of radium-223 [4]. The dose is 50 kBq/kg (1.35 μCi/kg). Administration of radium-223 is by IV push over 1 minute. The IV should be flushed with normal saline before and after injection. No dose adjustments are recommended for patients with moderate to severe liver dysfunction due to lack of clinical trial data but radium-223 is not metabolized in the liver or cleared through the bile, so hepatic impairment is unlikely to affect the body's ability to manage the drug [4]. There are also no dose adjustments recommended based on mild (creatinine clearance 60–89 mL/min) or moderate (creatinine clearance 30–59 mL/min) renal impairment [4]. There is insufficient data to recommend any dose adjustments for severe renal impairment (creatinine clearance less than 30 mL/min) [4].

## *Adverse Reactions and Warnings*

The most common side effects from radium-223, greater than 10%, include temporary bone marrow suppression, gastrointestinal side effects, and peripheral edema [4]. Less common side effects include renal insufficiency/failure, dehydration, injection site reactions, and rarely secondary malignant neoplasms [4]. Dehydration may be related to the gastrointestinal side effects from therapy. There was an increase in osteosarcomas in animal studies [4]. Radium-223 contributes to a patient's overall lifetime radiation dose, so this should also be taken into account when considering treatment.

In a clinical trial, 2% of patients experienced significant bone marrow suppression or ongoing pancytopenia compared to patients treated with placebo [4]. Patients to be treated with radium-223 should have an evaluation of blood counts prior to initiation of treatment and prior to each dose. Patients should have an absolute neutrophil count (ANC) greater or equal to $1.5 \times 10^9$/L, platelet count greater than or equal to $100 \times 10^9$/L, and hemoglobin greater than or equal to 10 g/dL [4] to begin treatment with radium-223. A complete blood count should be drawn prior to each dose of radium-223 and ANC should be greater than or equal to $1 \times 10^9$/L and platelet count greater than or equal to $50 \times 10^9$/L to continue treatment [4]. Treatment should be held if laboratory values are not adequate. If levels do not recover within 6–8 weeks, treatment with radium-223 should be terminated [4]. Chemotherapy should not be given concurrently outside of clinical trial [4, 8]. No comprehensive drug interaction studies have been done, but there have not been any clear interactions between radium-223 and bisphosphonates or calcium channel blockers in clinical trials [4].

## *Safety Precautions and Patient Education*

Precautions should be taken after administration of radium-223, and teaching should be done with patients and their families. Patients and family members should be advised to take precautions to avoid exposures for approximately 1–2 weeks after radium-223 injection. Patients should be instructed to remain well hydrated. Following micturition, patients should be instructed to flush toilets twice after each use and sit on the toilet for urination to avoid splashing of urine. Caregivers should wear gloves when handling bodily fluids, such as urine, feces, and emesis. Any clothing with bodily fluids should be washed immediately and separately. Patient should be instructed on good handwashing after urination. Radiation exposure is expected to be low given the low treatment activity range of radium-223, but precautions should be taken to minimize exposure in patient care. Men should be instructed to use condoms for sexual intercourse and female partners of childbearing age should use an effective contraceptive during radium-223 treatment and for at least 6 months after treatment to avoid pregnancy. While there are no clear data on the fertility effects of radium-223, it has the potential to inhibit fertility [4].

## *Background and Clinical Considerations*

The ALSYMPCA trial was a phase III, double-blind trial designed to assess the clinical benefit of radium-223 versus best supportive care. The trial enrolled 921 patients with castrate-resistant metastatic prostate cancer with known bone metastases with or without prior docetaxel treatment and randomized them to either treatment with radium-223 or placebo. The study was closed early, as interim analysis showed a significant improvement in overall survival for the radium-223 arm (overall survival 14.0 months vs. 11.2 months; hazard ratio, 0.70; 95% CI, 0.55–0.88; two-sided $P = 0.002$) [10]. Ultimately, the final analysis showed the median survival of patients receiving radium-223 was 3.6 months longer than those receiving placebo (14.9 months vs. 11.3 months; hazard ratio, 0.70; 95% CI, 0.58–0.83; $P < 0.001$) [10]. Patients treated with radium-223 also had a delay in symptomatic skeletal events, defined as symptomatic fractures, than patients treated with placebo [10]. There was no significant difference in adverse effects between the radium-223 and placebo arms of the trial. A subgroup analysis was later done to evaluate patients who had received docetaxel chemotherapy prior to radium-223 treatment. The analysis found that patients had improved overall survival regardless of prior docetaxel use and patients who had received prior docetaxel tolerated radium-223 well [13].

The ALSYMPCA trial was structured such that patients received six injections, though the optimal number of effective and tolerated doses has been in question. In a small study of 44 retreated patients with castrate-resistant metastatic prostate cancer with bone metastases who had previously undergone treatment with radium-223 without evidence of progression during treatment, the patients were given up to six additional infusions of radium-223 every 4 weeks. The retreated patients did not seem to have an increase in hematologic toxicities during therapy or for the 2 years of posttreatment follow-up [12]. Patients also had a low rate of radiographic progression [12]. Further studies are needed regarding retreatment or longer treatment durations with radium-223. Clinical trials are ongoing in diseases other than prostate cancer to see if radium-223 will be a benefit in patients with other tumor types, who have osteoblastic metastatic bone disease.

Studies have also been ongoing regarding combining radium-223 with other agents, including abiraterone, enzalutamide, docetaxel, olaparib, and immunotherapy [21, 22]. The ERA-223 trial was a large, double-blind, randomized, placebo-controlled phase III study in castrate-resistant metastatic prostate cancer patients with bone metastases, who were asymptomatic or mildly symptomatic and had not received prior chemotherapy that combined abiraterone and prednisone/prednisolone with radium-223 versus placebo [21]. This study was unblinded early due to interim findings of increased fractures and death [21]. It was determined that 28.6% of patients developed fractures in the radium-223 arm versus 11.4% in the placebo arm, and there was also an increase in the number of deaths on the radium-223 arm (38.5% versus 35.5%) [4]. These findings led to an updated warning in the package insert for radium-223, as well as warnings from the European Medicines Agency (EMA) and Health Canada [3, 4]. Therefore, concurrent use of abiraterone and prednisone with radium-223 is not currently recommended outside of a clinical trial.

Patients should have a baseline or updated nuclear medicine bone scan or sodium fluoride PET scan done prior to initiation of radium-223 to assess the state of the bony disease. Generally, patients with metastatic castrate-resistant prostate cancer, who have two or more bone metastases that are symptomatic, would be eligible for treatment with radium-223. Symptoms from bone disease could include pain or fracture. Patients with visceral disease, considered to be any evidence of cancer in the abdominal organs, lung, or brain, should not be considered for radium-223 therapy. In addition to blood work and side effect assessment, pain should be assessed at the start of therapy and monthly through the duration of therapy to assess for changes.

## New Directions and Conclusions

As discussed above, there are ongoing clinical trials assessing the use of radiopharmaceuticals in combination with other medications for metastatic prostate cancer, as well as investigations into radiopharmaceutical use in other cancers. There have also been new radiopharmaceuticals in development for the treatment of prostate cancer. Lutetium-177 PSMA radioligand is a medium-energy β-emitting radionuclide bound to a protein that binds with PSMA, which is a transmembrane glycoprotein highly expressed on prostate cancer cell membranes [22, 23]. PSMA has been found to be overexpressed in prostate cancer cells. Therefore, Lutetium-1777 PSMA radioligand targets both bone and soft tissue disease. It is also found in some other organ tissues, such as the small intestine and salivary glands, so there is the possibility of some radiation dose to these areas, as well [24]. The Lutetium-177 PSMA radioligand binds to PSMA on the cell surface and is taken into the cell where it emits radiation therapy causing DNA damage and cell death [23]. In early studies, Lutetium-177 PSMA has been found to decrease prostate-specific antigen levels, though measures such as overall survival have been limited to date due to the trials done [23]. The Lutetium-177 PSMA side effect profile so far has been favorable with some hematologic toxicities and mild nausea, fatigue, and xerostomia [23]. Thorium-227-labeled PSMA antibody is another alpha-emitting radionuclide that is beginning clinical trials and has shown promise in early preclinical studies [22].

Radiopharmaceuticals can play an important role in the treatment of bone metastases. Radium-223 is a treatment with category 1 evidence to support improvement in pain relief from prostate cancer with bone metastases and overall survival in men with bone metastases without known visceral involvement. The short active range of the alpha particles in radium-223 gives a higher dose of radiation to a more localized area than other radiopharmaceuticals, thereby decreasing the activity on normal tissue and myelosuppression. Radium-223 should not be used with combined chemotherapy or abiraterone and prednisone outside of clinical trials. Strontium-89 and samarium-153 have been shown to improve pain for bone metastases for patients who are not good candidates for traditional radiation therapy but have not shown any survival benefit. Because of the longer half-life of strontium-89, higher rates of myelosuppression are often seen in comparison to samarium-153. Myelosuppression with some of these agents may be prolonged, therefore inhibiting the ability to use chemotherapy options in the future. However, radiopharmaceuticals can be an effective means of treating pain related to bone metastases.

There are several considerations for the advanced practice provider (APP) related to radiopharmaceuticals in the treatment of bone metastases. While the APPs will not be involved in prescribing or administering these medications, often APPs are involved in the management of patients as they progress through treatment, as well as follow-up after treatment. Monitoring of labs prior to and after treatment is important in helping to identify patients who may not tolerate treatment or may be having adverse effects. APPs should be aware of the possible side effects of radiopharmaceuticals, as well as the precautions that patients should take immediately after administration. APPs can play an important role in patient education and reinforcement of teaching.

**Pearls for the Advanced Practice Provider**

- Only physicians and facilities with experience and licensing to handle and use these medications should administer radiopharmaceuticals.
- Strontium-89 and samarium-153 EDTMP have been shown to improve pain related to bone metastases in patients with metastatic cancer. Samarium-153 is generally the preferred of these two agents given its shorter half-life with better hematologic toxicity profile.
- Radium-223 has been shown to improve overall survival in patients with metastatic castrate-resistant prostate cancer to bone.
- Radium-223 should not be used with abiraterone and prednisone outside of clinical trial due to the increased risk for bone fracture and death. Use with other new-generation anti-androgen agents should likewise be limited to clinical trials.
- Blood counts should be monitored closely in patients receiving radiopharmaceuticals due to the risk for myelosuppression. The risk is highest with strontium-89.
- Advanced practice providers can play an important role in patient education regarding radiation safety after administration, possible side effects, and expectations around symptom management for patients undergoing treatment.

# References


1. Roodman GD. Mechanisms of bone metastasis [internet]. N Engl J Med. 2004;350:1655–64; [cited 9 Dec 2018]. Available from https://www.nejm.org/doi/full/10.1056/NEJMra030831.
2. Lewington VJ, McEwan AJ, Ackery DM, Bayly RJ, Keeling DH, Macleod PM, et al. A prospective, randomised double-blind crossover study to examine the efficacy of strontium-89 in pain palliation in patients with advanced prostate cancer metastatic to bone [internet]. Eur J Cancer Clin Oncol. 1991;27(8):954–8; [cited 7 Feb 2019]. Available from https://www.sciencedirect.com/science/article/pii/027753799190257E. https://doi.org/10.1016/0277-5379(91)90257-E.
3. European Medicines Agency. Xofigo [internet]. London: European Medicines Agency; 2018; [cited 7 Feb 2019]. Available from: https://www.ema.europa.eu/en/medicines/human/referrals/xofigo#all-documents-section.
4. Full prescribing information Xofigo (radium-223 dichloride) [internet]. Whippany: Bayer HealthCare Pharmaceuticals, Inc; c2013. Xofigo; [revised 2018 Aug; cited 10 Feb 2019]; [about 14 pages]. Available from: http://labeling.bayerhealthcare.com/html/products/pi/Xofigo_PI.pdf.
5. Metastron (strontium-89 chloride injection) [internet]. Arlington Heights: GE Healthcare; c2013. Metastron [revised 2013 Dec; cited 10 Feb 2019]; [about 7 pages]. Available from: https://www.accessdata.fda.gov/drugsatfda_docs/label/2013/020134s012lbl.pd.f
6. Quadramet (samarium sm-153 Lexidronam injection) [internet]. N. Billerica: Lantheus Medical Imaging, Inc; c2018. Quadramet; [revised 2018 Mar; cited 10 Feb 2019]; [about 2 pages]. Available from http://www.lantheus.com//assets/Quadramet-US-PI-513145-0318-mktg.pdf.
7. Lexicomp [internet]. Hudson: Wolters Kluwer; c2019. Samarium Sm-153 Lexidronam [updated 4 Dec 2018; cited 10 Feb 2019]; [about 9 pages]. Available from: http://online.lexi.com/lco/action/doc/retrieve/docid/patch_f/3509453?hl=480430.
8. Lexicomp [internet]. Hudson: Wolters Kluwer; c2019. Radium-223 [updated 24 Jan 2019; cited 10 Feb 2019]; [about 9 pages]. Available from: http://online.lexi.com/lco/action/doc/retrieve/docid/patch_f/4487822?hl=576710#.
9. Lexicomp [internet]. Hudson: Wolters Kluwer; c2019. Strontium-89 [updated 5 Jan 2019; cited 10 Feb 2019]; [about 8 pages]. Available from: http://online.lexi.com/lco/action/doc/retrieve/docid/patch_f/7705?hl=6990.
10. Parker C, Nilsson S, Heinrich D, Helle SI, O'Sullivan JM, et al. Alpha emitter Radium-223 and survival in metastatic prostate cancer [internet]. N Engl J Med. 2013;369:213–23; [cited 9 Dec 2018]. Available from https://www.nejm.org/doi/full/10.1056/NEJMoa1213755.
11. Tu SM, Millikan RE, Mengistu B, Delpassand ES, Amato RJ, Pagliaro LC, et al. Bone-targeted therapy for advanced androgen-independent carcinoma of the prostate: a randomised phase II trial [internet]. Lancet. 2001;357:336–41; [cited 7 Feb 2019]. Available from https://www.sciencedirect.com/science/article/pii/S0140673600036394?via%3Dihub. https://doi.org/10.1016/S0140-6736(00)03639-4.
12. Sartor O, Heinrich D, Mariados N, Mendez Vidal MJ, Keizman D, et al. Re-treatment with radium-223: first experience from an international, open-label, phase I/II study in patients with castration-resistant prostate cancer and bone metastases [internet]. Ann Oncol. 2017;28(10):2464–71; [cited 9 Dec 2018]. Available from https://academic.oup.com/annonc/article/28/10/2464/3978060.
13. Hoskin P, Sartor O, O'Sullivan JM, Johannessen DC, Helle SI, Logue J, et al. Efficacy and safety of radium-223 dichloride in patients with castration-resistant prostate cancer and symptomatic bone metastases, with or without previous docetaxel use: a prespecified subgroup analysis from the randomised, double-blind, phase 3 ALSYMPCA trial [internet]. Lancet Oncol. 2014;15(12):1397–406; [cited 15 Dec 2018]. Available from https://www.ncbi.nlm.nih.gov/pubmed/25439694. https://doi.org/10.1016/S1470-2045(14)70474-7.
14. Bruland O, Nilsson S, Fisher DR, Larson RH. High-linear transfer irradiation targeted to skeletal metastases by the α-emitter $^{223}$Ra: adjuvant or alternative to conventional modalities?

[internet]. Clin Cancer Res. 2006;12:6250s–7s; [cited 5 Jan 2019]. Available from http://clincancerres.aacrjournals.org/content/clincanres/12/20/6250s.full.pdf.
15. Das T, Pillai MRA. Options to meet future global demand of radionuclides for radionuclide therapy [internet]. Nucl Med Biol. 2013;40(1):23–32; [cited 5 Jan 2019]. Available from https://www.sciencedirect.com/science/article/pii/S0969805112002521.
16. Sartor O. Overview of samarium Sm 153 lexidronam in the treatment of painful metastatic bone disease [internet]. Rev Urol. 2004;6(Suppl 10):S3–S12; [cited 6 Jan 2019]. Available from https://www.ncbi.nlm.nih.gov/pmc/articles/PMC1472939/.
17. Serafini AN, Houston SJ, Resche I, Quick DP, Grund FM, et al. Palliation of pain associated with metastatic bone cancer using sarmarium-153 lexidronam: a double-blind placebo-controlled clinical trial [internet]. J Clin Oncol. 1998;16(4):1574–81; [cited 6 Jan 2019]. Available from http://ascopubs.org/doi/pdf/10.1200/JCO.1998.16.4.1574.
18. Sartor O, Reid RH, Hoskin PJ, Quick DP, Ell PJ, et al. Samarium-153-Lexidronam complex for treatment of painful bone metastases in hormone-refractory prostate cancer [internet]. Urology. 2004;63(5):940–5; [cited 6 Jan 2019]. Available from https://www.sciencedirect.com/science/article/pii/S0090429504001438?via%3Dihub.
19. Porter AT, McEwan AJB, Powe JE, Reid R, McGowan DG, Lukka H, et al. Results of a randomized phase-III trial to evaluate the efficacy of strontium-89 adjuvant to local field external beam irradiation in the management of endocrine resistant metastatic prostate cancer [internet]. Int J Radiat Oncol Biol Phys. 1993;25(5):805–13; [cited 30 Jan 2019]. Available from https://www.sciencedirect.com/science/article/pii/036030169390309J?via%3Dihub. https://doi.org/10.1016/0360-3016(93)90309-J.
20. James ND, Pirrie SJ, Pope AM, Barton D, Andronis L, Goranitis I, et al. Clinical outcomes and survival following treatment of metastatic castrate-refractory prostate cancer with docetaxel alone or with strontium-89, zoledronic acid, or both. The TRAPEZE randomized clinical trial [internet]. JAMA Oncol. 2016;2(4):493–9; [cited 30 Jan 2019]. Available from https://jamanetwork.com/journals/jamaoncology/fullarticle/2482917. https://doi.org/10.1001/jamaoncol.2015.5570.
21. van der Doelen MJ, Mehra N, Hemsen R, Janssen MJR, Gerritsen WR, van Oort IM. Patient selection for radium-223 therapy in patients with bone metastatic castration-resistant prostate cancer: new recommendations and future perspectives [internet]. Clin Genitourin Cancer. 17:79: Online 2018 November 22 [cited 7 Feb 2019]. Available from https://www.sciencedirect.com/science/article/pii/S1558767318307109#bib34. https://doi.org/10.1016/j.clgc.2018.11.008.
22. Nevedomskaya E, Baumgart SJ, Haendler B. Recent advances in prostate cancer treatment and drug discovery [internet]. Int J Mol Sci. 2018;19(5):1359; [cited 10 Feb 2019]. Available from https://www.ncbi.nlm.nih.gov/pmc/articles/PMC5983695/. https://doi.org/10.3390/ijms19051359.
23. Ferdinandus J, Violet J, Sandhu S, Hofman MS. Prostate-specific membrane antigen theranostics: therapy with lutetium-177 [internet]. Curr Opin Urol. 2018;28(2):197–204; [cited 10 Feb 2019]. Available from https://journals.lww.com/co-urology/fulltext/2018/03000/Prostate_specific_membrane_antigen_theranostics__.17.aspx. https://doi.org/10.1097/MOU.0000000000000486.
24. Emmett L, Willowson K, Violet J, Shin J, Blanksby A, Lee J. Lutetium $^{177}$ PSMA radionuclide therapy for men with prostate cancer: a review of the current literature and discussion of practical aspects of therapy [internet]. J Med Radiat Sci. 2017;64(1):52–60; [cited 10 Feb 2019]. Available from https://www.ncbi.nlm.nih.gov/pmc/articles/PMC5355374/. https://doi.org/10.1002/jmrs.227.

# Chapter 11
# Immunotherapy and Novel Agents on the Horizon for the Treatment of Prostate Cancer

**Suzanne Barron and Mark J. Mann**

## Therapeutic Vaccines

*Sipuleucel-T (Provenge™)* is an autologous cancer vaccine, approved by the FDA in April 2010 for patients with metastatic castrate-resistant prostate cancer (mCRPC). This is a patient-specific immunotherapy. It is designed to activate T cells in the body to attack prostate cancer cells. This process requires multiple steps which can take about 3 days. First, the patient's serum is obtained in a process called leukapheresis where the blood is filtered through a machine to collect white blood cells. Next, the white blood cells are activated in a laboratory by exposing them to specific protein antigens to orient them to attack prostate cancer cells. Finally, the activated cells are then transfused back into the patient [1].

Currently, Sipuleucel-T (Provenge™) is indicated in patients with mCRPC with little or no symptoms of prostate cancer such as bone pain. They should not have any evidence of metastatic disease to the liver. They should be relatively healthy with a life expectancy of greater than 6 months and have a good performance level. Studies have shown that patients who received the drug early in the course of their disease had a better survival benefit than those who received it later in the course of their disease [3]. The IMPACT (Immunotherapy for Prostate Adenocarcinoma Treatment) Trial 2010 showed a greater overall survival benefit was noted if Sipuleucel-T (Provenge™) was given in patients with a lower baseline PSA. It also revealed a 4.1-month survival benefit and a 22.5% reduction in risk of death [1].

The administration of Sipuleucel-T (Provenge™) can be timely and costly. Sipuleucel-T (Provenge™) treatments are given every 2 weeks for a total of three infusions. The cost is about $90,000 for three doses [12]. It is currently covered by Medicare for patients with asymptomatic or minimally symptomatic mCRPC. Vascular access is required prior to administration with either an 18-gauge peripheral intravenous

S. Barron (✉) · M. J. Mann
Thomas Jefferson University Hospital, Department of Urology, Philadelphia, PA, USA
e-mail: suzanne.barron@jefferson.edu; mark.mann@jefferson.edu



E. J. Trabulsi et al. (eds.), *Chemotherapy and Immunotherapy in Urologic Oncology*, https://doi.org/10.1007/978-3-030-52021-2_11

catheter or an alternative vascular access device such as an infusaport. Patients should be premedicated with acetaminophen and antihistamine 30 minutes prior to infusion. The drug is administered by intravenous infusion in about 250 mL of Lactated Ringer solution over 60 minutes. Once the PROVENGE™ infusion bag is removed from the insulated container, it should be given to the patient within 3 hours [4]. Most side effects occur during transfusion. Side effects include chills (53%), fatigue (41%), fevers (31%), back pain (34.3%), nausea (28.1%), and hypertension (7.4%) [2].

There are currently no markers to measure effectiveness of Sipuleucel-T (Provenge™). It does not affect or lower the PSA. Again, the benefit of Sipuleucel-T (Provenge™) is in patients early in the course of their disease with minimal symptoms [3].

*Prostvac-VF* is a vaccine that is currently undergoing clinical trials in men with asymptomatic mCRPC. Prostvac is a genetically engineered vaccine based upon the poxviral vaccine contained with a copy of the PSA (prostate-specific antigen) gene along with human T cell molecules. When administered, the vaccine stimulates an immune system response in which cells producing PSA are targeted. It has been well tolerated in clinical trials with the most common side effect being injection site irritation. Early clinical trials of Prostvac revealed an improvement in median survival rate but later studies not as promising. The future role of this vaccine may be as part of a more combined treatment approach [8].

## Immunomodulatory Drugs/Checkpoint Inhibitors

In mCRPC, the immune system has been disabled, thus not able to attack the invading cancer cells. Immune checkpoints are protein molecules made by the immune system that prevent destruction of cells which helps to control the immune response. Cancer cells are therefore saved and not attacked. Checkpoint inhibitors are targeted at blocking the immune system through immune checkpoint pathways such as CTLA-4 and PD-1 allowing T cells to kill cancer cells [10].

### *Treatments that Target CTLA-4 (Cytotoxic T-Lymphocyte-Associated Protein 4) Receptor*

CTLA-4 is a protein on some T cells that blocks the immune system from becoming overly aggressive.

Ipilimumab is a monoclonal antibody that targets CTLA-4. This medication was first used as a treatment for melanoma in 2011. Research studies have not been promising for prostate cancer, although there have been some rare reports of a few long-term responses [8].

Tremelimumab is a human IgG2 monoclonal antibody that targets CTLA-4. Phase I dose-escalation trial in PSA-recurrent prostate cancer demonstrated a prolongation in PSA doubling time in three of 11 patients several months after treatment with tremelimumab in combination with short-term androgen deprivation therapy [10].

## *Treatments that Target PD-1 (Programmed T-Cell Death 1) or PD-L1*

Medications in this category also target the immune response, but in a different pathway from CLA-4. PD-1 is a checkpoint protein on T cells. When attached to PD-L1, it prevents the immune system from attacking cancer cells. Certain cancer cells express a large amount of PD-L1, sparing them from being destroyed. PD-1 inhibitors and PD-L1 inhibitors are monoclonal antibodies that prevent this binding, allowing the immune system to work at killing cancer cells [5].

Nivolumab is a monoclonal antibody that blocks PD-L1 from binding on PD-1 (programmed T-cell death receptors) on activated T cells. This permits the immune system to attack cancer cells. Some responses were seen in other types of cancer, but no response was noted in prostate cancer. By combining treatments (nivolumab plus ipilimumab), there are small clinical trials that have found responses [8].

Pembrolizumab is an anti-PD-1 antibody. This immune checkpoint inhibitor has been used in combination therapy in early trials for mCRPC after progression of disease with enzalutamide alone. Results have shown some promise leading to the current KEYNOTE study ongoing at the time of this publication [8].

## *Adverse Effects of Immune Checkpoint Inhibitors*

Because these medications cause an increased immune response, they may lead to adverse autoimmune effects. Clinicians should monitor for diarrhea, colitis, rash, dermatitis, elevated liver function tests, adrenal insufficiency, hypophysitis, pancreatic dysfunction, thyroiditis, and pneumonitis. Severe adverse effects are treated by discontinuing the immune checkpoint inhibitor or by steroid induction. Steroid induction does not appear to affect the therapeutic effect of immune checkpoint inhibitors [6]. Because of the amount of side effects, it is important to determine which patients will respond to which type of treatment. Clinicians are now trying to check tumors for biomarkers such as PD-L1 markers. This will help to guide treatment to patients that will have a greater response.

### *Ongoing Studies of Immune Checkpoint Inhibitors*

There are multiple ongoing studies with these novel medications in combination with other treatments for prostate cancer. A phase II trial is under investigation combining ipilimumab, degarelix, and radical prostatectomy in men with mCRPC compared with ipilimumab and degarelix in men with biochemically recurrent hormone-sensitive prostate cancer after radical prostatectomy. A phase II trial examines the effect of ipilimumab with a GnRH agonist/antagonist on PSA levels. For patients that have mCRPC that have failed an androgen synthesis inhibitor and are inelegible for a taxane regimen, there is an ongoing phase III trial that is studying the effect of atezolizumab in combination with enzalutamide versus enzalutamide alone. The primary endpoint of the study is overall patient survival [8].

### *Administration of Immune Checkpoint Inhibitors*

These medications are given intravenously over 30–60 minutes. An infusaport or central venous access device is not needed. The number of treatments varies depending on the specific medication. Premedication is not usually required.

## PARP Inhibitors

PARP inhibitors aim treatment at the inhibition of PARP, poly(adenosine diphosphate ribose) polymerase, in patients with genetic mutations of DNA repair. PARP is a protein found in blood that helps damaged DNA cells repair themselves. DNA repair is necessary for cancer cells to live and thrive. By inhibiting PARP, cancer cells will not be able to repair themselves leading to cell death [11].

Prior to initiation with these medications, a tissue biopsy is needed in order to obtain genetic sequencing and information of the DNA makeup and changes of the cancer cell. This can be obtained from multiple core needle biopsies of metastatic prostate cancer tissue. A great deal of metastatic castrate-resistant prostate cancer spreads to the bone. However, bone tissue does not offer the best sample. Bone biopsies obtain tumor only 69% of time and may not be as successful at genetic sequencing offering 67% success rate compared to 80% success rate from non-bone metastatic sites [9]. A circulating cell-free DNA (via blood test) is currently under investigation as an option for identifying DNA repair mutations. However, a biopsy of tissue from a new metastatic site is the preferred approach [9].

At the time of this publication, PARP inhibitors are not currently on the market for treatment of prostate cancer. Ongoing clinical trials may lead to full FDA approval in the next few years. In clinical trials, PARP inhibitors are generally well tolerated. Common side effects include myelodysplastic syndrome, myelosuppression, anemia, nausea, nasopharyngitis, and fatigue. Less gastrointestinal side effects were noted if medication was taken with food.

The TOPARP trial investigated PARP inhibitors in mCRPC – a phase II clinical trial that studied olaparib tablets 400 mg twice daily. Patients were given this medication until progression of disease, unacceptable side effects, withdrawal of consent, or death. Of the 16 patients that had tumor aberrations in DNA-repair genes, 13 responded. In patients with BRCA2 loss, 100% showed response to therapy; in patients with truncated ATM, 80% patients showed response. Because of the excellent response in this study, in 2016, olaparib received FDA breakthrough designation for treatment in mCRPC patients with BRCA2, BRCA1, or ATM mutations who had received prior taxane and either enzalutamide or abiraterone. This was not full FDA approval but will lead to acceleration of clinical development [9].

Another study, currently under investigation, is the TRITON2 phase II study. The FDA granted breakthrough designation for rucaparib (Rubraca) for single-agent use in adult patients with BRCA 1/2-positive mCRPC following at least one androgen receptor-directed therapy and taxane-based chemotherapy [7].

More recently, the PROfound trial data published in the *New England Journal of Medicine* online ahead of print April 28, 2020, was a phase III trial of mCRPC men comparing olaparib to abiraterone or enzalutamide in men with BRCA 1/2 or ATM mutations that had progressed during treatment. Data analysis identified improved progression-free survival and overall survival [11].

## Combination Therapies

In the past decade, there have been many developments in the research and treatment of mCRPC. The greatest benefit of the newer agents may be seen in a more combined treatment plan. Multiple clinical trials are investigating using the combination of PARP inhibitors, Sipuleucel-T, immune checkpoint inhibitors, antiandrogens, and chemotherapy. This may provide synergistic effects in delaying the progression of metastatic castrate-resistant prostate cancer, thereby increasing the survival rate.

Research is also underway using combined treatment plans of these novel agents for the treatment of localized prostate cancer.

**Pearls for the Advanced Practice Provider**

- Patients receiving Sipuleucel-T (Provenge)™ should be premedicated prior to administration of treatment to help minimize side effects.
- Clinicians should monitor for new autoimmune-specific symptoms in patients that are undergoing treatment with immune checkpoint inhibitors. Steroids may be helpful in reducing side effects without altering treatment response.

- Tissue biopsy is still the standard for obtaining DNA to guide treatment. A biopsy of metastatic prostate cancer tissue is necessary prior to initiation of therapy with PARP inhibitors. This will help determine which patients will more likely respond to treatment.
- Patients on PARP inhibitors require frequent lab work (CBC) to monitor for myelosuppression.

## References

1. Kantoff PW, Higano CS, Shore ND, et al. Sipuleucel-T immunotherapy for castration-resistant prostate cancer. N Engl J Med. 2010;363:411–22.
2. Full prescribing information. Provenge package insert. Dendroen Pharmaceuticals LLC. 2017. http://www.provengehcp.com/Portals/5/Provenge-PI.pdf. Accessed 22 Jan 2019.
3. Presenters Gomella L, Delacruz A. Developing strategies for sequencing and combining therapies in advanced prostate cancer. Nursing considerations for implementing a tailored treatment approach. 2017. Sponsored by PleXus Communications [Power Point slides, Lecture Booklet]. Attended lecture 11 Jan 2017.
4. Provenge infusion checklist. Dendron Pharmaceuticals, LLC. 2014. https://www.provengehcp.com/Portals/5/PDF/Infusion_Checklist.pdf. Accessed 11 Jan 2019.
5. Patel A, Fong L. Immunotherapy for prostate cancer: where do we go from here?-Part 2: checkpoint inhibitors, immunotherapy combinations, tumor microenvironment modulation, and cell therapies. Oncology (Williston Park). 2018;32(6):65–73.
6. Goswami S, Aparicio A, Subudhi SK. Immune checkpoint therapies in prostate cancer. Cancer J. 2016;22(2):117–20.
7. Katz A. FDA grants rucaparib breakthrough designation for mCRPC. 2018. OncLive. https://www.onclive.com/web-exclusives/fda-grants-rucaparib-breakthrough-designation-for-mcrpc. Accessed 10 Feb 2019.
8. Nuhn P, De Bono JS, Fizazi K, Freedland SJ, Grilli M, Kantoff PW, Sonpavde G, Sternberg CN, Yegnasubramanian S, Antonarakis ES. Update on systemic prostate cancer therapies: management of metastatic castration-resistant prostate cancer in the era of precision oncology. Eur Urol. 2019;75:88–99.
9. Yentz S, Morgan T, Reichert Z. The potential role for PARP inhibitors in prostate cancer. Prostate Cancer Advisor, Renal and Urology News. 2018. August 10, 2018. https://www.renalandurologynews.com/home/news/urology/prostate-cancer/the-potential-role-for-parp-inhibitors-in-prostate-cancer/. Accessed 18 Feb 2019.
10. Modena A, Ciccarese C, Iacovelli R, Brunelli M, Montironi R, Fiorentino M, Tortara G, Massari F. Immune checkpoint inhibitors and prostate cancer: a new frontier? Oncol Rev. 2016;10(1):293. https://doi.org/10.4081/oncol.2016.293.
11. de Bono J, Mateo J, Fizazi K, et al. Olaparib for metastatic castration resistant prostate cancer. N Engl J Med. 2020;382;2091–102.
12. Anassi E, Ndefo U. Sipuleucel-T (Provenge) injection. The first immunotherapy agent (vaccine) for hormone-refractory prostate cancer. Pharm Ther. 2011;36(4):197–202.

# Part II
# Bladder Cancer

# Chapter 12
# Bladder Cancer: Overview, Epidemiology, Initial Presentation and Diagnosis

**Betsy M. Avinash, Jay D. Raman, and Matthew G. Kaag**

Bladder cancer, also known as urothelial carcinoma, is the most common malignancy of the genitourinary system. It is a highly aggressive and progressive disease with a high rate of incidence which is expensive to treat and can be lethal in nature. As the name suggests, urothelial carcinoma can occur anywhere along the urothelial lining, including the kidneys, ureters, bladder, and urethra. In this chapter, we mainly discuss urothelial carcinoma of the bladder. The lining of the bladder is mainly composed of transitional cells that can turn into various types of cells with the potential to become benign or malignant in nature. Urothelial carcinoma was previously known as "transitional cell carcinoma" as it primarily consists of transitional cells. This chapter will focus mainly on overview, epidemiology, initial presentation, and diagnosis of bladder cancer.

## Overview and Epidemiology of Bladder Cancer

Bladder cancer is the ninth most common cancer worldwide according to the Global Cancer Incidence Report [1]. In the United States, bladder cancer is the sixth most common cancer. According to the recent statistics from the American Cancer Society, there are about 81,190 new cases of bladder cancer (about 62,380 in men and 18,810 in women) and about 17,240 deaths from bladder cancer (about 12,520 in men and 4720 in women) each year [2]. With increasing awareness and early detection, the rates of new bladder cancer and cancer-related deaths have decreased slightly in recent years. Bladder cancer is considered the fourth most common

B. M. Avinash (✉) · J. D. Raman · M. G. Kaag
The Pennsylvania State University, College of Medicine, Department of Surgery,
Division of Urology, Hershey, PA, USA
e-mail: bavinash@pennstatehealth.psu.edu; jraman@pennstatehealth.psu.edu;
mkaag@pennstatehealth.psu.edu



E. J. Trabulsi et al. (eds.), *Chemotherapy and Immunotherapy in Urologic Oncology*, https://doi.org/10.1007/978-3-030-52021-2_12

cancer in men, and incidence rates have been decreasing and the rate of death has remained stable. Bladder cancer is comparatively less common in women [2].

The incidence and prevalence of urothelial carcinoma is seen to increase in the sixth decade of life and eventually peak between the seventh and eighth decade of life, as it is a cancer that is mainly affected by aging and environmental factors, including lifestyle [3]. Although in some areas the incidence of bladder cancer has risen in the last 60–70 years, in other geographical areas, the incidence has flattened off. The rise in incidence of bladder cancer is seen in underdeveloped countries, as there has been increased use of chemicals and pesticides with industrialization leading to increased exposure to environmental carcinogens [3]. When we look at the worldwide incidence rate of bladder cancer, it is highest in Egypt, Europe, and United States and lowest in Asian countries [4].

## Urothelial Carcinoma: Overview

The bladder wall is composed of three main histological layers. The innermost lining has urothelial or transitional cells called urothelium or transitional epithelium. Beneath the urothelium is the lamina propria containing connective tissue, blood vessels, and nerves. The next layer is the muscle layer of the bladder, also known as muscularis propria. The outer layer of the bladder is comprised of a fatty layer of connective tissue which separates the bladder from the other organs [5].

Transitional cell carcinoma is the most common type of urothelial carcinoma, and it occurs in the innermost layer of bladder and can occur anywhere along the site of the renal pelvis, ureters, bladder, and urethra [6]. Non-urothelial carcinoma is usually rare and more aggressive in nature and includes the squamous cell carcinoma (SCC) of the bladder, adenocarcinoma, clear cell carcinoma, and small cell cancer (neuroendocrine tumor of the bladder) [5, 6]. There are also rare non-epithelial carcinomas including sarcomas, carcinosarcomas, sarcomatoid cancers, paragangliomas, pheochromocytomas, primary bladder melanoma, and lymphomas [6]. The most common types of cancer that can metastasize into the bladder are lymphomas and melanomas [6].

## Staging

Staging of bladder cancer is important as it determines the modality of treatment after the biopsy of bladder or after transurethral resection of bladder tumor (TURBT). The most recent staging system has classified bladder cancer stages as Tcis, Ta, T1, T2a and T2b, T3, and T4. Table 12.1 gives a more definitive idea of how the tumors are staged (see Fig. 12.1).

The 2009 staging system is shown in Tables 12.1 and 12.2 [10]. Ta and CIS disease have no invasion of the basement membrane, but endophytic growth of

**Table 12.1** The TNM classification for bladder cancer [7]

| Stage (tumor) | Characteristics |
|---|---|
| Ta | Low grade and noninvasive papillary urothelial carcinoma |
| Tcis | Carcinoma in situ or flat tumor |
| T1 | Tumor invades subepithelial connective tissue |
| T2 | Tumor invades muscle<br>T2a – tumor invades superficial muscle (inner half)<br>T2b – tumor invades deep muscle (outer half) |
| T3 | Tumor invades perivesical tissue<br>T3a – invades perivesical tissue microscopically<br>T3b – invades perivesical tissue macroscopically (extravesical mass) |
| T4 | Tumor invades any of the adjacent organs: prostate, uterus, vagina, pelvic wall, and abdominal wall<br>T4a – tumor invades prostate or uterus or vagina<br>T4b – tumor invades pelvic wall or abdominal wall |
| Stage (node) | |
| N0 | No evidence of regional lymph node metastasis |
| N1 | Evidence of metastasis in a single lymph node ≤2 cm in greatest dimension |
| N2 | Evidence of metastasis in a single lymph node >2 cm but ≤5 cm in greatest dimension, or multiple lymph nodes, none >5 cm in greatest dimension |
| N3 | Evidence of metastasis in a lymph node >5 cm in greatest dimension |
| Stage (metastasis) | |
| M0 | No evidence of distant metastasis |
| M1 | Evidence of distant metastasis |

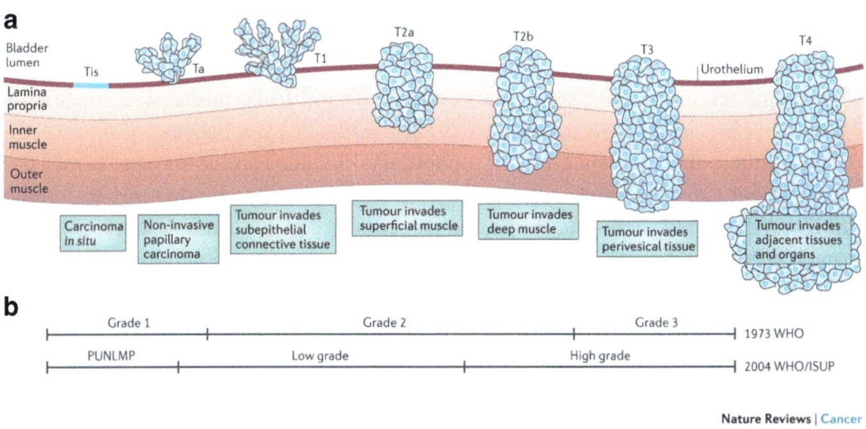


**Fig. 12.1** Staging and grading of bladder cancer. (**a**) Staging of bladder cancer; (**b**) Grading of bladder cancer. (Printed with permission from Knowles and Hurst [8])

low-grade tumors into the lamina propria is possible, and cancer can occur in von Brunn's nests [11, 12]. T1 disease, as mentioned earlier, can be divided into T1a and T1b disease [13]. The subdivision is based on the muscularis mucosa, which comprises thin wavy vesicles of muscle within the lamina propria that are associated with large vessels and lymphatics. The prognostic significance of T1a and T1b

**Table 12.2** The Jewett–Strong–Marshall classification for bladder tumors [9]

| Class | Characteristics |
|---|---|
| 0 | Preinvasive |
| A | Submucosal invasion |
| B1 | Superficial muscle |
| B2 | Deep muscle |
| C | Extravesical spread |
| D1 | Fixed to or invading prostate, uterus, vagina, or pelvic lymph nodes |
| D2 | Spread to extrapelvic lymph nodes or distant metastases |

disease is inconsistent because of the lack of muscularis mucosa in many bladder biopsy specimens. Essentially, the T1a and T1b stratifications suggest that the deeper the tumor invades the lamina propria, the worse the survival [5].

## Histologic Variants of Urothelial Carcinoma

In recent years, we have seen a rise in histologic variance of urothelial carcinomas, which are more aggressive and difficult to treat in comparison with traditional types. In this chapter, we briefly discuss the most common types of variant histology.

### *Micropapillary Urothelial Carcinoma*

Micropapillary urothelial carcinoma is usually found to be aggressive, since it is often found at a later stage, and due to its variant histology, it has poor prognosis. In recent studies, the incidence of micropapillary bladder carcinoma was 0.7%, the mean patient age at diagnosis was 69 years (range, 45–82), and the male-to-female ratio was 2.3:1 [14, 15]. Due to the advanced stage at the time of diagnosis, the overall survival rate of patients with micropapillary urothelial carcinoma at 5 and 10 years is 51% and 24%, respectively [13]. Due to the aggressive nature of this type of tumors, BCG is typically seen to be ineffective, and surgical resection with radical cystectomy is often warranted to provide the best chance of cure [15].

### *Nested Variant of Urothelial Carcinoma*

Nested variant is a rare but aggressive form of urothelial carcinoma which usually occurs as a benign lesion in the lamina propria, with a nested and tubular appearance [16]. Nested variant of urothelial carcinoma is usually similar in appearance to the hyperplastic von Brunn's nests, nephrogenic metaplasia, cystitis cystica, and inverted papilloma [5, 16]. The incidence of this cancer has a male to female ratio of 6:1 and has a 70% mortality within 3 years despite newer aggressive therapies [5].

### *Clear Cell Variant of Urothelial Carcinoma*

Clear cell variant is also a rare form of urothelial carcinoma and may be easily confused with the metastatic clear cell carcinoma of the kidney; however, it does not have a poor prognosis compared to the other variant histology. The clear cells contain glycogen-rich vacuoles and will have foci of clear cells within the tumor [5].

### *Glandular or Adenocarcinoma Differentiation*

Glandular differentiation is usually defined as the occurrence of two glandular spaces within the tumor and occurs in about 6% of urothelial cancer cases, but mixed tumor differentiation is most common with squamous cell cancer [17].

### *Plasmacytoid Tumor*

Plasmacytoid tumor is another variant of urothelial carcinoma that has been identified as a separate WHO classification since 2011 [5]. These tumors are usually diagnosed at an advanced stage, as the classical presentation of hematuria is delayed due to the presence of sessile and non-papillary tumor growth [18]. These tumors consist of plasmacytoid cells with the centric nuclei often invading through the bladder wall as well as the perivesical adipose tissue at the time of diagnosis, and hence, the average survival rate is about 27 months from the time of diagnosis. It has poor response to chemotherapy [19].

## Non-urothelial Malignancies

### *Squamous Cell Carcinoma*

The most common type of mixed differentiation is squamous cell carcinoma. Squamous cell carcinoma is usually seen in patients with chronic infection/irritation. Chronic infection with *Schistosoma haematobium* and other bacteria leads to squamous cell formation of the bladder [20]. The *Schistosoma* ova deposited in the wall of the bladder can cause chronic inflammation and cause inflammatory changes which then can turn into squamous cell epithelium. In patients with spinal cord injury, managing their bladder with either intermittent catheterization or chronic indwelling Foley can also cause chronic irritation to the bladder which can contribute to the development of squamous cell carcinoma of the bladder [21]. In the recent years, there has been less incidence of squamous cell carcinoma, most likely due to better catheter care [22].

### Sarcomas

Sarcomas consist of less than 1% of all bladder cancers and are the most common mesenchymal tumor of the bladder [5]. Sarcoma is subclassified based on the histologic variation, with leiomyosarcoma being the most common subtype, followed by rhabdomyosarcoma and then rarely angiosarcoma, osteosarcoma, and carcinosarcoma [23]. Grading of sarcoma is the primary prognostic factor and is incorporated into the staging system.

### Signet Ring Cell Carcinoma

Primary signet ring cell carcinoma of the bladder is very rare and constitutes less than 1% of all epithelial bladder neoplasms [24]. These can be urachal in origin and directly extend into the bladder. These tumors are generally high grade at presentation and have poor prognosis with radical cystectomy being the primary modality of treatment [5].

### Small Cell Carcinoma

Small cell carcinoma primarily occurs in the lungs but can occur in extrapulmonary sites such as bladder, prostate, and colon [25]. In patients with small cell carcinoma, these should be treated as metastatic disease even if there is no evidence of disease outside the bladder on imaging studies, and hence, the primary mode of treatment is chemotherapy followed by either radiation therapy or surgery with radical cystectomy [5].

## Risk Factors for Bladder Cancer Development

### Geographic Risk Factors

Various demographic areas have different risks factors for development of urothelial cancer. In Western countries and West Asia, smoking and occupational exposure to hazardous chemicals are considered major risk factors for the development of bladder cancer [26]. In Africa and other developing countries, almost 50% of the cancer is developed from chronic infections such as schistosomiasis. It is also noticed that in patients developing urothelial cancer as a result of schistosomiasis, the cancer is typically squamous cell carcinoma, whereas in patients who are smokers, urothelial cancer is primarily transitional cell carcinoma [26].

### *Environmental Risk Factors*

There are multiple environmental risk factors contributing to the development of bladder cancer. As discussed above, smoking is one of the major risk factors for the development of bladder cancer, and smokers are three times more susceptible to developing bladder cancer compared to nonsmokers [9, 27]. Secondhand smoke can also increase the risk of developing bladder cancer [9].

Workplace exposures also have an important role in the development of bladder cancer. Chemicals such as aromatic amines, including benzidine, 4-aminobiphenyl, beta-naphthylamine, and 4,4′- methylenebis(2-chloroaniline) used in the dye and rubber industries, are linked to the development of bladder cancer [28]. Another risk factor for development of bladder cancer is exposure to arsenic through drinking well water with concentrations greater than 300 μg/l [28]. Some of the other risk factors for bladder cancer include exposure to dyes, paint and paint products, and products used in leather making and textile work, and painters, machinists, printers, and hairdressers are exposed to these products. Truck drivers are also exposed due to diesel fumes, which are also a major risk factor [27].

## Medications/Chemicals Contributing to the Development of Bladder Cancer

Some medical therapies may also increase the risk of having urothelial cancer. Pioglitazone (Actos), an agonist of the peroxisome proliferator-activated receptor commonly used for treatment of type 2 diabetes mellitus, was thought to carry some risk for development of urothelial carcinoma [29]. Recent studies show that the risk of having bladder cancer is still being determined, and the most recent research shows that the outcome is usually dose and time dependent, and patients with long-term use (usually >2 years) and high dose exposure should be monitored more regularly for signs of bladder cancer [29]. Use of certain dietary pills, such as *Aristolochia fangchi*, a Chinese herb, is also considered a risk factor for development of bladder cancer [27].

Prior exposure to chemotherapy or radiation therapy can also increase the risk of developing urothelial carcinoma. Exposure to the chemotherapy drug cyclophosphamide (Cytoxan) for an increased amount of time can lead to bladder irritation, eventually increasing the risk of urothelial cancer ninefold [30]. In females who had treatment with radiation for cervical cancer and in males who had treatment with radiation for prostate cancer, any radiation exposure to pelvic region for cancer treatment is also seen to be a risk factor for development of urothelial cancer [30].

## Age, Gender, and Genetics as Risk Factors for Bladder Cancer

Risk factors that cannot be changed include age (>55), gender (more common in males than females), and chronic bladder irritations (including urinary tract infections, kidney and bladder stones, and indwelling Foley/suprapubic catheters), mainly causing development of squamous cell carcinoma of the bladder [27]. Other risk factors include personal history of bladder or urothelial carcinoma and bladder birth defects, especially urachus, a connection between the belly button and bladder; if this connection remains after birth, it can become cancerous [27]. Urachal carcinoma is a non-urothelial malignancy, which is almost always an adenocarcinoma that needs to be diagnosed accurately as the surgery and chemotherapy involved in this kind of carcinoma differ from those of the typical urothelial carcinoma [31]. Urinary bladder exstrophy is a rare congenital anomaly, and this can sometimes lead to adenocarcinoma requiring extensive abdominal reconstruction surgeries [32]. Genetics and family history also remain among the risk factors that cannot be changed. The family members may share a gene (like *GST* or *NAT*), which makes it harder for chemicals and toxins to be broken down, and family members may also be exposed to the same chemicals. In a very small number of people, mutation of the retinoblastoma gene and Lynch syndrome are linked to the development of urothelial carcinoma [27].

## Mortality

Recent studies have shown that the highest mortality rate is seen in Egypt due to the aggressive nature of the squamous cell carcinoma that is highly prevalent there. It is three times higher than in Europe, and eight times higher than in North America [33] (see Fig. 12.2). The global mortality rate among males is four per 100,000 versus 1.1 per 100,000 among females [34]. The mortality rate for urothelial cancer has decreased by 5% over the last decade mainly because of awareness, which helped with smoking cessation, changes in environmental carcinogens, and healthier lifestyles [5, 34]. The mortality rate for urothelial cancer has decreased by 5% during this period mainly because of awareness, which helped with smoking cessation, changes in environmental carcinogens, and healthier lifestyles [5]. Better access to treatments, better choice of chemotherapy for metastatic urothelial cancer patients, timely care, and advances in research have all led to an overall improvement in the survival rate [5].

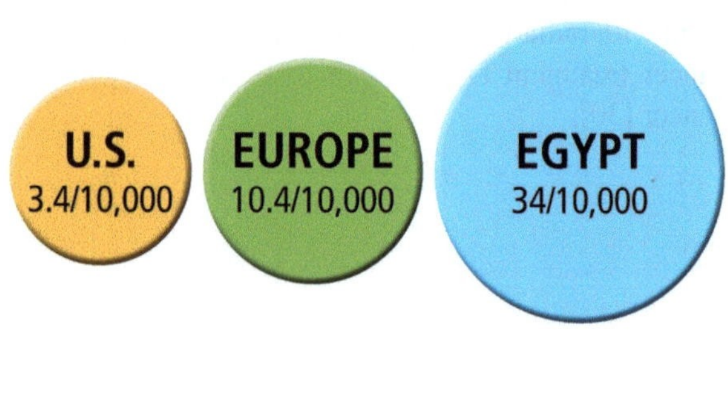


**Fig. 12.2** Comparison of estimated global mortality rates for bladder cancer

## Initial Presentation and Diagnosis

One of the key elements in diagnosing urothelial carcinoma is a complete urological evaluation with history and physical. This will help to identify various risk factors and assess signs and symptoms, which will aid in the diagnosis of urothelial carcinoma. It is notable that at diagnosis, majority of the patients (80%) present with non-muscle invasive disease, usually Ta or T1 papillary disease, which has a more favorable outcome for management than muscle invasive disease [35] (Table 12.3).

## Physical Exam

It is important to perform a complete head-to-toe physical exam. Assessing heart and lung sounds is essential for preoperative planning and also in cases where patients need to have anesthesia for diagnostic cystoscopy and to ensure there is no cardiopulmonary complication. An abdominal exam will help identify if there is any evidence of enlargement of the spleen or liver or the presence of any mass or tenderness/pain upon palpation. Females should have a pelvic exam to assess for masses or any abnormal finding of fullness. Males should have a rectal exam and a complete genitourinary exam to ensure there is no evidence of a mass extending into the prostate and to rule out rectal wall fullness, as well as direct inguinal palpation to rule out the presence of enlarged inguinal lymph nodes [6]. It is mainly when there is advanced bladder cancer disease that there is more prominent evidence of lymph nodes upon physical examination; otherwise, for early disease, physical exam is usually of low yield.

Recent studies support the use of ECOG (Eastern Cooperative Oncology Group) Performance Status Measure to assess how the disease affects one's quality of life and their activities of daily living, and it can help to determine provision of additional support and formulate appropriate treatment plan [37].

## Diagnostic Testing

### *Laboratory Data*

A complete evaluation with laboratory data will help in guiding the future steps in the management of urothelial carcinoma (Table 12.4). In patients with gross hematuria, no further microscopic analysis in necessary, but in patients with asymptomatic microscopic hematuria, a urinalysis should be performed to understand the total RBC count per HPF (>3 RBCs/HPF) to assess if it is considered a true microscopic hematuria [39]. A urine culture is an important test done to rule out the presence of a urinary tract infection [39]. Urine cytology is performed in patients with gross hematuria, but it is not routinely recommended to have urine cytology or tumor

**Table 12.3** Complete history for diagnosis of urothelial carcinoma [6]

| | |
|---|---|
| Medical history | A complete and thorough medical history is necessary for prescribing various medications, diagnostic testing, as well as treatment planning. It is also important to know of any previous history of radiation to the abdomen and pelvis [6] |
| Surgical history | It is important to be aware of any previous abdominal/pelvic surgery as it may change treatment planning as to whether the patient could have open or robotic/laparoscopic surgery [6] |
| Medication history | A complete medication history should be performed to evaluate for drug-to-drug interactions. Oftentimes, the patient may also be taking over-the-counter vitamins including fish oil, ibuprofen, and turmeric to name a few which have some anticoagulant properties that increase the risk of bleeding during the time of active disease process as well as during surgical intervention. It is also important know if the patient is anticoagulated/use of nicotine gum/ testosterone replacement or any recent use of antibiotics |
| Allergies | It is important to know if they have any allergies to contrast dye which is used to obtain a CT urogram to aid in the diagnosis of any filling defects which could be bladder tumor |
| Social history | A thorough social history will help us in determining tobacco use/alcohol use and illicit drug use. It is also important to assess the baseline sexual function, and for a lot of patients, it is important to counsel them about erectile dysfunction if they would require a cystoprostatectomy as a treatment for bladder cancer. It is also important to know if they have a good support system |
| Family history | It is also important to assess if there is any family history of bladder cancer or any other type of cancers as family members can possess the same genes which can increase the risk of having bladder cancer |
| Clinical presentation | Collecting a good history of their initial presentation is important. This include the onset, duration, frequency, severity, and other treatments or therapies used whether it be acute or chronic<br>Common signs and symptoms include:<br>Gross hematuria (usually painless) seen in 85% of population with a new diagnosis of bladder cancer<br>Presence of blood clots<br>Microscopic hematuria (>3 RBCs/HPF)<br>Lower urinary tract symptoms: urinary urgency, frequency, dysuria, nocturia, incomplete bladder emptying, and bladder pain<br>Urinary incontinence, abnormal urethral discharge<br>Recurrent UTI |
| Risk factors | Risk factors for malignancy in patients with hematuria [36]:<br>Older age<br>Male gender<br>History of cigarette smoking<br>History of chemical exposure (cyclophosphamide, benzenes, aromatic amines)<br>History of pelvic radiation<br>Irritative voiding symptoms (urgency, frequency, dysuria)<br>Prior urologic disease or treatment<br>History of chronic indwelling catheters<br>History of recurrent UTIs |

**Table 12.4** Evaluation of laboratory data [6]

| | |
|---|---|
| Comprehensive metabolic panel (CMP) | CMP will help in assessing any electrolyte imbalance, abnormal liver function and more importantly renal function. It is important to evaluate the renal function including BUN, creatinine, and GFR to determine if the patient can get a contrast-based CT scan or not |
| Complete blood count (CBC) | This will help evaluate if the blood count is within normal limits: decreased hemoglobin may indicate loss of blood, and elevated white count will indicate an infection that needs to be further worked up |
| PT/INR | This will help in evaluating for any bleeding disorders; especially if they are on any anticoagulation |
| Urinalysis | Urinalysis with a complete basic and microscopic evaluation should be done to detect the presence of bacteria and to determine if it is a true microscopic hematuria (>3 RBCs/HPF) |
| Urine culture and sensitivity | It is essential to send the urine for culture and sensitivity especially with the presence of gross hematuria or any other urinary symptoms to r/o an infection which can mimic bladder cancer symptoms and can be treated with antibiotics appropriately |
| Urine cytology | The voided urine sample is submitted to assess the presence of abnormal cells. The results can be negative or positive for malignant urothelial cells or atypical cells. Further tests need to be done based on the risk factors and urinary symptoms. Cytology is usually a good tool in detecting high-grade urothelial cancers and carcinoma in situ (CIS) |
| FISH (UroVysion Fluorescence In Situ Hybridization) | FISH test is a genetic test to detect the presence and for surveillance of bladder cancer cells done via urine test. This method helps in determining genetic alteration of urothelial cells found in the urine, using fluorescent DNA probes binding to the regions of chromosomes 3, 7, and 17 as well as on the 9p21 [38] |

markers done for patients with asymptomatic microscopic hematuria, but it could certainly be considered in patients with increased/high risk factors [36]. Other laboratory tests are performed for initial workup per Table 12.3 usually based on provider preference.

## *Diagnosis*

It is very important to diagnose urothelial cancer early, as delayed diagnosis can lead to adverse outcomes. Hence, it is important for clinicians to perform a thorough history and physical and basic tests to identify bladder cancer. One of the key presentations for bladder cancer is usually visible blood in the urine or gross hematuria and asymptomatic microhematuria, seen in urinalysis [39]. According to the AUA guidelines, patients presenting with gross hematuria or asymptomatic microscopic hematuria, who have high risk factors (see Table 12.3), should undergo complete urological evaluation [36]. Even though the risk of malignancy is low in patients with asymptomatic hematuria, or even if they have low risk factors, it is warranted that they have complete urological workup [36]. It is critical to pay attention to cues such as accompanying symptoms (see Table 12.3 for clinical presentation) as they may mimic the presence of urinary tract infection (UTI), pyelonephritis, or urinary stones (including kidney, ureteral, or bladder stones) [6]. By the time patients come to see the urologist, they may have had multiple courses of antibiotic without the evidence of true infection. Apart from painless gross hematuria, recurrent UTI with or without hematuria may also mimic bladder cancer.

## *Diagnostic Studies*

Computed tomography (CT) urogram should always be considered as the first choice of imaging in patients with hematuria [6], but with other urinary symptoms, sometimes, clinicians may start with a renal ultrasound (US) or a non-contrast CT to rule out urolithiasis or any other obstructive causes. A multi-detector row CT urogram (CTU) has become the choice of imaging for urinary tract abnormalities, since it is a single exam in its entirety that can be used to evaluate the kidneys, collecting systems, and ureters [40]. CTU is more expensive than an ultrasound but in the long run would save the patients from having to undergo multiple imaging modalities, so it can result in the overall reduction of health-care costs [40].

The non-contrast phase of the imaging study will show if there is any presence of hydronephrosis, which is usually due to the obstruction of urine flow from the kidneys through the ureter and bladder, any renal masses or urothelial lesions, or any obvious bladder masses. The presence of IV contrast during the 100-s phase and the 10-minute delayed phase will help in identifying the presence of any filling defects in the kidney (upper tract urothelial lesions), ureter, or bladder. An ultrasound or intravenous urography on its own is very likely to miss upper tract tumors [30]. CT urogram will also help in identifying any other tumors within the abdomen and pelvis and will show the presence of lymphadenopathy, which mostly may indicate metastatic disease [6] (see Fig. 12.3).

If the patient is unable to undergo CTU due to impaired renal function or due to dye allergies, a non-contrast CT or magnetic resonance (MR) urography or renal US can also be performed as a part of initial evaluation [36].

## *Cystoscopic Evaluation: Final Step for Hematuria Workup*

Cystoscopy is the gold standardized workup for detecting bladder cancer. AUA guidelines recommend that a complete cystoscopic evaluation needs to be done in all patients with gross hematuria and patients with asymptomatic microhematuria,

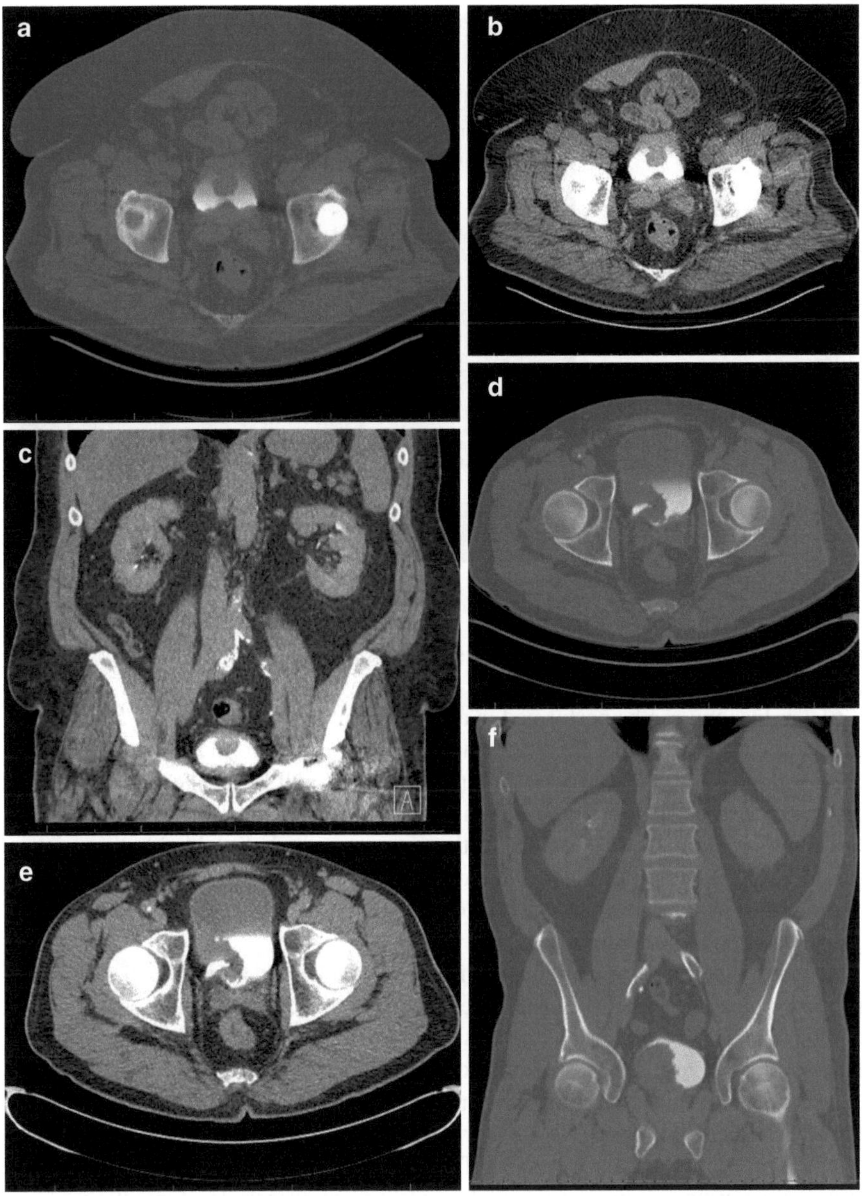


**Fig. 12.3** Filling defect suspicious for bladder cancer seen in the 10-minute delayed imaging of CT urogram. (**a**) 3–4 cm filling defect in the bladder in the 10 minute delayed phase on CT scan in the bone window in the axial phase; (**b**) 3–4 cm filling defect in the bladder in the 10 minute delayed phase on CT scan in the adominal window in the axial phase; (**c**) 3–4 cm filling defect in the bladder in the 10 minute delayed phase on CT scan in the adominal window in the coronal phase; (**d**) Large filling defect in the right bladder wall on the 10 minute delayed phase on CT scan in the bone window in the axial phase; (**e**) Large filling defect in the right bladder wall on the 10 minute delayed phase on CT scan in the abdominal window in the axial phase; (**f**) Large filling defect in the right bladder wall on the 10 minute delayed phase on CT scan in the bone window in the coronal phase

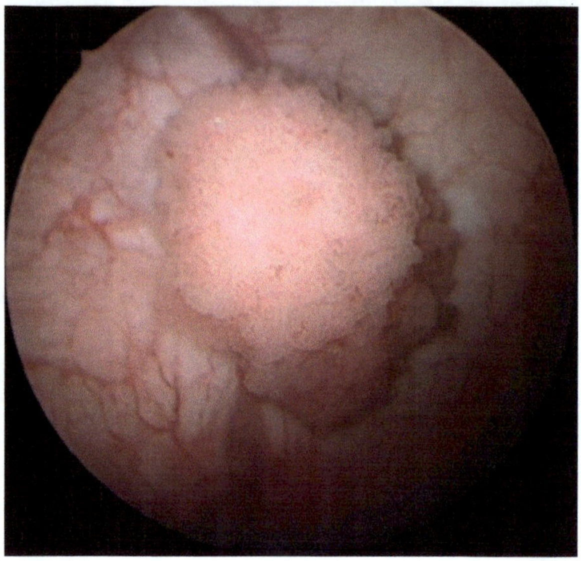

**Fig. 12.4** Cystoscopic surveillance showing evidence of tumor

especially in patients >35 years of age [36]. In patients presenting with asymptomatic microscopic hematuria with low risk factors and under 35 years of age, it is the provider's discretions on whether they should have a complete urologic evaluation [36]. Cystoscopy can be performed in a clinic under local anesthesia or at an outpatient surgical center under local anesthesia or light sedation. In most cases, cystoscopy is done under local anesthesia, and the patient will be awake during the time of the procedure. Cystoscopy will aid in detecting suspicious lesions and small and large tumors that will then require further treatment, including bladder biopsies or transurethral resection of bladder tumor (TURBT) [6] (see Fig. 12.4). These samples are then sent for further analysis to get an accurate tissue diagnosis, histology, grade, and depth of invasion [6].

It may sometimes be difficult to visualize the bladder in cases where there is increased bleeding or debris, or if there are flat urothelial lesions such as carcinoma in situ, which may sometimes be mistaken for inflammatory changes and which makes it harder to distinguish from normal bladder tissue [6]. Patients may often experience some urinary symptoms including gross hematuria, passing of clots, urinary frequency, urgency, and dysuria for a short period (usually for 2–3 days) after the procedure in most cases [6]. If urinary symptoms last longer, further evaluation with a urine culture is warranted to rule out any urinary tract infection.

After a complete workup, if patients have no evidence of malignancy, a yearly urinalysis should be done unless there is persistent gross hematuria. Patients with two negative urinalysis after 2 years do not need to be checked any further, but patients with continued asymptomatic microscopic hematuria should have a repeat urologic evaluation in 3–5 years especially if they have high risk factors [36].

**Clinical Pearls for the Advanced Practice Provider**

- Bladder cancer, also known as urothelial carcinoma, can occur anywhere along the urothelial lining, including the kidneys, ureters, bladder, and urethra.
- Bladder cancer is the ninth most common cancer worldwide and sixth most common cancer in the United States.
- Transitional cell carcinoma is the most common type of urothelial carcinoma.
- Histologic variants of bladder cancer are harder and aggressive to treat.
- Squamous cell carcinoma is the most common type of non-urothelial carcinoma.
- Smoking is one of the major risk factors for the development of bladder cancer, and smokers are three times more susceptible to developing bladder cancer compared to nonsmokers.
- Mortality rate for urothelial carcinoma has decreased due increasing awareness that led to smoking cessation, changes in environmental carcinogens, healthier lifestyles, better access to treatments, and better choice of chemotherapy for metastatic urothelial cancer patients to name a few.
- A complete urological evaluation with complete history and physical and laboratory tests including microscopic analysis, urine culture, and cytology is warranted for workup for urothelial carcinoma.
- Complete workup involves CT urogram and cystoscopy as the final steps of evaluation.
- Gross hematuria and asymptomatic hematuria are one of the key elements of clinical presentation, as well as other irritative urinary symptoms.
- Early detection of bladder cancer is the key to have a favorable prognosis and to prevent metastasis.

# References


1. Antoni S, Ferlay J, Soerjomataram I, Znaor A, Jemal A, Bray F. Bladder cancer incidence and mortality: a global overview and recent trends. Eur Urol. 2017;71(1):96–108.
2. American Cancer Society. Cancer facts and figures 2018. Atlanta: American Cancer Society; 2018. Available from: https://www.cancer.org/research/cancer-facts-statistics/all-cancer-facts-figures/cancer-facts-figures-2018.html.
3. Parkin DM. The global burden of urinary bladder cancer. Scand J Urol Nephrol Suppl. 2008;218:12–20.
4. Malats N, Real FX. Epidemiology of bladder cancer. Hematol Oncol Clin North Am. 2015;29(2):177–89, vii
5. Wein AJ, Kavoussi LR, Partin AW, Peters CA. Tumors of the bladder. In: McDougal WS, Wein AJ, Kavoussi LR, Partin AW, Peters CA, editors. Campbell-Walsh urology. 11th ed. Philadelphia: Elsevier; 2015.
6. Lajiness M, Quallich S. The nurse practitioner in urology. New York: Springer; 2016.

7. Tang H, Shi W, Fu S, Wang TW, Zhai S, Song Y, et al. Pioglitazone and bladder cancer risk: a systematic review and meta-analysis. Cancer Med. 2018;7(4):1070–80.
8. Knowles MA, Hurst CD. Molecular biology of bladder cancer: new insights into pathogenesis and clinical diversity. Nat Rev Cancer. 2015;15:25–41.
9. Freedman ND, Silverman DT, Hollenbeck AR, Schatzkin A, Abnet CC. Association between smoking and risk of bladder cancer among men and women. JAMA. 2011;306(7):737–45.
10. Edge SB, Compton CC. The American Joint Committee on Cancer: the 7th edition of the AJCC cancer staging manual and the future of TNM. Ann Surg Oncol. 2010;17(6):1471–4.
11. Jones TD, Zhang S, Lopez-Beltran A, Eble JN, Sung MT, MacLennan GT, et al. Urothelial carcinoma with an inverted growth pattern can be distinguished from inverted papilloma by fluorescence in situ hybridization, immunohistochemistry, and morphologic analysis. Am J Surg Pathol. 2007;31(12):1861–7.
12. Picozzi S, Casellato S, Bozzini G, Ratti D, Macchi A, Rubino B, et al. Inverted papilloma of the bladder: a review and an analysis of the recent literature of 365 patients. Urol Oncol. 2013;31(8):1584–90.
13. Smits G, Schaafsma E, Kiemeney L, Caris C, Debruyne F, Witjes JA. Microstaging of pT1 transitional cell carcinoma of the bladder: identification of subgroups with distinct risks of progression. Urology. 1998;52(6):1009–13; discussion 13-4
14. Klaile Y, Schlack K, Boegemann M, Steinestel J, Schrader AJ, Krabbe LM. Variant histology in bladder cancer: how it should change the management in non-muscle invasive and muscle invasive disease? Transl Androl Urol. 2016;5(5):692–701.
15. Johansson SL, Borghede G, Holmang S. Micropapillary bladder carcinoma: a clinicopathological study of 20 cases. J Urol. 1999;161(6):1798–802.
16. Terada T. Nested variant of urothelial carcinoma of the urinary bladder. Rare Tumors. 2011;3(4):e42.
17. Lopez-Beltran A, Cheng L. Histologic variants of urothelial carcinoma: differential diagnosis and clinical implications. Hum Pathol. 2006;37(11):1371–88.
18. Wang Z, Lu T, Du L, Hu Z, Zhuang Q, Li Y, et al. Plasmacytoid urothelial carcinoma of the urinary bladder: a clinical pathological study and literature review. Int J Clin Exp Pathol. 2012;5(6):601–8.
19. Keck B, Wach S, Stoehr R, Kunath F, Bertz S, Lehmann J, et al. Plasmacytoid variant of bladder cancer defines patients with poor prognosis if treated with cystectomy and adjuvant cisplatin-based chemotherapy. BMC Cancer. 2013;13:71.
20. Abol-Enein H. Infection: is it a cause of bladder cancer? Scand J Urol Nephrol Suppl. 2008;218:79–84.
21. Kaufman JM, Fam B, Jacobs SC, Gabilondo F, Yalla S, Kane JP, et al. Bladder cancer and squamous metaplasia in spinal cord injury patients. J Urol. 1977;118(6):967–71.
22. Bickel A, Culkin DJ, Wheeler JS Jr. Bladder cancer in spinal cord injury patients. J Urol. 1991;146(5):1240–2.
23. Spiess PE, Kassouf W, Steinberg JR, Tuziak T, Hernandez M, Tibbs RF, et al. Review of the M.D. Anderson experience in the treatment of bladder sarcoma. Urol Oncol. 2007;25(1):38–45.
24. Morelli O, Castellani D, Asciutti S, Baldoni M, Familiari L, Nardi E, et al. Colon and gastric metastases from a primary signet-ring cell carcinoma of the urinary bladder. Dig Liver Dis. 2006;38(8):609–11.
25. Thota S, Kistangari G, Daw H, Spiro T. A clinical review of small-cell carcinoma of the urinary bladder. Clin Genitourin Cancer. 2013;11(2):73–7.
26. Jemal A, Bray F, Center MM, Ferlay J, Ward E, Forman D. Global cancer statistics. CA Cancer J Clin. 2011;61(2):69–90.
27. American Cancer Society. Bladder cancer risk factors. Atlanta: American Cancer Society; 2016. Available from: https://www.cancer.org/cancer/bladder-cancer/causes-risks-prevention/risk-factors.html.
28. Letasiova S, Medve'ova A, Sovcikova A, Dusinska M, Volkovova K, Mosoiu C, et al. Bladder cancer, a review of the environmental risk factors. Environ Health. 2012;11 Suppl 1:S11.

29. Riesz P, Lotz G, Paska C, Szendroi A, Majoros A, Nemeth Z, et al. Detection of bladder cancer from the urine using fluorescence in situ hybridization technique. Pathol Oncol Res. 2007;13(3):187–94.
30. MacVicar AD. Bladder cancer staging. BJU Int. 2000;86(Suppl 1):111–22.
31. Nargund VH, Raghavan D, Sandler HM. Urological oncology. London: Springer-Verlag; 2015.
32. Siefker-Radtke A. Urachal adenocarcinoma: a clinician's guide for treatment. Semin Oncol. 2012;39(5):619–24.
33. Bhat S, Sathyanarayanaprasad M, Paul F. Primary squamous cell carcinoma of bladder exstrophy in an adult. Indian J Urol. 2015;31(2):142–3.
34. Parekh DJ, Jung C, O'Conner J, Dutta S, Smith ER Jr. Leiomyosarcoma in urinary bladder after cyclophosphamide therapy for retinoblastoma and review of bladder sarcomas. Urology. 2002;60(1):164.
35. Ploeg M, Aben KK, Kiemeney LA. The present and future burden of urinary bladder cancer in the world. World J Urol. 2009;27(3):289–93.
36. American Cancer Society. Early detection, diagnosis, and staging: bladder cancer signs and symptoms. Atlanta: American Cancer Society; 2019. Available from: https://www.cancer.org/cancer/bladder-cancer/detection-diagnosis-staging/signs-and-symptoms.html.
37. Goodison S, Rosser CJ, Urquidi V. Bladder cancer detection and monitoring: assessment of urine- and blood-based marker tests. Mol Diagn Ther. 2013;17(2):71–84.
38. Cha K, Hadjiiski L, Chan HP, Cohan RH, Caoili EM, Zhou C. Detection of urinary bladder mass in CT urography with SPAN. Med Phys. 2015;42(7):4271–84.
39. Oken MM, Creech RH, Tormey DC, Horton J, Davis TE, McFadden ET, et al. Toxicity and response criteria of the Eastern Cooperative Oncology Group. Am J Clin Oncol. 1982;5(6):649–55.
40. American Cancer Society. Medical student curriculum: hematuria. Linthicum: American Urological Association; 2016. Available from: https://www.auanet.org/education/auauniversity/for-medical-students/medical-student-curriculum/hematuria.

# Chapter 13
# Intravesical Therapy for Non-muscle Invasive Urothelial Carcinoma

**Waleed Hassen and Laura Motherway**

## Introduction

The majority of bladder cancer cases present as noninvasive disease [1]. Lower-grade disease tends to have a higher risk of recurrence, while higher-grade disease also carries the risk of disease progression (recurrence at a higher stage) [2]. The goal of intravesical therapy is to reduce the risks of recurrence and/or progression depending on the initial presenting pathological features.

Intravesical therapy is the administration of a medication directly into the bladder via the urethra through a urinary catheter. The goal of intravesical therapy is to maximize the exposure of malignant cells located within the bladder to therapeutic drugs while limiting a systemic response. The urothelium of the bladder is uniquely suited to limit a systemic response by minimizing absorption of the administered agent [3].

Intravesical agents are categorized into chemotherapeutic drugs and immunomodulators. These medications have different mechanisms of actions and side effects. The purpose of this chapter will be to outline the various available therapeutic options as well as their indications and methods of administration.

W. Hassen (✉)
Department of Urology, Cleveland Clinic Abu Dhabi, Abu Dhabi, UAE

Cleveland Clinic Lerner College of Medicine, Cleveland, OH, USA
e-mail: hassenw@ClevelandClinicAbuDhabi.ae

L. Motherway
Department of Urology, Cleveland Clinic Abu Dhabi, Abu Dhabi, UAE



E. J. Trabulsi et al. (eds.), *Chemotherapy and Immunotherapy in Urologic Oncology*, https://doi.org/10.1007/978-3-030-52021-2_13

## Intravesical Chemotherapy

Intravesical chemotherapy is the installation of chemotherapeutic agents that inhibit or slow cancer cell production [4].

### *Mitomycin*

Mitomycin C (MMC) is the most common chemotherapeutic agent used to treat non-muscle invasive bladder cancer (NMIBC) [5, 6]. It is an antibiotic that inhibits DNA synthesis and can be used in the perioperative setting to prevent tumor implantation or for induction and maintenance therapy [7, 8]. The typical dose of MMC is 40 mg in either 20 or 40 ml of saline. Side effects include cystitis and rarely bladder contraction (5%). Rash and desquamation may also occur if the drug comes in contact with skin. Increasing the concentration of MMC (40 mg/20 ml) [9] as well as urinary alkalinization has been shown to improve efficacy. Electromotive therapy has also been shown to improve the efficacy of MMC in some studies [10, 11].

### *Gemcitabine*

Gemcitabine is a deoxycytidine analogue that inhibits DNA synthesis [12]. It has been recently shown to be useful in the perioperative setting. The typical dosage is 2 gm/100 ml of normal saline [13]. Side effects are uncommon and include dysuria and hematuria.

### *Doxorubicin*

Doxorubicin is an antibiotic that inhibits protein synthesis by binding DNA pairs. It has been shown to reduce recurrences in the perioperative setting. The typical dose is 50 mg/50 ml of normal saline. Side effects include cystitis, fever, and rarely bladder contraction [14].

### *Epirubicin*

Epirubicin is an anthracycline chemotherapeutic agent and a derivative of doxorubicin that exerts its antineoplastic effect by intercalating DNA strands, thereby inhibiting replication and RNA synthesis. The typical dose is 50 mg/50 ml of normal saline. Side effects are similar to doxorubicin. It is also typically used in the perioperative setting but is not available in the United States [15].

## *Thiotepa*

Thiotepa was one of the first agents used for intravesical chemotherapy. It is an alkylating agent that acts to cross-link nucleic acids. The typical dose is 30 mg/30 ml of normal saline. Due to its low molecular weight, however, a significant amount of the drug can be systemically absorbed which may cause myelosuppression in up to 30% of patients [14]. It is because of this that thiotepa is not commonly used in most institutions.

## *Valrubicin*

Valrubicin is a semisynthetic analogue of doxorubicin and is the only therapy approved by the FDA for bacillus Calmette-Guerin (BCG) refractory carcinoma in situ (CIS) [12]. The dosage is 800 mg/75 ml of normal saline. Common side effects include cystitis and urinary frequency. Long-term disease-free survival rate remains poor, and it only has an 8% complete response rate at 30-month follow-up [16]. Its use therefore is rather limited.

## *Immunotherapy*

Intravesical immunotherapy is the installation of agents that work by triggering the body's immune response to destroy malignant cells that may be present in the bladder after a transurethral resection [17].

## *BCG*

Bacillus Calmette-Guerin (BCG) is a live strain of *Mycobacterium bovis* that was first used as a tuberculosis vaccine and later found to induce an immune response within the bladder [18]. BCG leads to the release of numerous cytokines that induces a Th1 immune response. BCG is supplied in various strains and is typically given as a vial diluted in 50 ml of normal saline. As it is a live attenuated bacterium, side effects can be more severe than intravesical chemotherapy and may include fever, irritative voiding symptoms, BCG sepsis, and rarely death [19].

Due to risks of systemic absorption, it is usually not given until 2–4 weeks after surgical resection to allow for bladder re-epithelialization. BCG should not be given in patients with a traumatic catheterization or hematuria. Caution should be used in immunosuppressed patients or patients with an active urinary tract infection (UTI) [20]. BCG has been shown to reduce the incidence of recurrence and progression of disease. BCG is typically given as an induction course of 6 weekly doses followed by a maintenance schedule. While maintenance schedules vary, the most effective schedule reported consists of a 6-week induction course followed by 3 weekly doses at 3, 6, 12, 18, 24, 30, and 36 months [21].

### *Interferon*

Interferon is an immunotherapeutic agent that can be used as an individual therapy or in combination with BCG. The mechanism of action is lymphocyte activation and potentiates a T-helper type I immune response [22]. Although it does have some efficacy as a single agent in BCG failure, it has most thoroughly been evaluated in combination with BCG [12, 23].

## Clinical Uses of Intravesical Therapy

### *Perioperative Intravesical Therapy*

Tumor seeding at the time of transurethral resection of bladder tumor (TURBT) is postulated to be one of the causes of recurrence [24]. Intravesical chemotherapy immediately after TURBT (within 24 hours) reduces tumor recurrence by 11% in patients with low-risk disease [25]. MMC is commonly used in the United States, while epirubicin is used in Europe. Gemcitabine, however, has recently been shown to decrease recurrences by 47% and is currently the preferred drug of choice per NCCN guidelines [6, 13]. Either medication is instilled for 1 hour into the bladder after resection or ideally within 6 hours [26]. Instillation should be avoided in cases of bladder perforation at the time of resection due to the increased risk of toxicity.

### *Reducing Recurrence and Progression*

Induction courses of 6 weekly doses of chemotherapy (MMC, doxorubicin, and epirubicin) have been shown to reduce the risk of recurrence in NMIBC by approximately 20–40% but have no appreciable effect on preventing disease progression [27]. They are typically used in low- to intermediate-risk disease and not recommended for use in high-risk disease unless there is a contraindication to BCG therapy. The value of maintenance therapy with chemotherapy is controversial. If given, the maintenance schedule typically involves monthly doses for 1 year [6].

Induction courses of BCG reduce recurrences by 20–60%; however, the main clinical utility of BCG is to reduce the impact of disease progression [28]. The impact of reduced progression is only seen with maintenance protocols. BCG has been reported to reduce rates of progression by approximately 20–30% [29]. About 25% of patients who fail an initial induction course may be salvaged by a second 6-week induction course; however, further courses are not recommended as there is a much higher chance of disease progression (up to 50%). Those patients should proceed to cystectomy or other salvage therapy [19].

## *Refractory Disease*

In general, patients with high-grade disease who fail intravesical therapy should proceed to cystectomy; however, salvage intravesical regimens may be attempted for patients who are not surgical candidates. Valrubicin is the only FDA-approved agent for BCG refractory disease. The complete response and disease-free survival rates are poor however (18% and 4%). Therefore, valrubicin is not commonly used [30].

Combination treatment with gemcitabine and docetaxel has been shown to have 49–54% complete response rate (CRR) after 1 year and 34% complete response rate after 2 years [31, 32]. Other therapies which have been shown to be safe and have achieved a complete response rate between 28% and 71% at 1 year include either gemcitabine as monotherapy [33] or in combination with mitomycin [34, 35] as well as nab-paclitaxel [36].

## *Complications of Intravesical Therapy*

Intravesical therapy can cause local reactions to the urothelium that can cause some patients significant symptoms. The most common symptoms experienced are dysuria, bladder pain, gross hematuria, low-grade fever, and malaise. These usually occur 24–48 hours post-treatment.

These symptoms can be treated with analgesics–nonsteroidal anti-inflammatory drugs (NSAIDs), anticholinergic medications, and antispasmodics. If the symptoms persist, a urine culture should be obtained to rule out a bacterial infection. If the urine culture is positive, treatment should be withheld, and the infection should be treated with an appropriate antibiotic. A negative urine culture should be obtained before intravesical treatment is continued.

A decrease in the dose of intravesical treatment can be appropriate if side effects become more severe over time and the patient can no longer tolerate the full dose. In some patients, chemical cystitis and urinary tract infection can occur.

## *Cystoscopic Follow-Up*

Cystoscopic follow-up is the standard tool for monitoring superficial bladder cancer. It is limited only to tumors that can be visualized, so therefore, urine cytology is used as an adjunct to detect high-grade disease [37]. Follow-up is imperative because of the high probability of tumor recurrence and the risk of progression. In general, the first cystoscopy should be 3 months after the initial transurethral resection. If the first cystoscopy is clear, follow-up was traditionally scheduled every 3 months for a period of 2 years, every 6 months until the end of the fifth year, and then yearly thereafter. However, this approach has been modified to individual risk using a scoring system (such as the EORTC) and risk tables for the prediction of short- and long-term risks of both recurrence and progression. The American Urological Association also recommends a more risk-adapted approach [37]. Fluorescent cystoscopy involves the intravenous injection of photoactive porphyrin precursors (commonly hexaminolevulinate) which preferentially accumulate in neoplastic tissue. Under blue light, they emit red fluorescence and aid in the diagnosis of subtle lesions. Blue light cystoscopy has been shown to reduce recurrences in multiple studies and should be considered if available [38, 39]. Narrow band imaging (NBI) utilizes two specific wavelengths (415 nm and 540 nm) that are specifically absorbed by hemoglobin and leads to improved visibility of blood vessels. Studies have been mixed, but the use of NBI may aid in the reduction of tumor recurrences [40, 41].

**Key Points**
**Intravesical Administration**
Intravesical chemotherapy has a clear impact on tumor recurrence when instilled immediately after TUR and as a maintenance protocol.

In general, side effects of chemotherapy tend to be less common and less severe than those with BCG.

Perform sterile catheterization using a sterile catheter kit and a 14F urethral catheter. Empty bladder completely.

Insert a catheter tip syringe or the primed tubing attached to the medication valve to the catheter and instill the agent per gravity flow or injection. Assess the patient for pain.

Remove syringe or medication vial with tubing intact using sterile gauze to help absorb any drops. If the patient has difficulty holding the solution, a Foley catheter may be used, and a catheter plug may be inserted onto the end of the catheter after installation so the chemotherapeutic agent remains in the bladder for a specified amount of time, usually 1–2 hours. Depending on the patient's mobility, the catheter can be removed and the patient can void, or the catheter can be connected to a urinary drainage bag to drain the chemotherapeutic agent.

Once the catheter is removed, dispose of the equipment appropriately. Repeat inspection of the perineal area for leaks and reassess for pain. Cleanse area as indicated.

Instruct the patient to retain the treatment for 1–2 hours [20, 24].

**Clinical Pearls**

- BCG is the only agent shown to delay or reduce high-grade tumor progression.
- A 6-week induction course alone is insufficient to obtain an optimal response in many patients and that maintenance therapy is requisite.
- Ideally, maintenance should be given for 1 year for intermediate-risk and 3 years for high-risk NMIBC.
- BCG should not be started until 2 weeks after a TURBT. It should be held in the setting of traumatic catheterization, bacteriuria, persistent gross hematuria, persistent severe local symptoms, or systemic symptoms. BCG is contraindicated in immunosuppressed patients.
- Patients should be instructed to not void for 1–2 hours following intravesical installation. Bleach should be added to the toilet during the first 6 hours.
- Sexually active patients should use condoms during the duration of therapy.
- Dose reduction may be considered if there are substantial local symptoms during maintenance therapy.
- Quinolones may affect the efficacy of BCG and should be avoided for the duration of the treatment if possible.
- Patients may experience flu-like symptoms that can last 48–72 (low-grade fever below 38.5°C, fatigue, and joint achiness) hours. Local symptoms such as frequency, urgency, and dysuria are common. Anticholinergics, analgesics, and NSAIDS are helpful.
- Symptoms lasting more than 48 hours:
  - Urine culture, chest X-ray, and liver function tests.
  - Hold therapy or consider dose reduction.
- Consider therapy with isoniazid (300 mg/day) and rifampin (600 mg/day) until symptoms resolve.
- Severe symptoms such as hemodynamic instability should be treated with isoniazid (300 mg/day) and rifampin (600 mg/day) for 3–6 months. Ethambutol (15 mg/kg/day) should be added for solid organ involvement [6, 12, 20, 21, 42–48].

## References

1. Ro JY, Staerkel GA, Ayala AG. Cytologic and histologic features of superficial bladder cancer. Urol Clin North Am. 1992;19(3):435–53.
2. Donat SM. Evaluation and follow-up strategies for superficial bladder cancer. Urol Clin North Am. 2003;30(4):765–76.
3. Packiam VT, Johnson SC, Steinberg GD. Non-muscle-invasive bladder cancer: intravesical treatments beyond Bacille Calmette-Guérin. Cancer. 2017;123(3):390–400.
4. Sexton WJ, Wiegand LR, Correa JJ, Politis C, Dickinson SI, Kang LC. Bladder cancer: a review of non-muscle invasive disease. Cancer Control. 2010;17(4):256–68.
5. Veeratterapillay R, Heer R, Johnson MI, Persad R, Bach C. High-risk non-muscle-invasive bladder cancer-therapy options during intravesical BCG shortage. Curr Urol Rep. 2016;17(9):68.
6. Network NCC. Bladder cancer 2018. Available from: https://www.nccn.org/professionals/physician_gls/PDF/bladder.pdf.
7. Zincke H, Utz DC, Taylor WF, Myers RP, Leary FJ. Influence of thiotepa and doxorubicin instillation at time of transurethral surgical treatment of bladder cancer on tumor recurrence: a prospective, randomized, double-blind, controlled trial. J Urol. 1983;129(3):505–9.
8. Klän R, Loy V, Huland H. Residual tumor discovered in routine second transurethral resection in patients with stage T1 transitional cell carcinoma of the bladder. J Urol. 1991;146(2):316–8.
9. Masters JR. Re: methods to improve efficacy of intravesical mitomycin C: results of a randomized phase III trial. J Natl Cancer Inst. 2001;93(20):1574–5.
10. Di Stasi SM, Giannantoni A, Stephen RL, Capelli G, Navarra P, Massoud R, et al. Intravesical electromotive mitomycin C versus passive transport mitomycin C for high risk superficial bladder cancer: a prospective randomized study. J Urol. 2003;170(3):777–82.
11. Riedl CR, Daniltchenko D, Koenig F, Simak R, Loening SA, Pflueger H. Fluorescence endoscopy with 5-aminolevulinic acid reduces early recurrence rate in superficial bladder cancer. J Urol. 2001;165(4):1121–3.
12. Brooks NA, O'Donnell MA. Treatment options in non-muscle-invasive bladder cancer after BCG failure. Indian J Urol. 2015;31(4):312–9.
13. Messing EM, Tangen CM, Lerner SP, Sahasrabudhe DM, Koppie TM, Wood DP Jr, et al. Effect of intravesical instillation of gemcitabine vs saline immediately following resection of suspected low-grade non-muscle-invasive bladder cancer on tumor recurrence: SWOG S0337 randomized clinical trial. JAMA. 2018;319(18):1880–8.
14. Thrasher JB, Crawford ED. Complications of intravesical chemotherapy. Urol Clin North Am. 1992;19(3):529–39.
15. Oosterlinck W, Kurth KH, Schroder F, Bultinck J, Hammond B, Sylvester R. A prospective European Organization for Research and Treatment of Cancer Genitourinary Group randomized trial comparing transurethral resection followed by a single intravesical instillation of epirubicin or water in single stage Ta, T1 papillary carcinoma of the bladder. J Urol. 1993;149(4):749–52.
16. Li R, Spiess PE, Kamat AM. Treatment options for patients with recurrent tumors after BCG therapy: are we ignoring the obvious? Eur Urol. 2018;74(4):405–8.
17. Shen Z, Shen T, Wientjes MG, O'Donnell MA, Au JL. Intravesical treatments of bladder cancer: review. Pharm Res. 2008;25(7):1500–10.
18. Smith SG, Zaharoff DA. Future directions in bladder cancer immunotherapy: towards adaptive immunity. Immunotherapy. 2016;8(3):351–65.
19. Catalona WJ, Hudson MA, Gillen DP, Andriole GL, Ratliff TL. Risks and benefits of repeated courses of intravesical bacillus Calmette-Guerin therapy for superficial bladder cancer. J Urol. 1987;137(2):220–4.
20. Association AU. Intravesical administration of therapeutic medication. 2015.
21. Lamm DL, Blumenstein BA, Crissman JD, Montie JE, Gottesman JE, Lowe BA, et al. Maintenance bacillus Calmette-Guerin immunotherapy for recurrent TA, T1 and carcinoma

in situ transitional cell carcinoma of the bladder: a randomized Southwest Oncology Group Study. J Urol. 2000;163(4):1124–9.
22. Naitoh J, Franklin J, O'Donnell MA, Belldegrun AS. Interferon alpha for the treatment of superficial bladder cancer. Adv Exp Med Biol. 1999;462:371–86; discussion 87-92.
23. O'Donnell MA, Luo Y, Chen X, Szilvasi A, Hunter SE, Clinton SK. Role of IL-12 in the induction and potentiation of IFN-gamma in response to bacillus Calmette-Guerin. J Immunol. 1999;163(8):4246–52.
24. Heney NM, Nocks BN, Daly JJ, Blitzer PH, Parkhurst EC. Prognostic factors in carcinoma of the ureter. J Urol. 1981;125(5):632–6.
25. Sylvester RJ, van der MA, Lamm DL. Intravesical bacillus Calmette-Guerin reduces the risk of progression in patients with superficial bladder cancer: a meta-analysis of the published results of randomized clinical trials. J Urol. 2002;168(5):1964–70.
26. Duque JL, Loughlin KR. An overview of the treatment of superficial bladder cancer. Intravesical chemotherapy. Urol Clin North Am. 2000;27(1):125–35, x.
27. O'Donnell MA. Practical applications of intravesical chemotherapy and immunotherapy in high-risk patients with superficial bladder cancer. Urol Clin North Am. 2005;32(2):121–31.
28. Han RF, Pan JG. Can intravesical bacillus Calmette-Guerin reduce recurrence in patients with superficial bladder cancer? A meta-analysis of randomized trials. Urology. 2006;67(6):1216–23.
29. Grossman HB, O'Donnell MA, Cookson MS, Greenberg RE, Keane TE. Bacillus Calmette-Guerin failures and beyond: contemporary management of non-muscle-invasive bladder cancer. Rev Urol. 2008;10(4):281–9.
30. Steinberg G, Bahnson R, Brosman S, Middleton R, Wajsman Z, Wehle M. Efficacy and safety of valrubicin for the treatment of Bacillus Calmette-Guerin refractory carcinoma in situ of the bladder. The Valrubicin Study Group. J Urol. 2000;163(3):761–7.
31. Milbar N, Kates M, Chappidi MR, Pederzoli F, Yoshida T, Sankin A, et al. Oncological outcomes of sequential intravesical gemcitabine and docetaxel in patients with non-muscle invasive bladder cancer. Bladder Cancer. 2017;3(4):293–303.
32. Steinberg RL, Thomas LJ, O'Donnell MA, Nepple KG. Sequential intravesical gemcitabine and docetaxel for the salvage treatment of non-muscle invasive bladder cancer. Bladder Cancer. 2015;1(1):65–72.
33. Skinner EC, Goldman B, Sakr WA, Petrylak DP, Lenz HJ, Lee CT, et al. SWOG S0353: phase II trial of intravesical gemcitabine in patients with nonmuscle invasive bladder cancer and recurrence after 2 prior courses of intravesical bacillus Calmette-Guérin. J Urol. 2013;190(4):1200–4.
34. Cockerill PA, Knoedler JJ, Frank I, Tarrell R, Karnes RJ. Intravesical gemcitabine in combination with mitomycin C as salvage treatment in recurrent non-muscle-invasive bladder cancer. BJU Int. 2016;117(3):456–62.
35. Lightfoot AJ, Breyer BN, Rosevear HM, Erickson BA, Konety BR, O'Donnell MA. Multi-institutional analysis of sequential intravesical gemcitabine and mitomycin C chemotherapy for non-muscle invasive bladder cancer. Urol Oncol. 2014;32(1):35.e15–9.
36. McKiernan JM, Holder DD, Ghandour RA, Barlow LJ, Ahn JJ, Kates M, et al. Phase II trial of intravesical nanoparticle albumin bound paclitaxel for the treatment of nonmuscle invasive urothelial carcinoma of the bladder after bacillus Calmette-Guérin treatment failure. J Urol. 2014;192(6):1633–8.
37. Soukup V, Babjuk M, Bellmunt J, Dalbagni G, Giannarini G, Hakenberg OW, et al. Follow-up after surgical treatment of bladder cancer: a critical analysis of the literature. Eur Urol. 2012;62(2):290–302.
38. Burger M, Oosterlinck W, Konety B, Chang S, Gudjonsson S, Pruthi R, et al. ICUD-EAU International Consultation on Bladder Cancer 2012: non-muscle-invasive urothelial carcinoma of the bladder. Eur Urol. 2013;63(1):36–44.
39. Stenzl A, Burger M, Fradet Y, Mynderse LA, Soloway MS, Witjes JA, et al. Hexaminolevulinate guided fluorescence cystoscopy reduces recurrence in patients with nonmuscle invasive bladder cancer. J Urol. 2010;184(5):1907–13.

40. Naselli A, Introini C, Timossi L, Spina B, Fontana V, Pezzi R, et al. A randomized prospective trial to assess the impact of transurethral resection in narrow band imaging modality on non-muscle-invasive bladder cancer recurrence. Eur Urol. 2012;61(5):908–13.
41. Naito S, Algaba F, Babjuk M, Bryan RT, Sun YH, Valiquette L, et al. The Clinical Research Office of the Endourological Society (CROES) multicentre randomised trial of narrow band imaging-assisted transurethral resection of bladder tumour (TURBT) versus conventional white light imaging-assisted turbt in primary non-muscle-invasive bladder cancer patients: trial protocol and 1-year results. Eur Urol. 2016;70(3):506–15.
42. Lamm DL, Dehaven JI, Riggs DR. Keyhole limpet hemocyanin immunotherapy of bladder cancer: laboratory and clinical studies. Eur Urol. 2000;37(Suppl 3):41–4.
43. Palou J, Laguna P, Millan-Rodriguez F, Hall RR, Salvador-Bayarri J, Vicente-Rodriguez J. Control group and maintenance treatment with bacillus Calmette-Guerin for carcinoma in situ and/or high grade bladder tumors. J Urol. 2001;165(5):1488–91.
44. Ehdaie B, Sylvester R, Herr HW. Maintenance bacillus Calmette-Guerin treatment of non-muscle-invasive bladder cancer: a critical evaluation of the evidence. Eur Urol. 2013;64(4):579–85.
45. Durek C, Rusch-Gerdes S, Jocham D, Bohle A. Interference of modern antibacterials with bacillus Calmette-Guerin viability. J Urol. 1999;162(6):1959–62.
46. Ehlers S. Why does tumor necrosis factor targeted therapy reactivate tuberculosis? J Rheumatol Suppl. 2005;74:35–9.
47. Herr HW. Intravesical bacillus Calmette-Guerin outcomes in patients with bladder cancer and asymptomatic bacteriuria. J Urol. 2012;187(2):435–7.
48. Durek C, Brandau S, Ulmer AJ, Flad HD, Jocham D, Bohle A. Bacillus-Calmette-Guerin (BCG) and 3D tumors: an in vitro model for the study of adhesion and invasion. J Urol. 1999;162(2):600–5.

# Chapter 14
# Bladder Cancer: Muscle-Invasive Disease, Neoadjuvant Chemotherapy, and Radical Cystectomy

**Mary W. Dunn and Matthew I. Milowsky**

## Neoadjuvant Chemotherapy

The preferred management of patients with muscle-invasive bladder cancer (MIBC) is neoadjuvant chemotherapy (NAC) followed by radical cystectomy (RC). Chemotherapy refers to cytotoxic drugs that are administered to inhibit or destroy the division and growth of cells. Neoadjuvant chemotherapy, a type of perioperative chemotherapy, is chemotherapy that is administered prior to surgery. There is level I evidence supporting the use of cisplatin-based chemotherapy in the neoadjuvant setting for the treatment of MIBC with the goal of reducing tumor burden, eradicating micrometastatic disease, and improving survival [1]. Although NAC improves survival when compared to locoregional treatment alone, it remains widely underutilized, with fewer than 20% of patients who undergo RC receiving NAC [2–4]. In a survey of 83 medical oncologists, 52% of whom practiced in academic medical centers, 79% reported offering NAC to all patients with MIBC, suggesting a shift toward adoption of recommendations that follow best evidence [5]. The European Association of Urology (EAU) developed guidelines for the management of MIBC, which the American Society of Clinical Oncology (ASCO) endorsed in 2016 [6]. These guidelines support the use of NAC followed by RC for patients who are eligible to receive cisplatin. For patient who are ineligible to receive cisplatin, RC is recommended.

Prior to the initiation of treatment for MIBC, patients must be clinically staged. In addition to transurethral resection of bladder tumor (TURBT), this includes

M. W. Dunn (✉)
Department of Urology, University of North Carolina Chapel Hill, Chapel Hill, NC, USA
e-mail: mwdunn@med.unc.edu

M. I. Milowsky
Department of Medicine, University of North Carolina Chapel Hill, Chapel Hill, NC, USA
e-mail: matt_milowsky@med.unc.edu



E. J. Trabulsi et al. (eds.), *Chemotherapy and Immunotherapy in Urologic Oncology*, https://doi.org/10.1007/978-3-030-52021-2_14

radiographic evaluation, typically with a computed tomography (CT) of the chest, abdomen, and pelvis. Baseline laboratory testing, including complete blood count (CBC) and comprehensive metabolic panel (CMP), should be obtained. A thorough review of systems should evaluate for any preexisting symptoms or medical conditions that may be exacerbated by chemotherapy (e.g., tinnitus, hearing loss, neuropathy).

There are no data to support using non-cisplatin-based regimens in the neoadjuvant setting. Specifically, carboplatin, another alkylating agent, should not be substituted for cisplatin in those who are ineligible to receive cisplatin. A 2003 meta-analysis of 11 randomized trials that compared cisplatin-based NAC and local therapy with local therapy alone demonstrated that NAC resulted in a survival benefit [7]. NAC plus local therapy resulted in an improvement in overall survival (OS) (5-year OS, 50% versus 45%; HR, 0.87, 95% CI, 0.78–0.98) and a lower risk of recurrence (HR, 0.81; 95% CI, 0.74–0.90). An update to the 2003 meta-analysis showed a significant survival benefit associated with cisplatin-based NAC (HR, 0.86, 95% CI, 0.77–0.95), translating to a 5% absolute improvement in survival at 5 years. In addition, there was a disease-free survival benefit (HR, 0.78, 95% CI, 0.71–0.86), which is equivalent to a 9% absolute improvement at 5 years [8].

There are several cisplatin-based chemotherapy regimens that are used in the neoadjuvant setting. Two of these regimens, classic methotrexate, vinblastine, doxorubicin, and cisplatin (MVAC) and cisplatin, methotrexate, and vinblastine (CMV), were studied in two large phase III randomized trials that each evaluated the effects of NAC versus no NAC on mortality. The phase III trial led by Southwest Oncology Group (SWOG) randomized patients ($n = 307$) with MIBC to either three cycles of neoadjuvant MVAC (given every 28 days) plus RC or RC alone [9]. The use of NAC followed by RC was associated with a decreased risk of all-cause mortality (59% versus 65%; HR, 0.75; 95% CI, 0.57–1.00) and bladder cancer mortality (35% versus 50%; HR, 0.60; 95% CI, 0.41–0.82) versus RC without NAC. In addition, MVAC was associated with a significant difference in the median overall survival (77 versus 46 months) as well as in pathologic complete response rates (38% versus 15%). Significant toxicities were seen with MVAC including grade 3 granulocytopenia ($n = 35$) and grade 4 granulocytopenia ($n = 50$), and 26 patients experienced gastrointestinal toxicity in the form of grade 3 nausea, vomiting, stomatitis, diarrhea, or constipation.

A larger trial of 976 patients compared three cycles of neoadjuvant CMV (given every 21 days) or no chemotherapy before RC, radiotherapy, or both [10]. Findings from this study demonstrated decreased risk of cancer-specific mortality for the combined approach of NAC plus RC versus RC or radiotherapy alone, or both without NAC. At the median follow-up of 4 years, the difference was not found to be statistically significant (HR, 0.85; 95% CI, 0.71–1.02). However, a longer follow-up (median, 8 years) of the same study demonstrated that NAC led to a significantly decreased risk of cancer-specific mortality (HR, 0.74; 95% CI, 0.57–0.96) [11]. In those patients who received CMV before RC or radiotherapy, there was a 16% reduction in cancer-specific mortality.

In an effort to shorten the duration of chemotherapy and reduce toxicities, studies have looked at the efficacy of high-dose MVAC (HDMVAC), which delivers MVAC every 2 weeks with growth factor support. Of note, this strategy to shorten the duration of MVAC is synonymously termed high dose, dose dense, or accelerated. In a phase III randomized controlled trial (RCT), patients were randomized to either 2-week cycles of HDMVAC ($n = 134$) or 4-week cycles of classic MVAC ($n = 129$) [12]. The study aimed to determine whether HDMVAC plus granulocyte colony-stimulating factor (G-CSF) improved overall survival in patients with advanced urothelial cancer. At a median follow-up of 38 months, a 50% difference in median overall survival (mOS) was not found. However, patients treated with HDMVAC had a benefit in progression-free survival (HR, 0.75; 95% CI, 0.58–0.98); complete response (CR) rates (21% versus 9%); and overall response (OR) rates (62% versus 50%). In addition, HDMVAC had fewer toxicities than classic MVAC including less white blood cell (WBC) toxicity (e.g., neutropenia and neutropenic fever) and mucositis. In a seven-year update to the initial EORTC 30924 trial, 24.6% of patients on the HDMVAC arm were alive, compared to 13.2% on the classic MVAC arm [13]. Median progression-free survival (mPFS) was 9.5 months with HDMVAC (95% CI, 7.6–12.2) and 8.1 months with MVAC (95% CI, 7.0–9.9); median survival was 15.1 months with HDMVAC and 14.9 months with MVAC, and mortality HR was 0.76 (95% CI, 0.58–0.99). More patients died from their urothelial carcinoma in the MVAC arm (76%) than in the HDMVAC arm (64.9%). Based on category 1 evidence that shows HDMVAC to be better tolerated and more effective than classic MVAC for advanced disease, it is preferred and recommended versus classic MVAC in the neoadjuvant setting.

While NAC dose-dense MVAC regimens have not been evaluated in randomized clinical trials, two small, single-arm studies suggest that this approach may be reasonable. A phase II trial tested the hypothesis that three cycles of accelerated MVAC (AMVAC) given over 6 weeks would be safe, shorten time to RC, and yield comparable pathologic response rates in the neoadjuvant setting [14]. Of the 40 patients evaluable for response, 15 showed pathologic complete response (pCR; pT0) at RC (95% CI, 23–53%), 82% experienced grade 1 to 2 chemotherapy-related toxicities, and the median time from the start of chemotherapy to RC was 9.7 weeks. Another study that included 39 patients who received four cycles of DDMVAC showed a pathologic response rate (pRR) of 49% and a pCR in ten patients. The disease-free rate was higher at 1 year for those patients who had achieved a pCR; 89% versus 67% among those without a pathologic response (95% CI, 0.80–8.1) [15].

Gemcitabine and cisplatin (GC) are used in the neoadjuvant setting based largely on category 1 data extrapolated from trials in the advanced and metastatic setting. In a phase III RCT, patients with advanced bladder cancer were randomized to either GC ($n = 203$) or classic MVAC ($n = 202$) for a maximum of six cycles [16]. OS, time to disease progression, time to treatment failure, and response rate data were similar between the two regimens. GC was associated with fewer toxicities and better tolerability than MVAC. More MVAC patients than GC patients had grade 3 neutropenia (82% versus 71%), neutropenic fever (14% versus 2%), neutropenic sepsis (12% versus 1%), and grade 3 mucositis (22% versus 1%). An update to this trial demonstrated similar long-term OS rates with GC and MVAC (9.8% and 11.3%, respectively) and similar mPFS rates, 7.7 months for GC and 8.3 months for MVAC [17]. A retrospective analysis of 42 patients who received four cycles of neoadjuvant GC was compared to a historical cohort who were treated with neoadjuvant MVAC [18]. This analysis demonstrated a pT0 proportion of 26% (95% CI, 14–42) and <pT2 of 36% (95% CI, 21–52) in the GC group. In comparison, the pT0 proportion in the MVAC cohort was 28% (95% CI, 16–42), and the pT2 proportion was 35% (95% CI, 23–49). If patients have borderline renal function, splitting the dose of cisplatin can be considered (e.g., 35 mg/m$^2$ on days 1 and 8, instead of 70 mg/m$^2$ on day 1). Results of a phase I/II trial where a split dose of cisplatin was used showed an overall response rate (ORR) of 65% and four CR [19].

Dose-dense MVAC has shown shortened time to surgery in the neoadjuvant setting. A small ($n = 31$) trial aimed to show that neoadjuvant dose-dense gemcitabine and cisplatin (DDGC) could also shorten time to cystectomy and yield a similar pCR compared with historical controls with standard GC [20]. Ten patients (95% CI, 16–49) achieved a pCR (pT0), and another four patients were downstaged to non-muscle-invasive disease (NMIBC). These findings are similar to those noted retrospectively with standard GC. This trial was closed early due to vascular events experienced in 23% of the patients that either precluded, delayed, or increased their risk for surgery. Another trial studying DDGC in the neoadjuvant setting enrolled 49 patients from three institutions with the primary endpoint of downstaging to non-muscle-invasive disease [21]. The majority of the patients (67%) completed all six cycles of chemotherapy, and 58% of patients were downstaged to NMIBC. While 39% of patients required a dose reduction due to toxicity, none failed to undergo RC due to toxicity. Pretreatment tumors underwent next-generation sequencing in order to identify predictors of chemosensitivity. The presence of a deleterious DNA damage repair (DDR) gene alteration was linked with chemosensitivity.

## Neoadjuvant Immunotherapy

As a result of an increased understanding of how the immune system interacts with cancers, a number of immune oncology drugs have been developed. Several checkpoint inhibitors (CPI) are approved for use in the metastatic bladder cancer setting, which has led to interest in how these immunotherapy agents may work in the neoadjuvant setting. To date, two anti-programmed cell death (PD)-1/ligand 1 (PD-L1) agents have been studied in the neoadjuvant space. An interim analysis of the phase II ABACUS trial of neoadjuvant atezolizumab in MIBC showed a pCR of 29% (95% CI, 18–42), and 39% of patients were downstaged to NMIBC [22]. The single-arm phase II PURE-01 trial of neoadjuvant pembrolizumab showed a pCR of 42% (95% CI, 28.2–56.8), and 54% of patients were downstaged to NMIBC [23]. A phase I/II study examining both neoadjuvant pembrolizumab alone in cisplatin-ineligible patients and pembrolizumab plus cisplatin and gemcitabine showed that of the 40 patients who received pembrolizumab and GC combination, 40% of those who had an RC ($n = 36$) had a pCR at the time of RC [24]. While these trials report high pathologic response rates, confirmation is needed in larger studies.

## Adverse Reactions

Common adverse events of chemotherapy depend on the specific regimen but can include myelosuppression, fatigue, nausea, vomiting, electrolyte imbalance, alopecia, stomatitis, and peripheral neuropathy, among others. Patients should be educated about the possibility of febrile neutropenia, which can be life-threatening when associated with infection, and given instructions on what to do in the event of a fever. In an effort to reduce potentially severe toxicities like neutropenia, regimens like DDMVAC are given with granulocyte-macrophage colony-stimulating factor (GM-CSF) [25]. Given the risk of ototoxicity associated with cisplatin, a baseline audiometry evaluation is recommended. The dose-limiting toxicity of cisplatin is nephrotoxicity, which is why pretreatment assessment of renal function is critical. Patients should receive adequate pre- and post-hydration with each dose of cisplatin [26]. Patients who receive MVAC should have a baseline assessment of left ventricular ejection fraction due to risk of cardiac toxicity with doxorubicin, such as cardiomyopathy leading to congestive heart failure, and be monitored for signs and symptoms of cardiotoxicity during treatment [27]. All NAC regimens include pretreatment antiemetics to prevent and/or lessen the degree of chemotherapy-induced nausea and vomiting. Patients should also be provided with a prescription for antiemetics (e.g., ondansetron, prochlorperazine) to have at home in the event they experience delayed nausea or vomiting.

Meta-analyses have demonstrated that platinum-based NAC yields both a significant survival benefit, which translates to an absolute benefit in survival of 5% at 5 years, and a disease-free survival benefit equivalent to a 9% absolute improvement at 5 years [8]. Despite this evidence, only a small percentage of patients receive NAC. There are several factors that may account for underuse of NAC, including fear of adverse events, delay to RC, and patients who may be deemed "unfit" to receive cisplatin [25]. Providers should offer NAC to patients who are eligible, while thoroughly explaining rationale, benefits, and risks. Additional information about the most common chemotherapy regimens used in the neoadjuvant setting can be found in Tables 14.1 and 14.2.

## Radical Cystectomy

Radical cystectomy is the surgical removal of the entire urinary bladder. For patients with non-metastatic MIBC, RC in combination with NAC is the standard of care [28]. This approach has been compared to bladder-sparing therapy in one RCT,

**Table 14.1** Chemotherapy regimens, schedules, and doses used in the neoadjuvant setting

| Neoadjuvant regimen | Schedule | Chemotherapy agent | Dose |
|---|---|---|---|
| Classic MVAC | Every 28 days for 3 cycles | Methotrexate | 30 mg/m$^2$ days 1, 15, and 22 |
| – | – | Vinblastine | 3 mg/m$^2$ days 2, 15, and 22 |
| – | – | Doxorubicin | 30 mg/m$^2$ day 2 |
| – | – | Cisplatin | 70 mg/m$^2$ day 2 |
| CMV | Every 21 days for 3 cycles | Cisplatin | 100 mg/m$^2$ day 2 |
| – | – | Methotrexate | 30 mg/m$^2$ days 1 and 8 |
| – | – | Vinblastine | 4 mg/m$^2$ days 1 and 8 |
| High-dose MVAC | Every 14 days for 3–4 cycles | Methotrexate | 30 mg/m$^2$ day 1 |
| – | – | Vinblastine | 3 mg/m$^2$ day 2 |
| – | – | Doxorubicin | 30 mg/m$^2$ day 2 |
| – | – | Cisplatin | 70 mg/m$^2$ day 2 |
| GC | Every 21 days for 4 cycles | Gemcitabine | 1000 mg/m$^2$ days 1 and 8 |
| – | – | Cisplatin | 70 mg/m$^2$ day 1 |

**Table 14.2** Classes of commonly used chemotherapeutic agents used for urothelial carcinoma

| Chemotherapy agent | Category |
|---|---|
| Methotrexate | Antimetabolite; folic acid antagonist |
| Vinblastine | Vinca alkaloid |
| Doxorubicin | Antitumor antibiotic; anthracycline |
| Cisplatin | Alkylating agent; metal salt |
| Gemcitabine | Antimetabolite; pyrimidine antagonist |

several retrospective cohort studies, and one non-RCT [29]. One population-based cohort study of 1843 patients showed that bladder-preserving therapy was associated with decreased 5-year survival as compared to RC (27.9% vs. 46.5%) [30]. Of note, bladder-sparing therapy will be discussed in another chapter.

Radical cystectomy and bilateral pelvic lymph node dissection (PLND) provide locoregional control and pathologic staging. Bilateral PLND includes removal of external and internal iliac and obturator nodes. There is some evidence to suggest that an extended template dissection may be indicated, which includes removal of presacral and common iliac nodes up to the aortic bifurcation. In a study of 290 patients who had an extended lymph node dissection, 28% of patients had positive lymph nodes, of which only 25% had positive nodes in the standard template [31]. In a prospective phase III trial of extended versus limited lymph node dissection, 203 patients were randomized to limited dissection (obturator and internal and external nodes), and 198 patients were randomized to extended dissection (limited plus deep obturator, common iliac, presacral, paracaval, interaortocaval, and para-aortal nodes) [32]. The primary endpoint of the study was recurrence-free survival (RFS). Secondary endpoints included cancer-specific survival (CSS), OS, and complications. Extended dissection did not show superiority over limited dissection with regard to RFS (5-year RFS 65% vs 59%), CSS (5-year CSS 76% vs 65%), and OS (5-year OS, 59% vs 50%). Additional larger studies are needed in order to determine the benefit of extended lymph node dissection.

In addition to RC and PLND, surgical management of MIBC entails removal of adjacent organs that have the highest risk of containing cancer outside of the bladder. In males, this includes the prostate and seminal vesicles, and in females, the uterus, cervix, ovaries, fallopian tubes, and anterior vaginal wall. However, given the significant sexual dysfunction that occurs with this technique, select patients who desire preservation of sexual function may be eligible for sexual function preserving procedures, as long as cancer control is not compromised [33]. Potential candidates for sexual function preserving techniques should have organ-confined disease without involvement of the bladder neck, urethra, and prostate and no preexisting erectile dysfunction (ED). Damage to the neurovascular bundle can lead to ED in men; thus, prostate-sparing and nerve-sparing approaches have been studied, though robust data on safety of these approaches is lacking [34]. Men with a suspicion of prostate adenocarcinoma (i.e., elevated prostate-specific antigen) should not have prostate-sparing surgery. In women, a vaginal sparing RC can be considered in certain instances, such as absence of tumor in the trigone or bladder base [35]. The effectiveness of nerve-sparing surgery in women to prevent vaginal dryness and dyspareunia has not been established.

## Approaches

Surgical approaches to RC include open, laparoscopic, and robotic. Many high-volume bladder cancer centers utilize a minimally invasive or robotic approach, but currently, there is insufficient evidence to recommend for or against robotic cystectomy. Several small RTs and observational and systemic reviews have found that robotic cystectomy is associated with longer operative time, higher cost, less intraoperative blood loss, and no significant difference in major postoperative complications [36]. One single-center RCT compared open with robotic cystectomy in 118 patients. At postoperative day 90, grade 2–5 complications were observed in 62% of patients in the robotic arm and 66% of patients who had an open RC [37]. There were no significant differences in length of stay, patient-reported quality of life, or pathologic outcomes. The robotic cohort had less intraoperative blood loss but longer operative time than the open cohort. The RAZOR trial is a non-inferiority study that randomly assigned 350 patients to either robotic or open cystectomy. The aim of this trial was to compare PFS in patients treated with open or robotic cystectomy [38]. Two-year PFS was 71.6% (95% CI, 63.6–78.2) in the open group and 72.3% (95% CI, 64.3–78.8) in the robotic group (difference, 0.7%, 95% CI, −9.6–10.9%, $p = 0.001$), demonstrating non-inferiority of robotic cystectomy. The decision whether or not to use an open or robotic technique should take into account surgeon experience and individual patient variables. Relative contraindications to minimally invasive surgery include prior abdominal or pelvic radiation due to potential for scarring and adhesions, abdominal hernia repair with mesh, colon resection that may limit the selection of urinary diversion, and obesity due to body size in relationship to the length and configuration of the laparoscopic instruments [39]. Trials comparing long-term cancer control rates will be helpful in gathering more data about open versus minimally invasive cystectomy.

## Perioperative Teaching

Patients who smoke should undergo smoking cessation counseling prior to RC. In addition to the known health benefits of smoking cessation, patients who stop smoking prior to RC have a reduced risk of postoperative complications (e.g., wound healing, infection) and improved long-term oncologic control [40]. Patients may also benefit from a preoperative nutritional assessment. Preoperative malnutrition is associated with increased risk of postoperative mortality for patients undergoing major surgery. In a study of 538 patients undergoing RC, 103 patients (19%) met criteria for malnutrition, which included preoperative albumin less than 3.5 gm/dl, body mass index (BMI) less than 18.5 kg/m$^2$, or weight loss greater than 5% of body weight [41]. The 90-day mortality rate was 7.3% (39 deaths), 16.5% in patients identified as having a nutritional deficiency and 5.1% in patients without nutritional deficiency. There are no consensus recommendations for referral to a registered dietitian, and more prospective studies are needed in order to determine the best markers of preoperative malnutrition.

## Select Surgical Complications

Prior to RC, patients should be educated about potential short- and long-term complications. Patients should also be counseled on the impact of age and gender as they relate to postoperative complications. Older patients and women experience higher complication rates compared to younger patients and men [29]. It is important for providers to establish realistic expectations with patients with regard to postoperative pain, expected length of stay in the hospital, and return to baseline functional status.

Postoperative ileus (POI) is the most commonly reported postoperative complication and is usually defined as delay of return of bowel function greater than 4 days [42]. Symptoms of POI include abdominal pain, abdominal distention, nausea, and vomiting. Eliminating preoperative mechanical bowel preparation and fasting prior to surgery with early nutritional support have shown some positive impact on bowel activity. This approach means that patients are less likely to be volume depleted on the day of surgery and require less aggressive intraoperative fluid resuscitation [43].

Patients should ambulate early in the postoperative setting, and normal electrolyte levels should be maintained. Management of POI is usually conservative but may require nasogastric tube decompression in cases of severe pain or prolonged ileus. Bowel obstruction can be ruled out with a CT scan. Thromboembolic events (e.g., deep vein thrombosis [DVT] and pulmonary embolism [PE]) are potentially life-threatening complications of major pelvic surgery. Signs of DVT include calf tenderness and edema. Prevention strategies include early ambulation; use of lower extremity compression stockings or sequential compression devices in the preoperative holding area through 72 hours postop; and use of prophylactic low-molecular-weight heparin (LMWH) [44]. There is evidence to suggest that continuing LMWH for up to 4 weeks in the perioperative setting may be beneficial [45].

## Urinary Diversions

Following radical cystectomy, the lower urinary tract is reconstructed, and urinary flow is redirected through either an incontinent or continent urinary diversion. Continent urinary diversions (CUDs) can be further subdivided into orthotopic and nonorthotopic diversions. Factors that influence choice of urinary diversion include patient and surgeon preference, extent of cancer, comorbidities, and renal function, among others. It is imperative that providers obtain and clarify the patient's expectations prior to undergoing a urinary diversion and extensively counsel patients about the advantages and disadvantages of each type of diversion.

### *Incontinent Diversion*

An incontinent urinary diversion is a surgical conduit constructed from a segment of terminal ileum. The ureters are connected to the proximal end of the bowel segment, and urine is diverted through peristalsis from the upper tracts through the abdominal wall stoma, where it drains into an external urostomy. Ileal conduits (IC) have become the gold standard of incontinent diversions given the relatively straightforward surgical technique and lower complication risks than other incontinent diversions [46]. The formation of an IC also tends to have the shortest operative time when compared to other types of diversions [25].

Oftentimes, IC is chosen for patients who have significant comorbidities in order to reduce risk of postoperative complications. Because of the tendency of patients who undergo IC to have higher risk factors than patients who are healthier and undergo a continent diversion, rate of surgical complications between the two groups may be similar [47]. Common complications associated with IC include renal dysfunction, bowel complications (e.g., ileus, obstruction, and anastomotic leak), stomal problems, urinary tract infections (UTIs), ureteral obstruction, ureteroenteric anastomotic obstruction, and urolithiasis [46].

Stomal complications may be seen in upwards of 50% of patients who undergo IC and can be related to surgical technique, location of the stoma, lifestyle factors that impair subcutaneous healing (e.g., smoking, alcohol abuse), and obesity [48]. Complications related to the stoma include stomal retraction, stenosis, and less likely obstruction, necrosis, and prolapse [49]. A parastomal hernia (PH) is an incisional hernia related to an abdominal wall stoma and is one of the most common stomal related complications. One retrospective study of 433 patients found the risk of developing a PH following RC with IC creation was 27% (95% CI, 22–32%) at 1 year and 48% (95% CI, 42–55%) at 2 years [50]. Risk factors for developing PH include higher BMI, female gender, and lower preoperative albumin.

Generally, the terminal 10–15 cm of ileum is preserved in order to maintain adequate absorption of vitamin $B_{12}$, fat-soluble vitamins, and bile salts [47]. Nonetheless, metabolic complications such as electrolyte abnormalities and vitamin deficiencies can be seen as a result of malabsorption. The incidence of vitamin $B_{12}$ deficiency after IC is not well documented, but patients should be monitored for symptoms. Ileal diversions are associated with an increased risk of hyperchloremic-hypokalemic metabolic acidosis, though severity is lessened in newer reconstructive procedures that decrease the amount of time that urine is in contact with bowel mucosa [51]. Patients should have lab work checked periodically to evaluate for acidosis, which is usually treated with sodium bicarbonate ($NaHCO_3$).

Patients should have the opportunity to meet with an enterostomal nurse prior to his or her cystectomy in order to receive additional education about IC and to be marked for the stoma. An enterostomal nurse will also follow the patient after RC in the hospital and at postoperative visits for appliance fitting and additional teaching. In addition, enterostomal nurses are experts in educating patients about body image issues, problem-solving around leaking and appliance fitting, and treating skin breakdown around the stoma. It is important for patients with ICs to be taught about symptoms of a urinary tract infection (e.g., fever, chills, and flank pain) and to not accept antibiotics in the absence of symptoms and a positive urine culture.

## *Continent Urinary Diversions*

### Orthotopic Diversion

Orthotopic diversions (ODs) are created of detubularized bowel, formed into a pouch to which the ureters are rerouted, and anastomosed to the native urethral stump. The most commonly used OD is the ileal orthotopic neobladder (ONB), which is created from 40 to 50 cm of terminal ileum [46]. Unlike an IC with stoma, the ONB allows preserved body image and allows for more natural volitional voiding that relies on the external striated sphincter [47].

Neobladders are ideal for patients who are interested in maintaining physical appearance by avoiding a stoma or ostomy appliance, as it most closely resembles the storage function of a urinary bladder. ODs also allow for a more "normal" voiding pattern after a period of postoperative rehabilitation, where patients must learn to contract his or her abdominal muscles in order to empty the ONB. In general, surgery is longer and more technically challenging for patients who undergo ONB creation and is associated with higher complication rates and prolonged postoperative catheterization [52]. Since advanced age has been associated with higher complication rates, ONBs are usually performed in healthier, younger patients, though physiologic age seems to be more closely associated with outcomes than chronological age. As such, there is no age-related absolute contraindication to ONB. Instead, providers should take into consideration performance status, surgical fitness, and motivation when evaluating candidacy for ONB [53].

It is important to recognize both absolute and relative contraindications to continent urinary diversions. Absolute contraindications include the following: insufficient bowel length; poor motor function and/or psychological issues that limit the ability to self-catheterize; inadequate renal or hepatic function that would increase the risk of metabolic abnormalities; and uncorrectable urethral stricture. An absolute contraindication specific to ONB is a positive urethral margin [47]. Relative contraindications to CUDs include the following: advanced age, multiple comorbidities, prior pelvic radiation, bowel disease, and need for adjuvant chemotherapy. Relative contraindications specific to ONB include extensive local disease with soft tissue extension and high risk of local recurrence, neurologic diseases that impair continence, and planned adjuvant radiation [46].

Early complications of ONB are usually related to the RC and not the diversion itself. Urine leaks are more common in ODs given the multiple suture lines, tapered limbs, and anti-incontinence mechanisms that increase the operative time [47]. Urine leaks are usually managed with catheter drainage. In cases that cannot be managed conservatively, percutaneous nephrostomy (PCN) tubes or drain placement may be necessary. The most common late complications associated with ODs include urinary incontinence (UI), hypercontinence, UTIs, urethral stricture, urolithiasis (including calculi in the pouch), and pouch rupture [54].

Urinary incontinence following ONB is common and may last up to 6 months after RC. However, there are patients who experience some degree of permanent daytime and/or nighttime UI. Daytime continence is usually recovered more quickly than nighttime continence. Daytime UI is a consequence of reduced urethral outlet resistance heightened by low ONB capacity, diminished compliance, or elevated ONB pressure. Nighttime UI is a result of diminished or absent sensation that allows disproportionate nocturnal volumes to overcome the impaired continence mechanisms of the bladder outlet, coupled with the loss of physiological storage reflexes. A review of over 2000 patients with ONB found that 13% reported daytime UI and 15–40% experienced nocturnal enuresis [55]. Urinary retention requiring clean intermittent catheterization (CIC) can affect 16–25% of patients with ONBs, which is why it is imperative that patients be willing to learn CIC. Techniques to prevent voiding dysfunction include using an adequate length of bowel, avoiding pelvic floor injury, using an appropriate urethral length, and positioning the neobladder neck in the most dependent portion of the pelvis. Time voiding every 3–4 hours during the day and setting an alarm clock to awaken at least twice during the night may be helpful strategies [55].

Patients who undergo ONB must be willing to commit to intensive neobladder training early in the postoperative period. In the immediate postoperative setting, an indwelling catheter will remain in the neobladder to allow for healing. Scheduled flushing of 100 mL of normal saline every 8 hours reduces the risk of catheter obstruction. Two to 3 weeks after surgery, a cystogram should be performed to assess for leaking [56]. Strategies to teach patients to help with emptying their ONB include sitting, relaxing the sphincter and pelvic floor muscles, and using Valsalva. Leaning forward or exerting gentle pressure over the lower abdomen can increase intra-abdominal pressure and assist with more complete emptying. Another important consideration is gradual increase in ONB capacity from 150–200 mL initially to 400–500 mL in the longer term. Voiding every 2–3 hours during the day and every 3 hours during the night can help with this [57]. These intervals can be gradually increased with a goal of voiding every 5–6 hours during the day and once at night. Failing to be compliant with recommendations for neobladder training may result in increased risk of complications such as UI, retention, and bladder stones.

## Nonorthotopic Diversion

Continent cutaneous urinary diversions (CCUDs) are nonorthotopic reservoirs that use a low-pressure pouch created from detubularized bowel with either ileum or the right colon, which includes a piece of aperistaltic bowel with a functional mechanism that prevents involuntary urine flow. These reservoirs differ depending on the type of valve and catheterizable stoma created and segment of intestine used [47]. The ureters are connected to the bowel segment, and the distal bowel terminates in a stoma within the umbilicus or lower abdomen. The stoma is small and does not require an external drainage bag and instead can be covered with a bandage. CCUDs must be catheterized every 4–6 hours in order to empty the urine from the reservoir and prevent buildup of mucus. As such, patients must be able to self-catheterize the stoma. Types of catheterizable CCUDs include the Indiana, Kock, and Miami pouches, among others.

Continent cutaneous urinary diversions have largely been replaced by ONBs, but some patients prefer this approach, especially if they are not candidates for ONB and wish to avoid an IC. CCUDs have the same absolute contraindications as ONBs, minus the ones previously mentioned as specific to ONB. Preoperative education is crucial for these patients, as the importance of compliance with a catheterization schedule cannot be overemphasized. Failure to maintain a strict CIC schedule can result in pouch rupture, UTIs, upper tract deterioration, stomal stenosis, and calculi [46]. In a similar fashion to the ONB, CCUDs require postoperative indwelling catheter followed by cystogram and pouch cycling.

The risk of UI is less than with ONB, ranging from 2% to 10% [58]. This benefit should be weighed against the disadvantage of longer operative time and lifelong around-the-clock catheterization. The most common complications include urine leaks, difficulty with catheterization, and pouch calculi. Less common complications include recurrent UTIs, small bowel obstruction, pouchitis, and anastomotic strictures. Most of these complications do not require major intervention and can be managed conservatively [49].

A primary reason that patients desire a CUD, either orthotopic or nonorthotopic, is for preservation of "normal" body image and better quality of life (QoL). Defining QoL is highly subjective. There have been some reports that have noted improvements in specific health-related quality of life (HRQoL) areas; there are few formal studies that have demonstrated improvement in overall HRQoL [47]. While some studies have reported better HRQoL outcomes with ONBs than other diversions, most studies show that patients who are well counseled about their diversion have equivalent levels of satisfaction [59].

The main goals in selecting a type of urinary diversion is to attain a high QoL and low complication rates. The decision-making process can be complex and overwhelming for patients. While patient preference is important, providers must also take into consideration comorbidities, functional status, and absolute and relative contraindications when counseling patients on the optimal urinary diversion. Establishing realistic expectations prior to surgery regarding diversion-specific risks, side effects, postoperative rehabilitation, and long-term care is critical. In addition, it is important to recognize that each type of diversion is associated with its own learning curve and lifestyle adjustment, which can vary drastically between patients.

## Posttreatment Survivorship

A diagnosis of cancer can be a life-changing experience. Cancer survivors have unique health needs given the risks of long-term side effects of cancer treatments, the risk of recurrence, and the risk of secondary cancers. Patients may report a feeling of loss of control. Talking to patients about things over which they can take control to improve their overall health can be helpful during times of uncertainty. Examples include maintaining a balanced diet, incorporating physical activity in daily routines, getting restorative sleep, tobacco cessation, minimal alcohol consumption, and following up with health-care providers as directed. A small study of 30 patients examined the unmet needs of patients with MIBC who underwent RC [60]. Prior to RC, unmet informational needs consisted of insufficient discussion related to urinary diversions, self-care, recovery, and health insurance. Postoperative unmet needs included physical recovery and instrumental needs. In the 6–72 months after surgery, unmet needs centered around psychological concerns (e.g., depression, body image, sexual dysfunction) and support adjusting to the new normal. Providers can encourage participation in support groups, whether in-person or online, and refer to a mental health specialist if patients disclose difficulty with coping or other emotional or psychological concerns. In addition to assessing for long-term side effects from treatment, posttreatment survivorship visits consist of monitoring for cancer recurrence. Providers should reiterate the importance of compliance with follow-up to include diagnostic tests (e.g., radiographic tests, labs, urine cytology) and office visits. Recommendations for surveillance schedules can be found at the National Comprehensive Cancer Network (NCCN) website. A Survivorship Care Plan (SCP) can serve as a useful tool to outline aspects of the treatment and surveillance plan as well as provide information about support organizations.

## Summary

Bladder cancer is one of the most common cancers in the world, affecting mostly older people, which can pose unique challenges if patients have preexisting medical comorbidities. Treatment of muscle-invasive bladder cancer requires a multidisciplinary team approach including urologists, medical oncologists, radiation oncologists, advanced practice providers, nurses, dietitians, social workers, etc. It is imperative that patients are educated about their treatment options, potential early and late side effects of treatment, and importance of posttreatment surveillance.

**Clinical Pearls**

- The standard of care for muscle-invasive bladder cancer is radical cystectomy.
- Alternative treatment for those patients who refuse radical cystectomy or who are not good surgical candidates includes radiation and chemotherapy.
- Patients who are to undergo a radical cystectomy should be considered for neoadjuvant chemotherapy.
- Immunotherapy treatment with checkpoint inhibitors has shown much improved outcomes when given in the neoadjuvant setting.
- Continent diversion should be reserved for relatively healthier, younger, and motivated patients.

## References

1. Patel A, Campbell S. Current trends in the management of bladder cancer. J Wound Ostomy Continence Nurs. 2009;31(3):91–3.
2. Miles BJ, Fairey AS, Eliasziw M, Estey EP, Venner P, Finch D, et al. Referral and treatment rates of neoadjuvant chemotherapy in muscle-invasive bladder cancer before and after publication of a clinical practice guideline. Can Urol Assoc J. 2010;4(4):263–7.
3. Porter MP, Kerrigan MC, Donato BM, Ramsey SD. Patterns of use of systemic chemotherapy for medicare beneficiaries with urothelial bladder cancer. Urol Oncol. 2011;29(3):252–8.
4. Raj GV, Karavadia S, Schlomer B, Arriaga Y, Lotan Y, Sagalowsky A, et al. Contemporary use of perioperative cisplatin-based chemotherapy in patients with muscle-invasive bladder cancer. Cancer. 2011;117(2):276–82.
5. Apolo AB, Kim JW, Bocher BH, Steinburg SM, Bajorin DF, Kelly WK, et al. Examining the management of muscle-invasive bladder cancer by medical oncologists in the United States. Urol Oncol. 2014;32(5):637–44.

6. Milowsky MI, Rumble RB, Booth CM, Gilligan T, Eapern LJ, Hauke RJ, et al. Guideline on muscle-invasive and metastatic bladder cancer (European Association of Urology Guideline): American Society of Clinical Oncology Clinical Practice Guideline Endorsement. J Clin Oncol. 2016;34(16):1945–54.
7. Advanced Bladder Cancer Meta-analysis Collaboration. Neoadjuvant chemotherapy in invasive bladder cancer: a systemic review and meta-analysis. Lancet. 2003;361(9373):1927–34.
8. Advanced Bladder Cancer Meta-analysis Collaboration. Neoadjuvant chemotherapy in invasive bladder cancer: update of a systemic review and meta-analysis of individual patient data. Eur Urol. 2005;45:202–6.
9. Grossman HB, Natale RB, Tangen CM, Speights VO, Vogelzang NJ, Trump DL, et al. Neoadjuvant chemotherapy plus cystectomy compared with cystectomy alone for locally advanced bladder cancer. N Engl J Med. 2003;349(9):859–66.
10. International Collaboration of Trialists. Neoadjuvant cisplatin, methotrexate and vinblastine chemotherapy for muscle-invasive bladder cancer: a randomized controlled trial. Lancet. 1999;354(9178):533–40.
11. International Collaboration of Trialists. International phase III trial assessing neoadjuvant cisplatin, methotrexate, and vinblastine chemotherapy for muscle-invasive bladder cancer: long-term results of the BA06 30894 trial. J Clin Oncol. 2011;29(16):2171–7.
12. Sternberg CN, de Mulder PHM, Schornagel JH, Theodore C, Fossa SD, van Oosterom AT, et al. Randomized phase III trial of high-dose-intensity methotrexate, vinblastine, doxorubicin, and cisplatin (MVAC) chemotherapy and recombinant human granulocyte colony-stimulating factor versus classic MVAC in advanced urothelial tract tumors: European organization for research and treatment of cancer protocol no. 30924. J Clin Oncol. 2001;19(10):2638–46.
13. Sternberg CN, de Mulder PHM, Schornagel JH, Theodore C, Fossa SD, van Oosterom AT, et al. Seven year update of an EORTC phase III trial of high-dose intensity M-VAC chemotherapy and G-CSF versus classic MVAC in advanced urothelial tract tumours. Eur J Cancer. 2006;42:50–4.
14. Plimack ER, Hoffman-Censits JH, Viterbo R, Trabulsi EJ, Ross EA, Greenberg RE, et al. Accelerated methotrexate, vinblastine, doxorubicin, and cisplatin is safe, effective, and efficient neoadjuvant treatment for muscle-invasive bladder cancer: results of a multicenter phase II study with molecular correlates of response and toxicity. J Clin Oncol. 2014;32(18):1895–901.
15. Choueiri TK, Jacobus S, Bellmunt J, Qu A, Appleman LJ, Tretter C, et al. Neoadjuvant dose-dense methotrexate, vinblastine, doxorubicin, and cisplatin with pegfilgrastim support in muscle-invasive urothelial cancer: pathologic, radiologic, and biomarker correlates. J Clin Oncol. 2014;32(18):1889–94.
16. der Maase H, Hansen SW, Roberts JT, Dogliotti L, Oliver T, Moore MJ, et al. Gemcitabine and cisplatin versus methotrexate, vinblastine, doxorubicin, and cisplatin in advanced or metastatic bladder cancer: results of a large, randomized, multinational, multicenter, phase III study. J Clin Oncol. 2000;17(17):3068–77.
17. Von der Maase H, Senglev L, Roberts JT, Ricci S, Dogliotti L, Oliver T. Long-term survival results of a randomized trial comparing gemcitabine plus cisplatin, with methotrexate, vinblastine, doxorubicin, plus cisplatin in patient with bladder cancer. J Clin Oncol. 2005;23(21):4602–8.
18. Dash A, Pettus JA, Herr H, Bochner BH, Dalbagani G, Donat SM, et al. A role for neoadjuvant gemcitabine plus cisplatin in muscle-invasive urothelial carcinoma of the bladder: a retrospective experience. Cancer. 2008;113(9):2471–7.
19. Hussain SA, Stocken DD, Riley P, Palmer DH, Peake DR, Geh JI, et al. A phase I/II study of gemcitabine and fractionated cisplatin in an outpatient setting using a 21-day schedule in patients with advanced and metastatic bladder cancer. Br J Cancer. 2004;91(5):844–9.
20. Anari F, O'Neill J, Choi W, Chen D, Haseebuddin M, Kutikov A, et al. Neoadjuvant dose-dense gemcitabine and cisplatin in muscle-invasive bladder cancer: results of a phase II trial. Eur Urol Oncol. 2018;1(1):54–60.
21. Iyer G, Balar AV, Milowsky MI, Bochner BH, Dalbagni G, Donat SM, et al. Multicenter prospective phase II trial of neoadjuvant dose-dense gemcitabine plus cisplatin in patient with muscle-invasive bladder cancer. J Clin Oncol. 2018;36(19):1949–56.

22. Powles T, Rodriguez-Vida A, Duran I, Crabb SJ, van Der Heijden M, Pous A, et al. A phase II study investigating the safety and efficacy of neoadjuvant atezolizumab in muscle invasive bladder cancer (ABACUS) [abstract]. J Clin Oncol. 2018;36 Suppl 15:4506.
23. Necchi A, Anichini A, Raggi D, Briganti A, Massa S, Luciano R, et al. Pembrolizumab as a neoadjuvant therapy before radical cystectomy in patients with muscle-invasive urothelial bladder carcinoma (PURE-01): an open-label, single-arm, phase II study. J Clin Oncol. 2018;36(34):3353–63.
24. Hoimes C. Neoadjuvant therapy with pembrolizumab alone or in combination with cisplatin plus gemcitabine for locally advanced urothelial cancer, a phase 1b/2 study. Proceedings of the European Society for Medical Oncology Congress; 2018 Oct 19–23; Munich, Germany.
25. Tyler A, Profusek P. Bladder cancer. In: Yarboro CH, Wujcik D, Gobel BH, editors. Cancer nursing: principles and practice. Burlington: Jones & Bartlett; 2018. p. 1227–42.
26. Tortorice PV. Cytotoxic chemotherapy: principles of therapy. In: Yarboro CH, Wujcik D, Gobel BH, editors. Cancer nursing: principles and practice. Burlington: Jones & Bartlett; 2018. p. 375–416.
27. Floyd JD, Perry MC. Cardiotoxicity of cancer therapy: antitumor antibiotics. In: Perry MC, Doll DC, Freter CE, editors. Perry's: the chemotherapy sourcebook. Philadelphia: Lippincott, Williams & Wilkins; 2012. p. 194–6.
28. Witjes JA, Comperat E, Cowan NC, De Santis M, Gakis G, Lebret T, et al. EAU guidelines on muscle-invasive and metastatic bladder cancer: summary of the 2013 guidelines. Eur Urol. 2014;65(4):778–92.
29. Chang SS, Bochner BH, Chou R, Dreicer R, Kamat AM, Lerner SP. Treatment of non-metastatic muscle-invasive bladder cancer: AUA/ASCO/ASTRO/SUO guideline. [Internet]. American Urological Association [Cited 2019 Feb 7]. Available from https://www.auanot.org/guidelines/bladder-cancer-non-metastatic-muscle-invasive-(2017).
30. Bekelman JE, Handorf EA, Guzzo T, Pollack E, Christodouleas J, Resnick MJ, et al. Radical cystectomy versus bladder-preserving therapy for muscle-invasive urothelial carcinoma: examining confounding and misclassification bias in cancer observational comparative effectiveness research. Value Health. 2013;16(4):610–8.
31. Leissner J, Ghoneim MA, Abol-Enein H, Thuroff JW, Franzaring L, Fisch M, et al. Extended radical lymphadenectomy in patient with urothelial bladder cancer: results of a prospective multicenter study. J Urol. 2004;171(1):139–44.
32. Gschwend JE, Heck MM, Lehmann J, Rubben H, Albers P, Wolff JM, et al. Extended versus limited lymph node dissection in bladder cancer patients undergoing radical cystectomy: survival results from a prospective, randomized trial. Eur Urol. 2019;75(4):604–11.
33. Schoenberg MP, Walsh PC, Breazeale DR, Marshall FF, Mostwin JL, Brendler CB. Local recurrence and survival following nerve sparing radical cystoprostatectomy for bladder cancer: 10-year follow up. J Urol. 1996;155:490–4.
34. Jacobs BL, Daignault S, Lee CT, Hafez KS, Montgomery JS, Montie JE, et al. Prostate capsule sparing versus nerve sparing radical cystectomy for bladder cancer: a randomized, controlled trial. J Urol. 2015;193(1):64–70.
35. Bhatta DN, Kessler TM, Mills RD, Burkhard F, Studer UE. Nerve-sparing radical cystectomy and orthotopic bladder replacement in female patients. Eur Urol. 2007;52(4):1006–114.
36. Yuh B, Wilson T, Bochner B, Chan K, Palou J, Stenzl A, et al. Systemic review and cumulative analysis of oncologic and functional outcomes after robotic-assisted radical cystectomy. Eur Urol. 2015;67(3):402–22.
37. Bochner BH, Dalbagni G, Sjoberg DD, Silberstein J, Keren Paz G, Donat M, et al. Comparing open radical cystectomy and robot-assisted laparoscopic radical cystectomy: a randomized clinical trial. Eur Urol. 2015;67:1042–50.
38. Parekh DJ, Reis IM, Castle EP, Gonzalgo ML, Woods ME, Svatek RS, et al. Robot-assisted radical cystectomy versus open radical cystectomy in patients with bladder cancer (RAZOR): an open-label, randomized, phase 3, non-inferiority trial. Lancet. 2018;391(10139):2525–36.

39. Overstreet D, Sims T. Care of the patient undergoing radical cystectomy with a robotic approach. Urol Nurs. 2006;26(2):117–22.
40. Crivelli JJ, Xylinas E, Kluth LA, Rieken M, Rink M, Shariat SF. Effect of smoking on outcomes of urothelial carcinoma: a systemic review of the literature. Eur Urol. 2014;65(4):742–54.
41. Gregg JR, Cookson MS, Phillips S, Salem S, Chang SS, Clark PE. Effect of preoperative nutritional deficiency on mortality after radical cystectomy for bladder cancer. J Urol. 2011;185(1):90–6.
42. Chang SS, Baumgartner RG, Wells N, Cookson MS, Smith JA Jr. Causes of increased hospital stay after radical cystectomy in a clinical pathway setting. J Urol. 2002;167(1):208–11.
43. Maffezzini M, Campodonico F, Canepa G, Parodi D. Current perioperative management of radical cystectomy with intestinal urinary reconstruction for muscle-invasive bladder cancer and reduction of the incidence of postoperative ileus. Surg Oncol. 2008;17(1):41–8.
44. Forrest JB, Clemens JQ, Finamore P, Leveillee R, Lippert M, Pisters L, et al. AUA best practice statement for the prevention of deep vein thrombosis in patients undergoing urologic surgery. J Urol. 2009;181(3):1170–7.
45. Rasmussen MS, Jorgensen LN, Willie-Jorgensen P. Prolonged thromboprophylaxis with low molecular weight heparin for abdominal or pelvic surgery. Cochrane Database Syst Rev. 2009;1:CD004318.
46. Spencer ES, Lyons MD, Pruthi RS. Patient selection and counseling for urinary diversions. Urol Clin N Am. 2018;24:1–9.
47. Lee RK, Abol-Enein H, Artibani W, Bochner B, Dalbagni G, Daneshmand S, et al. Urinary diversion after radical cystectomy for bladder cancer: options, patient selection, and outcomes. BJU Int. 2014;113:11–23.
48. Kouba E, Sands M, Lentz A, Wallen E, Pruthi RS. Incidence and risk factors of stomal complications in patients undergoing cystectomy with ileal conduit urinary diversion for bladder cancer. J Urol. 2007;178(3 Pt 1):950–4.
49. Farnham SB, Crookson MS. Surgical complications of urinary diversion. World J Urol. 2004;22(3):157–67.
50. Donahue TF, Bochner BH, Sfakinos JP, Kent M, Bernstein M, Hilton WH, et al. Risk factors for the development of parastomal hernia after radical cystectomy. J Urol. 2014;191(6):1708–13.
51. Mills RD, Studer UE. Metabolic consequences of continent urinary diversion. J Urol. 1999;161:1057–66.
52. Gore JL, Saigal CS, Hanley JM, Schonlau M, Litwin MS. Variations in reconstruction after radical cystectomy. Cancer. 2006;107(4):729–37.
53. Clark PE, Stern JP, Groshen SG, Cai J, Miranda G, Lieskovsky G, et al. Radical cystectomy in the elderly: comparison of clinical outcomes between younger and older patients. Cancer. 2005;104(1):36–43.
54. Skinner E, Daneshmand S. Orthotopic urinary diversion. In: Wein AJ, Kavoussi LR, Partin AW, editors. Campbell-Walsh urology. Philadelphia: Elsevier; 2016. p. 2344–86.
55. Steers WD. Voiding dysfunction in the orthotopic neobladder. World J Urol. 2000;18:330–7.
56. Chang DTS, Lawrentschuk N. Orthotopic neobladder reconstruction. Urol Ann. 2015;7(1):1–7.
57. Herdiman O, Ong K, Johnson L, Lawrentschuk N. Orthotopic bladder substitution (neobladder): part II: postoperative complications, management and long term follow up. J Wound Ostomy Continence Nurs. 2013;40:171–80.
58. Bihrle R. The Indiana pouch continent urinary reservoir. Urol Clin North Am. 1997;24(4):773–9.
59. Ghosh A, Somani BK. Recent trends in post cystectomy health-related quality of life (qol) favors neobladder diversion: systemic review of the literature. Urology. 2016;93:22–6.
60. Mohamed NE, Choaprang HP, Hudson S, Revenson TA, Lee CT, Quale DZ, et al. Muscle invasive bladder cancer: examining survivors' burden and unmet needs. J Urol. 2014;191(1):48–53.

# Chapter 15
# Chemoradiation Bladder Preservation

**Adele Marie Caruso and Thomas Joseph Guzzo**

## Indications and Mechanisms

Bladder cancer is the ninth most common cancer in the world [1]. In the United States, it is estimated that there will be 81,400 new bladder cancer cases and an estimated 17,980 cancer-specific deaths [2]. Twenty to 30% of these individuals will have muscle-invasive bladder cancer (MIBC). The survival rate at 5 years approaches zero when muscle-invasive disease is left untreated [3].

Chemoradiation is a potential treatment option for muscle-invasive bladder cancer for low-volume focal disease or limited disease, those individuals who desire bladder preservation, or those who are medically unfit for cystectomy. Ideal candidates are patients with an organ-confined solitary tumor, therefore without multifocal disease, or carcinoma in situ, hydronephrosis, or mixed histology [4]. Renal function is also a consideration as part of the selection criteria and choice of chemotherapy regimens as the prevalence of renal insufficiency is high in this patient population.

Trimodal therapy (TMT) is the most supported chemoradiation bladder preservation approach. In the setting of TMT, chemotherapy is administered concurrently with radiation therapy (RT) as a radiosensitizer. Long-term outcomes of the BC2001 phase III trial have shown that MIBC patients treated with radiation plus concurrent 5FU + mitomycin had higher cancer-specific survival, locoregional disease control, and lower rate of salvage cystectomy compared to those treated with RT alone with a median follow-up of 18 months [5–7]. There is no level 1 evidence comparing radiosensitizing chemotherapy agents. Most of the clinical trials have used either

A. M. Caruso (✉) · T. J. Guzzo
Urology Division, Department of Surgery, University of Pennsylvania,
Philadelphia, PA, USA
e-mail: Adele.caruso@pennmedicine.upenn.edu; Thomas.guzzo@pennmedicine.upenn.edu



E. J. Trabulsi et al. (eds.), *Chemotherapy and Immunotherapy in Urologic Oncology*, https://doi.org/10.1007/978-3-030-52021-2_15

cisplatin alone or in combination with 5FU and mitomycin or paclitaxel [8]. Gemcitabine is well tolerated and also associated with good oncologic outcomes. Gemcitabine is useful when nephrotoxicity is a concern and patients do not have adequate renal function to receive cisplatin safely. Overall, cisplatin, gemcitabine, and 5-FU/mitomycin are effective options as radiosensitizers in patients treated with TMT.

RT alone, although seldom used as a single modality option, may play a curative role in patients who are frail and with multiple comorbidities which preclude the use of chemotherapy.

In selected patients, transurethral resection of bladder tumor (TURBT) alone is capable of curing some invasive bladder tumors [9]. Chemotherapy alone for those who have not gone on to cystectomy due to other comorbidities or by patient choice has shown that a percentage of these individuals can achieve P0 status. The durability of this effect is still uncertain [10].

Patient selection for TMT eligibility constitutes two groups: those that are the ideal TMT patient and the non-ideal TMT patient. The ideal TMT candidate is defined as one who has T2N0M0 cancer, underwent a visibly complete TURBT, has a unifocal tumor, is without hydronephrosis or carcinoma in situ (CIS), and has good baseline bladder function. A non-ideal TMT candidate is defined as one who has T3-T4a, N0M0 cancer, has diffuse multifocal disease, and has hydronephrosis and CIS. Variant histology (other than urothelial cell carcinoma) has not been associated with response to TMT or survival [11].

Two strategies for TMT include a continuous course of trimodal treatment, generally the method of choice, and a split course of trimodal treatment. The continuous strategy employs a maximal safe TURBT followed by continuous radiation therapy and cystoscopic evaluation with biopsy performed at 6 months after the completion of therapy to allow time for and assess adequate response. The split course approach was developed within the Radiation Therapy Oncology Group (RTOG) and involves a maximal safe TURBT, induction chemoradiotherapy, radiation to 40Gy, mid-treatment restaging, and ultimately consolidation chemoradiotherapy to 64Gy [12].

Complications of bladder preservation regimens or TMT include adverse effects from radiation therapy as related to urinary, bowel, and sexual function. Acute genitourinary and gastrointestinal toxicity can occur in 30–40% of patients. However, many of these symptoms resolve within a few months in most patients [13].

Patients who receive TMT and experience recurrent or persistent MIBC should proceed to salvage cystectomy. Salvage cystectomy is reserved for patients that fail TMT or those with greater than or equal to T1 recurrence post-treatment. In these cases, neobladder reconstruction is generally avoided due to technical difficulties and an increase in functional complications. The data is less clear for non-muscle-invasive recurrence. Patients may be treated in the usual fashion with intravesical therapies reserved for that stage of the disease.

## *Quality of Life*

Maintenance of bladder function and the goal of treatment response is key in choosing a management strategy. TMT is an alternative to mitigate bladder cancer undertreatment [14]. Often, those patients with ≥T2 disease only undergo repeat TURBT. While effective for low-volume disease, it is palliative in most cases. Additionally, for those patients suited for TMT, it allows for adequate therapy while avoiding the complications associated with cystectomy. The benefit of this alternative to surgery is maintaining a functional genitourinary system with better urinary and sexual quality of life (QOL). Preservation of QOL is often a motivating factor for patients in choosing TMT.

## Algorithms

See Fig. 15.1. Algorithm for Trimodal Therapy – Continuous Course.
See Fig. 15.2. Algorithm for Trimodal Therapy – Follow up.

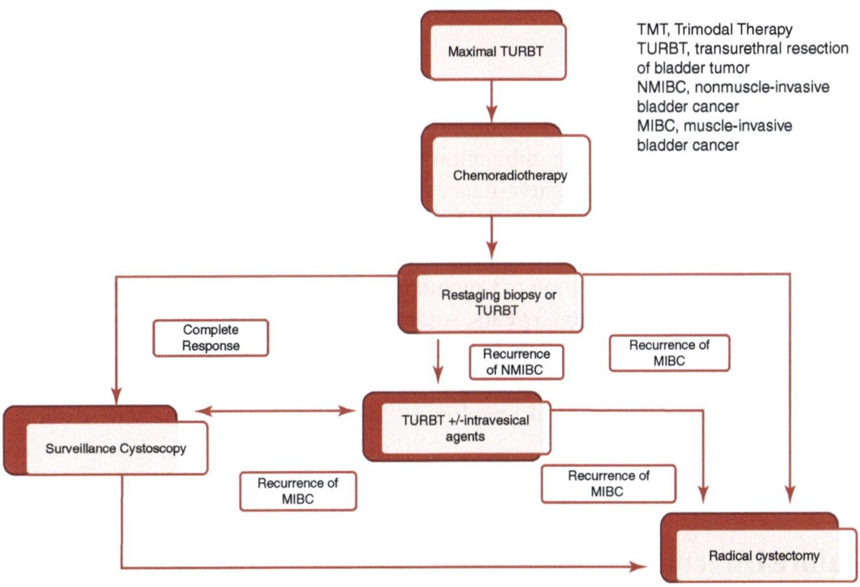


**Fig. 15.1** Algorithm for Trimodal Therapy – Continuous Course

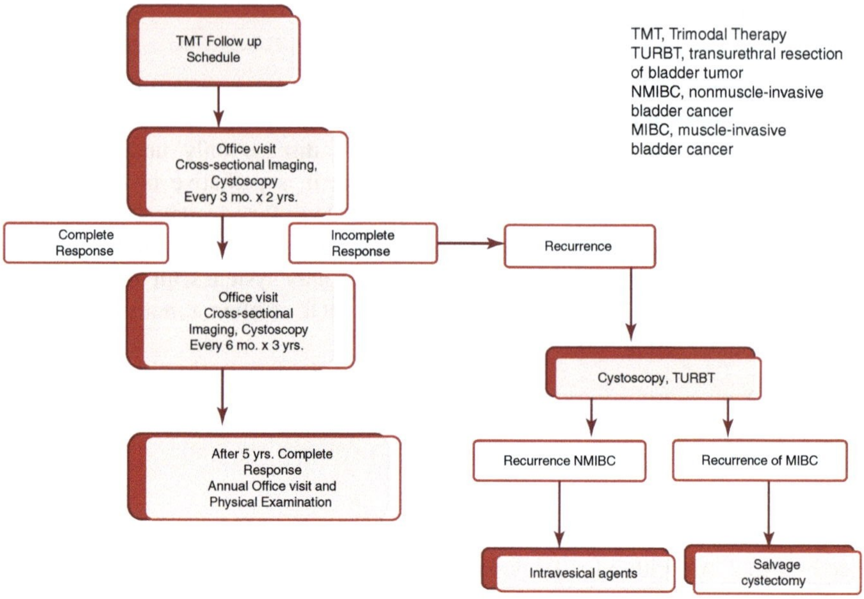


**Fig. 15.2** Algorithm for Trimodal Therapy – Follow up

## Survivorship

Survivorship encompasses a combination of established guidelines and a personalized plan. Additionally, close surveillance of the upper tracts and bladder is required. There is the also burden of recurrent disease and also that of bladder dysfunction. The surveillance pathway involves regular clinic visits, cross-sectional imaging, and cystoscopic examination on a 3-month basis for the first 2 years and then on a 6-month schedule for the next 3 years, sometimes a negotiation with the patient. At the end of 5 years, an annual clinic visit with physical examination is recommended [15]. Survivorship care is managed collaboratively by the genitourinary disciplines inclusive of urologists, medical oncologists, radiation oncologists, and advanced practice providers.

## Future Directions

Currently, there are no established tumor markers for radio responsiveness. As they emerge, they may provide some insight in selecting patients for TMT. Checkpoint inhibitors are a new approach in the treatment of genitourinary cancers. The use of checkpoint inhibitors is being readily incorporated in the treatment of metastatic bladder cancer as second-line therapies and for platinum-ineligible patients. Future trials are anticipated to evaluate TMT with immune checkpoint inhibition.

**Clinical Pearls**

- Chemoradiation is a potential treatment option for muscle-invasive bladder cancer for low-volume focal disease or limited disease, those individuals who desire bladder preservation, or those who are medically unfit for cystectomy.
- Ideal candidates for bladder preservation are patients with an organ-confined solitary tumor, therefore without multifocal disease, or carcinoma in situ, hydronephrosis, or mixed histology.
- Trimodal therapy (TMT) is the most supported chemoradiation bladder preservation approach.
- In the setting of TMT, chemotherapy is administered concurrently with radiation therapy (RT) as a radiosensitizer.
- Cisplatin, gemcitabine, and 5-FU/mitomycin are effective options as radiosensitizers in patients treated with TMT.
- In selected patients, usually those who are very frail, radiation or transurethral resection of bladder tumor (TURBT) alone is capable of curing some invasive bladder tumors.
- The ideal TMT candidate is defined as one who has T2N0M0 cancer, underwent a visibly complete TURBT, has a unifocal tumor, is without hydronephrosis or CIS, and has good baseline bladder function.
- The continuous strategy of TMT employs a maximal safe TURBT followed by continuous radiation therapy and cystoscopic evaluation with biopsy performed at 6 months after the completion of therapy to allow time for and assess adequate response.
- Complications of bladder preservation regimens or TMT include adverse effects from radiation therapy as related to urinary, bowel, and sexual function.
- Patients who receive TMT and experience recurrent or persistent MIBC should proceed to salvage cystectomy.

## References


1. Antoni S, Ferlay J, Soejomataram I, Znaor A, Jemal A, Bray F. Bladder cancer incidence and mortality: a global overview and recent trends. Eur Urol. 2017;71(1):96–108.
2. Siegel RL, Miller KD, Jemel A. Cancer statistics, 2020. Cancer J Clin. 2020;70(1):7–30. https://doi.org/10.3322/caac.21590.
3. Prout GR, Marshall VF. The prognosis with untreated bladder tumors. Cancer. 1956;9:551–8.
4. Pietzak EJ, Sterling ME, Smith ZL, Malkowicz SB, Guzzo TJ. Outcomes of radical cystectomy in potential candidates for bladder preservation therapy. Oncology. 2015;85(4):869–75. https://doi.org/10.1016/j.urology.2015.01.001.
5. Hall E, Hussain SA, Porta N, et al. BC2011 long-term outcomes: a phase III randomized trial of chemoradiotherapy versus radiotherapy alone and standard RT versus reduced high-dose volume RT in muscle-invasive bladder cancer. J Clin Oncol. 2017;35(Suppl 6S):280.

6. James ND, et al. Radiotherapy with or without chemotherapy in muscle-invasive bladder cancer. N Engl J Med. 2012;366(16):1477–88.
7. El-Achkar A, Souhami L, Kassouf W. Bladder preservation therapy: review of literature and future directions of trimodal therapy. Curr Urol Rep. 2018;19(108):1–10. https://doi.org/10.1007/s11934-018-0859-z.
8. Ploussard G, Daneshmand S, Efstathiou JA, Herr HW, James ND, Rodel CM, et al. Critical analysis of bladder sparing with trimodal therapy in muscle-invasive bladder cancer: a systematic review. Eur Urol. 2014;66(1):120–37.
9. Herr H. Transurethral resection of muscle-invasive bladder cancer: 10-year outcome. J Clin Oncol. 2001;19(1):89–93.
10. Mazza P, Moran GW, Li G, Robins DJ, Matulay JT, Herr HW, Decastro GJ, McKiernan JM, Anderson CB. Conservative management following complete clinical response to neoadjuvant chemotherapy of muscle invasive bladder cancer: contemporary outcomes of a multi-institutional cohort study. J Urol. 2018;200(5):1005–2013. https://doi.org/10.1016/j.juro.2018.05.078.
11. Krasnow RE, Drumm M, Roberts HJ, Niemierko A, Wu CL, Wu S, et al. Clinical outcomes of patients with histologic variants of urothelial cancer treated with trimodality bladder-sparing therapy. Eur J Urol. 2017;72(1):54–60.
12. Zeitman AL, Hunt D, Kauffman DS, et al. Preliminary results of RTOG 0233: a phase II randomized trial for muscle-invading bladder cancer treated by transurethral resection and radiotherapy comparing two forms of concurrent induction chemotherapy. Int J Radiat Oncol Biol Phys. 2010;78(3Suppl):S31–2.
13. Mirza A, Choudhury A. Bladder preservation for muscle invasive bladder cancer. Bladder Cancer. 2016;2:151–63. https://doi.org/10.3233/BLC-150025.
14. Cahn DB, Ristau BT, Ghiraldi EM, Churilla TM, Geynisman DM, Horwitz EM, Uzzo RG, Smaldone MC. Bladder preservation therapy: a review of the literature and future directions. Urology. 2016;96:54–61. https://doi.org/10.1016/j.urology.2016.05.041.
15. Smith Z, Christoudouleas JP, Keefe SM, Malkowicz SB, Guzzo TJ. Bladder preservation in the treatment of muscle-invasive bladder cancer (MIBC): a review of the literature and a practical approach to therapy. BJU Int. 2013;112:13–25. https://doi.org/10.1111/j.1464-410X.2012 11762.x.

# Chapter 16
# Metastatic Bladder Cancer and the Use of Cisplatin Chemotherapy

**Patrick Mille and Janice Carsello**

## Introduction

Bladder cancer accounted for 4.6% of all cancer diagnoses and 2.9% of cancer-related deaths in the United States in 2019. Approximately 2.4% of men and women will be diagnosed with bladder cancer during their lifetime [1]. While only 5% of new bladder cancer patients present with metastatic disease at the time of diagnosis, nearly 25% will develop locally advanced or metastatic disease during the course of their illness. Without treatment, patients with metastatic bladder cancer (MBC) have a life expectancy of approximately 3–6 months [2]. The last decade has seen rapid development of new treatment options for these patients. This expanded arsenal now includes FDA-approved checkpoint inhibitors, fibroblast growth factor receptor inhibitors, and antibody-drug conjugates. However, multidrug cisplatin-containing regimens remain the preferred first-line treatment option.

## Diagnosis/Initial Evaluation

The initial evaluation for locally advanced and/or metastatic bladder cancer requires collaboration between a multidisciplinary team comprised of specialists in urology, medical oncology, radiation oncology, pathology, and radiology [3]. Tissue must be obtained via cystoscopy or biopsy of a metastatic site. This serves to confirm the diagnosis and to provide tissue for molecular, genomic, and programmed death-ligand 1 (PD-L1) characterization, which is increasingly important in guiding therapy. Initial imaging should include contrast-enhanced chest and abdominal and

P. Mille (✉) · J. Carsello
Department of Medical Oncology, Thomas Jefferson University, Philadelphia, PA, USA
e-mail: Patrick.mille@jefferson.edu; Janice.carsello@jefferson.edu



E. J. Trabulsi et al. (eds.), *Chemotherapy and Immunotherapy in Urologic Oncology*, https://doi.org/10.1007/978-3-030-52021-2_16

pelvic computed tomography (CT) or magnetic resonance imaging (MRI) if there is renal compromise. A nuclear medicine bone scan should be considered for those patients with elevated alkaline phosphatase or bony pain. A neurological history and examination should also be performed and neuro-imaging considered if any neurologic symptom is identified. The initial imaging evaluation allows for accurate staging and documents baseline index lesions that can subsequently be followed to assess treatment response.

## Treatment Selection

Although cisplatin-containing regimens are our preferred first-line treatment, selecting the patients most likely to benefit from their use has remained a challenge. A 2011 consensus statement by Gaslky et al. remains the standard used to identify cisplatin-eligible patients [4]. These criteria, which are applied in clinical trial design and in clinical practice, require a thorough evaluation of medical comorbidities, determination of the patient's functional performance status, assessment of renal function, and presence of pretreatment neuropathy and hearing loss. Patients are deemed ineligible for cisplatin-based chemotherapy if one or more of the criteria listed in Table 16.1 are met.

Using the above criteria, as many as 50% of patients with MBC are considered cisplatin ineligible [5, 6]. Eligible patients should receive multidrug cisplatin-based chemotherapy as the standard approach [1, 3, 7]. While numerous cisplatin-containing regimens have been evaluated, two have become established as preferred first-line options (Table 16.2) [2, 8].

## Treatment-Related Toxicities

Chemotherapeutic agents primarily exert their anticancer effects by disrupting cancer cells' cellular division machinery. It is the increased rate of replication and rapid division in cancer cells that make them more susceptible to chemotherapy than normal tissue. However, the cellular machinery of rapidly dividing cells in healthy

**Table 16.1** Criteria for determining ineligibility for cisplatin-based treatment

| |
|---|
| Eastern Cooperative Oncology Group (ECOG) performance status of 2 or Karnofsky Performance Status of 60–70% |
| Creatinine clearance (calculated or measured) <60 ml/min |
| Common Terminology Criteria for Adverse Events (CTCAE) Gr ≥2 audiometric hearing loss |
| CTCAE Gr ≥2 peripheral neuropathy |
| New York Heart Association class III heart failure |

Galsky et al. [5]

**Table 16.2** Systemic therapy for metastatic bladder cancer

| Regimen | Schedule |
|---|---|
| Gemcitabine and cisplatin | Days 1, 8, and 15: Gemcitabine<br>Day 2: Cisplatin<br>Repeat every 4 weeks for a maximum of 6 cycles |
| DDMVAC with growth factor support | Day 1: Methotrexate<br>Day 2: Vinblastine + Adriamycin + cisplatin<br>Day 4: G-CSF[a] daily for 7 consecutive days (days 4–10)<br>Repeat cycle every 2 weeks for 6 cycles<br>*OR*<br>Day 1: Methotrexate<br>Day 2: Vinblastine + adriamycin + cisplatin<br>Day 3: G-CSF[a] daily for 5 consecutive days (days 3–7)<br>Repeat cycle every 15 days for 6 cycles |

[a]Granulocyte-colony-stimulating factor is used to prevent or mitigate neutropenia

tissue (e.g., bone marrow, epithelial lining) may be similarly affected. Toxicities commonly seen with cisplatin-containing regimens include myelosuppression (e.g., anemia, thrombocytopenia, leukopenia), renal failure, neurotoxicity, gastrointestinal side effects (mucositis, nausea, vomiting), and hearing loss and are detailed in Table 16.3.

Chemotherapy-induced cytopenias are frequently encountered during treatment with multidrug cisplatin-containing regimens. Patients should have a complete blood count (CBC) prior to each therapeutic cycle. Clinical exam should focus on signs of infection, severe anemia, and signs of bleeding or bruising. Dose modifications or therapy delays are indicated if patients experience significant myelosuppression. Growth factor can be used at the discretion of the ordering clinician, although it is required with DDMVAC as rates of neutropenia exceed 20% [10]. Transfusion support with platelets and packed red blood cells may also be needed. Vigilance for rare but serious hematologic complications such as thrombotic thrombocytopenic purpura or hemolytic-uremic syndrome is important, as these can be seen in patients receiving gemcitabine. These conditions manifest with microangiopathic hemolytic anemia and renal dysfunction. With close surveillance of blood counts, most patients are able to safely complete chemotherapy. Patients who are receiving chemotherapy should be counseled to seek immediate evaluation for any concerning symptom, including temperature greater than 100.4 °F, rigors, bleeding, or unexplained bruising.

Cisplatin-related nephrotoxicity is a well-described multifactorial phenomenon. Cisplatin can cause tubular injury, thrombotic microangiopathy, distal renal tubular acidosis, and most commonly electrolyte wasting (hypomagnesemia). Patients receiving cisplatin require serial serum creatinine and electrolyte measurements. Adequate pre- and post-hydration are essential to reduce rates of nephrotoxicity. Electrolyte replacement with oral or intravenous agents should be used judiciously. Dose modifications or treatment delays are essential to preventing permanent damage if a change in renal function is identified. Patients should additionally be

**Table 16.3** Commonly occurring MBC chemotherapy treatment toxicities [9]

| Adverse event | Grade 1 | Grade 2 | Grade 3 | Grade 4 | Grade 5 |
|---|---|---|---|---|---|
| Anorexia | Loss of appetite without alteration in eating habits | Oral intake altered without significant weight loss or malnutrition; oral nutritional supplements indicated | Associated with significant weight loss or malnutrition (e.g., inadequate oral caloric and/or fluid intake); IV fluids, tube feedings or TPN indicated | Life-threatening consequences | Death |
| Constipation | Occasional or intermittent symptoms; occasional use of stool softeners, laxatives, dietary modification, or enema | Persistent symptoms with regular use of laxatives or enemas as indicated | Symptoms interfering with ADL; obstipation with manual evacuation indicated | Life-threatening consequences (e.g., obstruction, toxic megacolon) | Death |
| Diarrhea | Increase of <4 stools per day over baseline; mild increase in ostomy output compared to baseline | Increase of 4–6 stools per day over baseline; IV fluids indicated <24 hours; moderate increase in ostomy output compared to baseline; not interfering with ADL | ≥7 or more stools per day over baseline; incontinence; IV fluids ≥24 hours; hospitalization; severe increase in ostomy output compared to baseline; interfering with ADL | Life-threatening consequences (e.g., hemodynamic collapse) | |
| Fatigue (asthenia, lethargy, malaise) | Mild fatigue over baseline | Moderate or causing difficulty performing some ADL | Severe fatigue interfering with ADL | Disabling | -- |
| Hearing | – | Hearing loss not requiring hearing aid or intervention (i.e., not interfering with ADL) | Hearing loss requiring hearing aid or intervention (i.e., interfering with ADL) | Profound bilateral hearing loss (>90 dB) | -- |

**Table 16.3** (continued)

| Adverse event | Grade 1 | Grade 2 | Grade 3 | Grade 4 | Grade 5 |
|---|---|---|---|---|---|
| Nausea | Loss of appetite without alteration in eating habits | Oral intake decreased without significant weight loss, dehydration, or malnutrition; IV fluids indicated | Inadequate oral caloric or fluid intake; IV fluids, tube feedings, or TPN indicated | Life-threatening consequences | Death |
| Sensory neuropathy (CIPN) | Asymptomatic: loss of deep tendon reflexes or paresthesia (including tingling) but not interfering with function | Sensory alteration or paresthesia (including tingling), interfering with function but not interfering with activities of daily living | Sensory alteration or paresthesia interfering with activities of daily living | Disabling | Death |
| Vomiting | 1 episode in 24 hours | 2–5 episodes in 24 hours; IV fluids indicated | ≥6 episodes in 24 hours; IV fluids or TPN indicated | Life-threatening consequences | Death |

counseled to avoid nephrotoxic agents like nonsteroidal anti-inflammatory drugs (NSAIDs) [11].

Chemotherapy-induced peripheral neuropathy (CIPN) is common and can have a profound impact on quality of life and survivorship [12]. Cisplatin is among the agents with the highest prevalence of CIPN, reported to be as high as 68%, and its occurrence is dose dependent and cumulative [13]. CIPN has a distinct pattern of symmetrical peripheral neuropathy in the hands and feet known as the "stocking and glove distribution" [14]. Symptoms are generally sensory with preserved motor function and typically improve with discontinuation of therapy. Cisplatin-related CIPN may develop weeks after therapy and may persist for months after chemotherapy has been discontinued. Though most patients see an improvement in symptoms, recovery from cisplatin-induced CIPN is often incomplete. Physical therapy and rehabilitation can improve posture and balance. Pharmacologic treatment using duloxetine, pregabalin, or gabapentin is endorsed by the American Society of Clinical Oncology, but effectiveness is limited [14]. Appropriate assessment and prompt recognition are critical to mitigating long-term neurotoxicity. Additionally, oncologic outcomes may be impacted by dose reductions or premature discontinuation of treatment [15]. Treatment plan changes are always made after comprehensively weighing the risks of treatment-mediated side effects against the benefits of continuing to administer the cytotoxic agent.

Cisplatin is highly emetogenic. Proactive antiemetic support including premedication with steroids (e.g., dexamethasone), serotonin receptor antagonist (e.g., ondansetron), and neurokinin-1 receptor antagonist (e.g., aprepitant) is recommended to ensure tolerability of the regimen [16]. Oral antiemetics (e.g., ondansetron, prochlorperazine) should be empirically prescribed. Furthermore, patients are encouraged to promptly report symptoms that do not respond to oral agents as rehydration and intravenous antiemetic support may be required.

Even with excellent control of nausea and vomiting, anorexia is a common treatment-related side effect and can be challenging to manage. MBC patients are at high risk for malnutrition because both the disease and treatment pose a threat to nutritional status [17]. Patients should be encouraged to eat small meals on a more frequent schedule. Breaking up a large meal into smaller sections and eating something every 2–3 hours is an effective way to maintain adequate caloric intake. Nutritional supplements are recommended for patients as a complement to meals and not a replacement whenever possible [13]. When severe, pharmacologic interventions are warranted.

Fatigue, asthenia, and malaise are among the most commonly reported chemotherapy treatment side effects. Psychological intervention and/or increased physical activity have a positive impact on cancer and treatment-related fatigue. Pharmacologic treatments are often ineffective and are not recommended [18].

Pretreatment physical assessment along with a comprehensive review of systems and side effects (ROSS) should occur before each chemotherapy treatment commences. Recent laboratory values should be evaluated prior to treatment. Chemotherapy doses may be reduced depending upon the results of the physical examination, ROSS, and/or laboratory test results.

## Monitoring Disease Response

Periodic surveillance imaging should be obtained at regular intervals to assess for disease response. Contrast-enhanced CT of the chest, abdomen, and pelvis and MRI with and/or without contrast for patients with renal dysfunction remain the modalities of choice. Clinical trials, second-line therapies, and best supportive care should be promptly discussed if disease progression is identified. Fortunately, there are a growing number of treatment options for patients with disease progression on a cisplatin-based regimen.

**Clinical Pearls**

- Cisplatin-based chemotherapy regimens remain the standard first-line treatment for advanced or metastatic bladder cancer.
- Identifying a patient as cisplatin eligible continues to be a challenge.
- As a general rule, cisplatin-ineligible patients are those patients who have any one or more of the following: poor performance status, poor renal function, hearing loss, existing neuropathy, and heart disease.
- Patients who are placed on a cisplatin-based chemotherapy regimen must be monitored closely for treatment-related toxicities.

# References

1. Siegel RL, Miller KD, Jemal A. Cancer statistics, 2019. CA Cancer J Clin. 2019;69(1):7–34.
2. von der Maase H, Sengelov L, Roberts JT, Ricci S, Dogliotti L, Oliver T, Moore MJ, Zimmermann A, Arning M. Long-term survival results of a randomized trial comparing gemcitabine plus cisplatin, with methotrexate, vinblastine, doxorubicin, plus cisplatin in patients with bladder cancer. J Clin Oncol. 2005;23(21):4602–8.
3. Lue TF, JW MA, editors. Smith & Tanagho's general urology. New York: McGraw-Hill Medical; 2013.
4. Galsky MD, Hahn NM, Rosenberg J, Sonpavde G, Hutson T, Oh WK, Dreicer R, Vogelzang N, Sternberg C, Bajorin DF, Bellmunt J. A consensus definition of patients with metastatic urothelial carcinoma who are unfit for cisplatin-based chemotherapy. Lancet Oncol. 2011;12(3):211–4.
5. Galsky MD, Hahn NM, Rosenberg J, Sonpavde G, Hutson T, Oh WK, Dreicer R, Vogelzang N, Sternberg CN, Bajorin DF, Bellmunt J. Treatment of patients with metastatic urothelial cancer "unfit" for cisplatin-based chemotherapy. J Clin Oncol. 2011;29(17):2432–8.
6. Bellmunt J, Mottet N, De Santis M. Urothelial carcinoma management in elderly or unfit patients. EJC Suppl. 2016;14(1):1.
7. De Santis M, Bellmunt J, Mead G, Kerst JM, Leahy M, Maroto P, Gil T, Marreaud S, Daugaard G, Skoneczna I, Collette S. Randomized phase II/III trial assessing gemcitabine/carboplatin and methotrexate/carboplatin/vinblastine in patients with advanced urothelial cancer who are unfit for cisplatin-based chemotherapy: EORTC study 30986. J Clin Oncol. 2012;30(2):191.
8. Sternberg CN, De Mulder PH, Schornagel JH, Theodore C, Fossa SD, Van Oosterom AT, Witjes F, Spina M, Van Groeningen CJ, De Balincourt C, Collette L. Randomized phase III trial of high–dose-intensity methotrexate, vinblastine, doxorubicin, and cisplatin (MVAC) chemotherapy and recombinant human granulocyte colony-stimulating factor versus classic MVAC in advanced urothelial tract tumors: European Organization for Research and Treatment of Cancer Protocol No. 30924. J Clin Oncol. 2001;19(10):2638–46.
9. Colevas AD, Setser A. The NCI common terminology criteria for adverse events (CTCAE) v 3.0 is the new standard for oncology clinical trials. J Clin Oncol. 2004;22(14_suppl):6098.
10. Crawford J, Althaus B, Armitage J, Balducci L, Bennett C, Blayney DW, Cataland SR, Dale DC, Demetri GD, Erba HP, Foran J. Myeloid growth factors: clinical practice guidelines in oncology™. JNCCN J Natl Compr Canc Netw. 2007;5(2):188–202.

11. Manohar S, Leung N. Cisplatin nephrotoxicity: a review of the literature. J Nephrol. 2018;31(1):15–25.
12. Mols F, Beijers T, Vreugdenhil G, van de Poll-Franse L. Chemotherapy-induced peripheral neuropathy and its association with quality of life: a systematic review. Support Care Cancer. 2014;22(8):2261–9.
13. Seretny M, Currie GL, Sena ES, Ramnarine S, Grant R, MacLeod MR, Colvin LA, Fallon M. Incidence, prevalence, and predictors of chemotherapy-induced peripheral neuropathy: a systematic review and meta-analysis. Pain. 2014;155(12):2461–70.
14. Hershman DL, Lacchetti C, Dworkin RH, Lavoie Smith EM, Bleeker J, Cavaletti G, Chauhan C, Gavin P, Lavino A, Lustberg MB, Paice J. Prevention and management of chemotherapy-induced peripheral neuropathy in survivors of adult cancers: American Society of Clinical Oncology clinical practice guideline. J Clin Oncol. 2014;32(18):1941–67.
15. Albers JW, Chaudhry V, Cavaletti G, Donehower RC. Interventions for preventing neuropathy caused by cisplatin and related compounds. Cochrane Database Syst Rev. 2014;3:CD005228.
16. Berger MJ, Ettinger DS, Aston J, Barbour S, Bergsbaken J, Bierman PJ, Brandt D, Dolan DE, Ellis G, Kim EJ, Kirkegaard S. NCCN guidelines insights: antiemesis, version 2.2017. J Natl Compr Cancer Netw. 2017;15(7):883–93.
17. Arends J, Baracos V, Bertz H, Bozzetti F, Calder PC, Deutz NE, Erickson N, Laviano A, Lisanti MP, Lobo DN, McMillan DC. ESPEN expert group recommendations for action against cancer-related malnutrition. Clin Nutr. 2017;36(5):1187–96.
18. Mustian KM, Alfano CM, Heckler C, Kleckner AS, Kleckner IR, Leach CR, Mohr D, Palesh OG, Peppone LJ, Piper BF, Scarpato J. Comparison of pharmaceutical, psychological, and exercise treatments for cancer-related fatigue: a meta-analysis. JAMA Oncol. 2017;3(7):961–8.

# Chapter 17
# Immunotherapy for Metastatic Urothelial Cancer

**Javaughn Corey R. Gray and Jean Hoffman-Censits**

## General Overview of Systemic Immunotherapy for Urothelial Cancer

Cancer immunotherapy aims to reinvigorate the immune system to control cancer through targeting of the immune cell-tumor cell interaction. The goal of immunotherapy is to trigger a patient's immune cells to recognize and destroy cancer cells through restoration of immune function. Ideally, tumor-reactive T cells would be generated after being stimulated by tumor antigens, and T cells would infiltrate tumor sites exhibiting cytotoxic activity to destroy cancer cells [1, 2]. There are several immunotherapy strategies being investigated to stimulate this antitumor immune response in patients. In solid tumor oncology, the most successful to date has been the use of the checkpoint inhibitors through anti-PD-1/L1 and anti-CTLA4 inhibition. Checkpoint blockade involves the use of antibodies to block the activation of immune suppressive mechanisms and enhance immune activation [3].

In urothelial cancer, humanized monoclonal antibodies to PD-1 and PD-L1 are FDA approved. These and other immunotherapy agents are currently being investigated in various disease states [4]. In normal physiology, PD-1 and PD-L1 interactions balance the immune system by preventing autoimmunity and damage to healthy tissue while allowing stimulated T cells to fight infections, viruses, and cancer. However, cancer cells can manipulate this inhibition system to their advantage. These are targets of interest because PD-1 is highly expressed by antigen-activated T cells and at the same time is often upregulated by tumor cells to counteract the immune response and suppress T cell infiltration into tumor sites. The interaction between PD-1 and PD-L1 triggers immune suppressive mechanisms

J. C. R. Gray · J. Hoffman-Censits (✉)
The Greenberg Bladder Cancer Institute, Sidney Kimmel Comprehensive Cancer Center at Johns Hopkins, Baltimore, MD, USA
e-mail: jgray51@jhmi.edu; jhoffm57@jhmi.edu



E. J. Trabulsi et al. (eds.), *Chemotherapy and Immunotherapy in Urologic Oncology*, https://doi.org/10.1007/978-3-030-52021-2_17

when T cells encounter tumor cells. In this way, PD-L1 checkpoint blockade can for some tumors interfere with tumor/immune cell interactions and thus improve anti-tumor immune responses.

# Treatment of Metastatic Urothelial Cancer with Immunotherapeutic Agents

## *Overview*

The treatment of metastatic urothelial cancer has evolved over the last several years. Systemic chemotherapy has been the standard treatment for patients initially diagnosed with unresectable or metastatic urothelial cancer. For eligible patients, based on adequate performance status, organ function, and lack of neuropathy or hearing loss, standard cisplatin-based regimens are accelerated MVAC (methotrexate, vinblastine, doxorubicin, and cisplatin) and GC (gemcitabine and cisplatin) [5, 6].

Historically, carboplatin-based chemotherapy is administered to patients that are ineligible to receive cisplatin in the first-line setting [7]. In the last few years, multiple clinical trials have been conducted to evaluate the role of immune checkpoint inhibitors in metastatic urothelial cancers that are refractory to platinum, and as a result, several new agents (Table 17.1) have been approved by the US Food and Drug Administration (FDA) for urothelial cancer.

## *First-Line Treatments in Platinum-Ineligible Patients*

Systemic cisplatin-based combination chemotherapy is the standard of care for patients with metastatic urothelial bladder cancer [7]. However, patients with chronic kidney disease with impaired renal function (GFR <50–60), Eastern Cooperative Oncology Group (ECOG) performance status of $\geq 2$, hearing loss, peripheral neuropathy, heart failure, and creatinine clearance less than 60 mL/min

**Table 17.1** Approved checkpoint inhibitors for metastatic or locally advanced urothelial carcinoma post-platinum chemotherapy

| Target | Drug | Indication |
|---|---|---|
| PD-1 | Pembrolizumab | Cisplatin-ineligible first line or progression on or post platinum therapy |
| | Nivolumab | Progression on or post platinum therapy |
| PD-L1 | Atezolizumab | Cisplatin-ineligible first line or progression on or post platinum therapy |
| | Avelumab | Progression on or post platinum therapy |
| | Durvalumab | Progression on or post platinum therapy |

are generally ineligible for cisplatin-based therapies [8]. Though cisplatin-based chemotherapy is associated with an excellent response rate, toxicity and general lack of response durability have long posed a dire need for effective treatments beyond, or as alternatives to platinum chemotherapy.

For patients with advanced urothelial cancer that are not candidates for platinum-based therapy due to comorbidities listed above, immunotherapy has been studied. The toxicity profile for immunotherapy treatments is, in general, more manageable than cisplatin in the first-line setting. Two trials demonstrated the efficacy of immunotherapy as a first-line treatment for metastatic urothelial cancer. The first was atezolizumab reported in 2016 and the second was pembrolizumab reported in 2017 [9, 10]. These trials demonstrated the significant potential of immunotherapy as a first-line treatment in metastatic urothelial bladder cancer.

## Atezolizumab

In a single-arm, multicenter phase II trial, atezolizumab was investigated as a first-line treatment in 119 patients with advanced or metastatic urothelial cancer who were ineligible for platinum-based chemotherapy due to comorbidities [10]. Eligible patients included those who met the following criteria: inoperable, locally advanced or metastatic urothelial cancer, measurable disease per RECIST v1.1, and ECOG status of 2 or less. Subjects were required to be cisplatin ineligible due to one or more of the following criteria: GFR >30 and <60 based on Cockcroft-Gault formula, grade 2 or higher hearing loss or peripheral neuropathy, or ECOG of 2.

These subjects received 1200 mg of atezolizumab every 21 days until progression and were followed up for a median of 17.2 months. The study met its primary endpoint, with an objective response rate of 23%, with complete responses being observed in 9% of patients. A median overall survival of 15.9 months is noteworthy when compared to historical data from platinum-based chemotherapy trials that have a median overall survival of 9.3 months with carboplatin [11] and 15.5 months with cisplatin [6, 12]. There were manageable adverse events experienced among the cohort, with the most common events being fatigue (30%), diarrhea (12%), pruritus (11%), and decreased appetite (9%) [10]. Additionally, high-grade (grade ≥3) adverse events were uncommon and experienced by 16% of study subjects. These findings suggest that atezolizumab was well tolerated in this population, with more manageable toxicity than historically reported with cisplatin chemotherapy. Based on these data, atezolizumab was FDA approved in the first-line setting for cisplatin-ineligible patients with metastatic urothelial cancer.

## Pembrolizumab

Pembrolizumab was studied in the first-line setting in the phase II KEYNOTE-052 study. In this study, 370 subjects with metastatic or advanced urothelial cancer, who were not eligible for a platinum-based treatment regimen, were treated with pembrolizumab [9]. Eligible patients included those with locally advanced and unresectable or metastatic urothelial cancer, no previous systemic chemotherapy for advanced disease within 12 months, and cisplatin ineligible based on one of the following criteria: ECOG ≤2, creatinine clearance 30–60 mL/min, grade ≥2 audiometric hearing loss, grade ≥2 peripheral neuropathy, or New York Heart Association Class III heart failure.

These subjects received pembrolizumab 200 mg every 21 days until progression or for up to 2 years and were followed for a median of 5 months following completion. The objective response rate for the entire cohort was 29%, with 7% experiencing complete responses. As with the first-line atezolizumab study, modest adverse events were reported. Sixty-two percent of patients experienced a treatment-related adverse event, and 16% were high grade. The most common adverse events were fatigue (15%), pruritus (14%), rash (9%), decreased appetite (8%), diarrhea (7%), and nausea (7%). The most common high-grade adverse events (grade 3 or higher) were decreased appetite (<1%), fatigue (2%), alkaline phosphatase increase (1%), colitis (1%), and muscle weakness (1%). These findings indicated that pembrolizumab was well tolerated in the platinum-ineligible patient population and ultimately led to the approval of pembrolizumab as a frontline agent in the cisplatin-ineligible population.

In August 2018, the FDA updated its label for the first-line use of atezolizumab and pembrolizumab in urothelial cancer. In addition to approving companion diagnostic tests to assay PD-L1 tumor status, the FDA recommended that for cisplatin-ineligible but chemotherapy-eligible (carboplatin) patients, chemotherapy sequenced prior to checkpoint should be considered for patients with PD-L1 low tumors. This label change reminds clinicians that although carboplatin as a first-line agent has an inferior response rate compared to cisplatin, carboplatin chemotherapy remains active and may be suitable for some patients who are not cisplatin eligible. Furthermore, the label change indicated that for patients who were not chemotherapy eligible at all (the parameters for which were not defined), with low or undefined PD-L1 tumor status, immunotherapy remains a standard first-line option [13]. Gupta and colleagues recently presented a consensus recommendation on ineligibility to platinum/chemotherapy at GU ASCO 2019 to better define this population.

This change in label was based on interim data safety monitoring committee analyses of two ongoing phase III trials comparing frontline chemotherapy, chemotherapy plus immunotherapy (atezolizumab or pembrolizumab), and immunotherapy alone. In these trials, KEYNOTE-361 and IMvigor130, cisplatin-eligible patients in the immunotherapy alone arms whose tumors had low PD-L1 expression had inferior survival outcomes compared to patients in the chemotherapy alone arms. Thus, enrollment of cisplatin-eligible patients to the immunotherapy-alone arms with low tumor PD-L1 expression was halted.

## *Second-Line Treatments in Patients with Disease Progression Post-platinum*

### Pembrolizumab

KEYNOTE-045 is the only randomized phase III trial which demonstrates that immunotherapy is superior to second-line chemotherapy in patients who progressed after platinum-based chemotherapy. Patients were deemed eligible for this study if they met the following criteria: confirmed urothelial carcinoma of the renal pelvis, ureter, bladder, or urethra that exhibited predominantly transitional-cell features; progression after platinum-based chemotherapy for advanced disease or recurrence within 12 months after receiving platinum-based adjuvant or neoadjuvant therapy; received two or less lines of systemic chemotherapy; had at least one measurable lesion per RECIST v1.1; and had tumor samples that could be evaluated for PD-L1 expression.

In this study of 542 subjects, 270 were randomized to the pembrolizumab arm and 272 were randomized to an investigator-choice chemotherapy arm (docetaxel, paclitaxel, or vinflunine) [14]. Subjects in the pembrolizumab arm received 200 mg every 3 weeks for up to 2 years, while those in the chemotherapy arm received investigator's choice of chemotherapy with paclitaxel, docetaxel, or vinflunine. Overall survival on the pembrolizumab arm was significantly longer compared to the chemotherapy arm, with a median overall survival of 10.3 months versus 7.4 months (HR for death, 0.73; 95% CI, 0.59–0.91; $p$=0.002). Subjects that received pembrolizumab had higher objective response rates 21.1% versus 11.4% for chemotherapy.

In this study, PD-L1 expression was characterized as a PD-L1 combined positive score (CPS), which was defined as the percentage of PD-L1 expressing tumor and infiltrating immune cells relative to the total number of tumor cells. In patients with tumor CPS ≥10%, the pembrolizumab group had significantly longer overall survival compared to the chemotherapy arm (hazard ratio for death, 0.57; 95% CI, 0.37–0.88; $p$=0.005). Survival benefit of pembrolizumab over chemotherapy was also seen in those with low CPS, as well as with visceral disease. Patients in this study had no significant between-group difference in the duration of progression-free survival among patients who had a tumor PD-L1 combined positive score of 10% or more (hazard ratio for disease progression or death, 0.89; 95% CI, 0.61–1.28; $p$=0.24). Though the median time to response (2.1 months) was similar, overall objective response was higher in the pembrolizumab arm compared to the chemotherapy arm.

Consistent with other pembrolizumab studies, treatment-related high-grade adverse events were uncommon [14]. Grade ≥3 treatment-related adverse events were seen in 15% of patients in the pembrolizumab arm compared to 49.4% in the chemotherapy arm. Notably, health-related quality of life was either stable or improved in those subjects who received pembrolizumab, compared to a decline seen in those assigned to chemotherapy [15].

### Atezolizumab

In the phase II, single-arm IMvigor210 study reported by Rosenberg et al., atezolizumab was tested in subjects with inoperable locally advanced or metastatic urothelial carcinoma whose disease had progressed after platinum-containing chemotherapy regimens. Three hundred and ten received at least one dose of atezolizumab and were evaluable for safety and efficacy [16]. The primary endpoint of this study was objective response rate assessed independently and by investigators. In this study, patient tumor samples were prospectively and centrally assessed for PD-L1 expression by tumor-infiltrating immune cells (IC) and were classified as being IC0 (indicating less than 1% expression), IC1 (greater than 1% but less than 5%), and IC2/3 (greater than 5%). Patient samples were evenly distributed between the PD-L1 IC groups: IC0 (33%), IC1 (35%), and IC2/3 (32%).

For all evaluable patients, the objective response rate was 15%, with complete responses being observed in 15 of 310 patients. In the high PD-L1 expression group (IC2/3), the objective response rate was 26%, with 11% of those patients experiencing a complete response. In the intermediate and low PD-L1 expression group (IC1/2/3), the objective response rate was 18%, with a complete response being observed in 13 patients (6%). Additionally, during the follow-up period, median survival was found to be highest in the IC2/3 group at 11.4 months, lower in the IC1/2/3 group at 8.8 months, and 7.9 months for the entire cohort of patients. Sixty-nine percent of patients had a treatment-related adverse event of any grade, and 16% experienced a high-grade (grade 3–4)-related adverse event. The most common adverse events of any grade were fatigue, nausea, and decreased appetite. Based on these data, the FDA granted atezolizumab accelerated approval for treatment of patients with urothelial cancer progression post-platinum.

In subjects who maintained good functional status and adequate laboratory parameters, treatments on this and other ≥2 line immunotherapy trials were allowed post-progression. During IMvigor210 follow-up evaluation, 137 subjects continued on atezolizumab for more than one dose after progression, while 19 received other systemic therapy, and 63 received no further systemic therapy at progression [17]. The median survival for the group that continued with atezolizumab after progression was 8.6 months, compared to 6.8 and 1.2 months of the other systemic therapy and no systemic therapy, respectively. Interestingly, patients who continued on atezolizumab after PD were more likely to have high baseline PD-L1 expression on tumor-infiltrating cells, highlighting PD-L1 as a potential biomarker that may be predictive of better overall survival, among other measures, for atezolizumab.

Furthermore, among the 137 patients, post-PD overall survival (OS) was numerically longer in those with baseline ECOG PS 0, no visceral metastases, or only lymph node disease, suggesting the possibility that atezolizumab may work more effectively in the earlier stages of PD or simply in those who are healthier during progression. Similarly, subjects treated with atezolizumab beyond progression were more likely to have an ECOG status of 0, less likely to have had baseline liver metastases, and more likely to have had an initial response to atezolizumab. Adverse event frequencies were similar before and after progression and comparable with the safety profile of the overall study population.

The open-label, phase III randomized-controlled IMvigor211 trial compared the safety and efficacy of atezolizumab to chemotherapy in patients with locally advanced or metastatic urothelial carcinoma after progression with platinum-based chemotherapy. Subjects received either 1200 mg of atezolizumab or chemotherapy intravenously every 3 weeks. Within the intention to treat (ITT) population, patients receiving atezolizumab numerically had better overall survival (OS) than those undergoing chemotherapy (39.2% vs. 32.4%). However, this outcome was not statistically significant and was not the primary endpoint of the trial. Unlike the similar phase III design which showed that pembrolizumab demonstrated improved OS compared with chemotherapy in the same population, IMvigor211 was a negative trial. In this study, the primary endpoint was based on patients with high PD-L1 expression (IC 2/3), who had no significant difference in OS compared to those assigned to receive chemotherapy.

Assessment of the ITT group by chemotherapy subgroups revealed that patients on atezolizumab showed better comparative OS than patients on taxanes (8.3 months vs. 7.5 months), but not when compared to those on vinflunine (8.3 months vs. 9.2 months). Furthermore, patients assigned to atezolizumab had fewer grade 3–4 treatment-related adverse events (AE) than those with chemotherapy (20% vs. 43%) and fewer adverse events that prompted discontinuation of treatment (7% vs. 18%). Interestingly, within the IC2/3 group, the overall survival (OS) did not significantly differ between treatment groups (11.1 months vs. 10.6 months). Confirmed objective response rates were lower for both atezolizumab-treated patients and chemotherapy-treated patients in the ITT group than those in the IC2/3 subgroup. In patients with samples with a high tumor mutation burden, OS was better at 11.3 months for atezolizumab-treated subjects than those treated with chemotherapy at 8.3 months. For patients with samples with a low tumor mutational burden (TMB), there was no discernable OS difference between patients treated with atezolizumab and patients treated with chemotherapy.

To further highlight the significance of PD-L1 as a biomarker, authors of this study also evaluated PD-L1 as a predictor of survival advantage in patients with a high tumor mutation burden—finding that patients with a high tumor mutation burden and PD-L1 IC2/3 had a median survival of 17.8 months if treated with atezolizumab and 10.6 months if treated with chemotherapy.

## Durvalumab

In a phase I/II trial, durvalumab was evaluated for safety and efficacy in subjects with urothelial cancer that had progressed on platinum-based chemotherapy [18]. This trial initially enrolled 61 patients, and they were treated with 10 mg/kg every 2 weeks for up to 12 months or until progression, intolerable adverse effects, or withdrawal. The first 20 patients were enrolled regardless of PD-L1 expression status, but subsequent patients were required to have greater than 5% expression in their tumor cells to be eligible for enrollment. This allowed for assessment of response in PD-L1-positive and PD-L1-negative subgroups. PD-L1 was defined as positive if ≥25% of tumor cells (TC) or immune cells (IC) expressed PD-L1, and negative was defined as <25% of TC and IC. The overall objective response rate was 31.0%, with 46.4% in the PD-L1-positive subgroup and 0% in the PD-L1-negative subgroup. Subjects on this trial experienced minimal adverse events with 39 patients reporting a treatment-related AE of any grade. The most frequently reported AEs were low-grade fatigue, diarrhea, and decreased appetite. The median follow-up of response-evaluable patients was 6.5 months, and there were 12 of 13 patients that had an ongoing response at the time of the last follow-up. In a study update including 191 patients, the objective response rate (ORR) was 17.8% (34 of 191; 95% CI, 12.7–24.0%), with seven patients achieving complete response, and the median overall survival was 18.2 months [19].

**Nivolumab**

CheckMate 275, a single-arm phase II study, measured the activity and safety of nivolumab in subjects with urothelial carcinoma that progressed during or after platinum-based chemotherapy [20]. In this study, 270 patients were enrolled and treated with nivolumab at 3 mg/kg every 2 weeks until disease progression, unacceptable toxicity, or other protocol-defined discontinuation reasons, with 265 reported. Confirmed objective response was achieved in 19.6% of patients (52 of 265). In patients with PD-L1 expression >5%, the confirmed objective response rate (ORR) was 28.4% (23 of 81); for those with PD-L1 expression >1%, the ORR was 23.8% (29 of 122), and for those with PD-L1 expression <1%, the ORR was 16.1% (23 of 143). Nivolumab was well tolerated, with treatment-related adverse events in 64% of subjects (174 of 270). The most common adverse events were fatigue, pruritus, diarrhea, and decreased appetite, with high-grade events occurring in 18% of patients [20]. The median overall survival was 8.74 months in the treated population, 11.3 months in subjects with tumors harboring PD-L1 expression >1%, and 5.95 months in those with PD-L1 expression <1%.

**Avelumab**

In a phase Ib study, 44 subjects with disease progression post-platinum were enrolled and evaluated for safety and efficacy with avelumab 10 mg/kg once every 2 weeks until progression or unacceptable toxicity [21]. Similar to the other immunotherapy trials, this trial performed immunohistochemistry to assign PD-L1 expression levels across patients. The trial used ≥5% staining threshold in tumor cells to assign positivity or negativity, and using these criteria, 13 subjects had PD-L1-positive tumors. At the time of data analysis, among the patients evaluable for response, the confirmed ORR was 18.2% overall and was 53.8% in those with PD-L1-positive tumors compared to 4.2% in the subjects with PD-L1-negative tumors.

Avelumab was generally well tolerated in this patient population. The most frequent treatment-related adverse events in this trial were fatigue, infusion-related reaction, asthenia, and nausea, with high-grade events occurring in 6.8% of subjects. In the follow-up period, the median overall survival was found to be 13.7 months, and the median progression-free survival was 11.6 weeks [21]. This phase Ib study illustrated that avelumab was well tolerated and showed great clinical promise as it had minimal treatment-related adverse events and prolonged overall survival of patients. Ultimately, avelumab received accelerated FDA approval for patients with locally advanced or metastatic urothelial carcinoma in the post-platinum chemotherapy patient population.

JAVELIN Solid Tumor, a phase I open-label trial, assessed the safety profile in platinum-naive and post-platinum patients [22]. Two hundred and forty-nine patients were eligible and received treatment with avelumab for a median of 12 weeks and were followed up for a median of 9.9 months. These patients were unselected for PD-L1 expression and received avelumab at a dose of 10 mg/kg every 2 weeks until disease progression or other protocol-defined withdrawal criteria. In 161 of the post-platinum patients with at least 6 months of follow-up, the ORR was 17% including 6% complete response rate. During the follow-up period, median progression-free survival was 6.3 weeks with a median overall survival of 6.5 months.

Avelumab was generally well tolerated among all patients with the rate of high-grade adverse events similar to that previously reported at 8%, the most common events being fatigue, asthenia, elevated lipase, and pneumonitis.

## *Summary*

In conclusion, PD-1 and PD-L1 inhibitors have revolutionized urothelial cancer therapy since their initial approval by the FDA in 2017. There are five agents with approval in the post-platinum setting, and thus, they can be used within 12 months of progression following perioperative chemotherapy, or beyond platinum in the second line. There is one randomized phase III trial which demonstrates superior overall survival of pembrolizumab compared to second-line single-agent chemotherapy, with improved toxicity compared to chemotherapy in both second-line phase III studies (Table 17.2). Ongoing late phase trials will continue to inform the use of these agents, including in the first-line cisplatin-eligible population, with and without combination chemotherapy. Perioperative trials assessing safety and efficacy in noninvasive bladder cancer will inform the use of these agents in even earlier settings.

**Table 17.2** Summary of trials which led to FDA approval of checkpoint inhibitors for urothelial cancer

| Trial | Drug | Phase | OS (months) | ORR (%) |
|---|---|---|---|---|
| Metastatic urothelial carcinoma – first-line therapy in cisplatin- or chemotherapy-ineligible patients | | | | |
| NCT02335424 [9] | Pembrolizumab | II | N | 24% (89/370) |
| NCT02108652 [10] | Atezolizumab | II | 15.9 | 23% (27/119) |
| Metastatic urothelial carcinoma – second-line therapy in post-platinum therapy patients | | | | |
| NCT02108652 [16] | Atezolizumab | II | 7.9 | 15% (45/310) |
| NCT01693562 [18] | Durvalumab | I/II | 18.2 | 31% (13/42) |
| NCT02256436 [14] | Pembrolizumab | III | 10.3 (P)<br>7.4 (C) | 21.1% (P, 57/270)<br>11.4% (C, 31/272) |
| NCT02387996 [20] | Nivolumab | II | 8.7 | 19.6% (52/265) |
| NCT01772004 [21] | Avelumab | Ib | 13.7 | 18.2% (8/44) |
| NCT01772004 [22] | Avelumab | Ib | 6.5 | 17% (27/161) |
| NCT02108652 [17] | Atezolizumab | II | 8.6[a] 6.8[b], 1.2[c] | 11.7% (16/137) |
| NCT02302807 [23] | Atezolizumab | III | 11.1 (A)<br>10.6 (C) | 23.0% (A, 26/116)<br>21.6% (C, 25/118) |

*ORR* unselected objective response rate, *OS* overall survival, *N* not reported, *A* atezolizumab arm, *P* pembrolizumab arm, *C* chemotherapy arm

[a]Median post-progression overall survival in patients continuing atezolizumab

[b]Median post-progression overall survival in patients receiving another treatment

[c]Median post-progression overall survival in patients receiving no treatment

In the first-line setting, both pembrolizumab and atezolizumab are FDA approved based on efficacy and toxicity data. For patients who are chemotherapy eligible, PD-L1 tumor testing may inform treatment choice, as carboplatin remains a reasonable first-line therapy. For those refusing or not chemotherapy eligible, atezolizumab or pembrolizumab can still be used in the absence of PD-L1 tumor testing. Understanding predictors of toxicity, overcoming resistance, and combination strategies will continue to be areas of research interest for years to come.

**Pearls for Advanced Practice Providers**

- *Role of PD-L1 Testing in Clinical Practice*
- Currently, PD-L1 testing is recommended for chemotherapy-eligible, but cisplatin-ineligible, patients undergoing treatment in the first line [24]. Completed and ongoing trials have incorporated measurement of PD-L1 as a means of correlating response with PD-L1 expression status [4, 25]. However, despite being assessed in all trials, there is no standardization of how and when biopsy specimens are collected for PD-L1 testing. Furthermore, PD-L1 status is likely a heterogeneous and evolving biomarker that can potentially change based on therapy. Other biomarkers such as tumor mutation burden, TCGA subtype, and CD8 T cell infiltration, combined with PD-L1 status, may prove to be a more robust biomarker of response than any one of these factors alone [26].

- *Managing Immune-Related Toxicity*
- Immune-related toxicity differs from chemotherapy-related toxicity substantially. While chemotherapy-related toxicity tends to be cumulative and dose limiting, the side effects of immunotherapy can be variable and not dose dependent. As with chemotherapy, toxicities fall into mild, moderate, severe, life-threatening, and fatal outcomes. Thus, close follow-up and supportive care to mitigate toxicity are important. Unlike chemotherapy, often, the mainstay of supportive therapy other than treatment hold and supportive care is immune suppression with steroids. Thorough workup to differentiate infectious, cancer progression-related, or comorbid causes of adverse events on immunotherapy is important, as severe toxicity necessitates permanent discontinuation of immunotherapy. Several published guidelines are available for guidance, and many academic centers have now assembled multidisciplinary teams throughout internal medicine subspecialties to develop expertise in immune-related toxicity diagnosis and management [27–29].

## References

1. Pardoll DM. The blockade of immune checkpoints in cancer immunotherapy. Nat Rev Cancer. 2012;12(4):252–64.
2. Kim J. Immune checkpoint blockade therapy for bladder cancer treatment. Investig Clin Urol. 2016;57(Suppl 1):S98–S105.
3. Drakaki A, McDermott DF. Novel immunotherapies in GU malignancies. Curr Oncol Rep. 2013;15(3):224–31.
4. Alsaab HO, Sau S, Alzhrani R, Tatiparti K, Bhise K, Kashaw SK, et al. PD-1 and PD-L1 checkpoint signaling inhibition for cancer immunotherapy: mechanism, combinations, and clinical outcome. Front Pharmacol. 2017;8:561.
5. Sternberg CN, de Mulder PH, Schornagel JH, Theodore C, Fossa SD, van Oosterom AT, et al. Randomized phase III trial of high-dose-intensity methotrexate, vinblastine, doxorubicin, and cisplatin (MVAC) chemotherapy and recombinant human granulocyte colony-stimulating factor versus classic MVAC in advanced urothelial tract tumors: European Organization for Research and Treatment of Cancer Protocol no. 30924. J Clin Oncol. 2001;19(10):2638–46.
6. von der Maase H, Sengelov L, Roberts JT, Ricci S, Dogliotti L, Oliver T, et al. Long-term survival results of a randomized trial comparing gemcitabine plus cisplatin, with methotrexate, vinblastine, doxorubicin, plus cisplatin in patients with bladder cancer. J Clin Oncol. 2005;23(21):4602–8.
7. Necchi A, Pond GR, Raggi D, Giannatempo P, Vogelzang NJ, Grivas P, et al. Efficacy and safety of gemcitabine plus either taxane or carboplatin in the first-line setting of metastatic urothelial carcinoma: a systematic review and meta-analysis. Clin Genitourin Cancer. 2017;15(1):23–30.. e2
8. Galsky MD, Hahn NM, Rosenberg J, Sonpavde G, Hutson T, Oh WK, et al. Treatment of patients with metastatic urothelial cancer "unfit" for Cisplatin-based chemotherapy. J Clin Oncol. 2011;29(17):2432–8.
9. Balar AV, Castellano D, O'Donnell PH, Grivas P, Vuky J, Powles T, et al. First-line pembrolizumab in cisplatin-ineligible patients with locally advanced and unresectable or metastatic

urothelial cancer (KEYNOTE-052): a multicentre, single-arm, phase 2 study. Lancet Oncol. 2017;18(11):1483–92.
10. Balar AV, Galsky MD, Rosenberg JE, Powles T, Petrylak DP, Bellmunt J, et al. Atezolizumab as first-line treatment in cisplatin-ineligible patients with locally advanced and metastatic urothelial carcinoma: a single-arm, multicentre, phase 2 trial. Lancet. 2017;389(10064):67–76.
11. De Santis M, Bellmunt J, Mead G, Kerst JM, Leahy M, Maroto P, et al. Randomized phase II/III trial assessing gemcitabine/carboplatin and methotrexate/carboplatin/vinblastine in patients with advanced urothelial cancer who are unfit for cisplatin-based chemotherapy: EORTC study 30986. J Clin Oncol. 2012;30(2):191–9.
12. Bellmunt J, von der Maase H, Mead GM, Skoneczna I, De Santis M, Daugaard G, et al. Randomized phase III study comparing paclitaxel/cisplatin/gemcitabine and gemcitabine/cisplatin in patients with locally advanced or metastatic urothelial cancer without prior systemic therapy: EORTC Intergroup Study 30987. J Clin Oncol. 2012;30(10):1107–13.
13. Administration USFaD. FDA updates prescribing information for Keytruda and Tecentriq 2018. Available from: https://www.fda.gov/Drugs/InformationOnDrugs/ApprovedDrugs/ucm617378.htm.
14. Bellmunt J, de Wit R, Vaughn DJ, Fradet Y, Lee JL, Fong L, et al. Pembrolizumab as second-line therapy for advanced urothelial carcinoma. N Engl J Med. 2017;376(11):1015–26.
15. Vaughn DJ, Bellmunt J, Fradet Y, Lee JL, Fong L, Vogelzang NJ, et al. Health-related quality-of-life analysis from KEYNOTE-045: a phase III study of pembrolizumab versus chemotherapy for previously treated advanced urothelial cancer. J Clin Oncol. 2018;36(16):1579–87.
16. Rosenberg JE, Hoffman-Censits J, Powles T, van der Heijden MS, Balar AV, Necchi A, et al. Atezolizumab in patients with locally advanced and metastatic urothelial carcinoma who have progressed following treatment with platinum-based chemotherapy: a single-arm, multicentre, phase 2 trial. Lancet. 2016;387(10031):1909–20.
17. Necchi A, Joseph RW, Loriot Y, Hoffman-Censits J, Perez-Gracia JL, Petrylak DP, et al. Atezolizumab in platinum-treated locally advanced or metastatic urothelial carcinoma: post-progression outcomes from the phase II IMvigor210 study. Ann Oncol. 2017;28(12):3044–50.
18. Massard C, Gordon MS, Sharma S, Rafii S, Wainberg ZA, Luke J, et al. Safety and efficacy of durvalumab (MEDI4736), an anti-programmed cell death ligand-1 immune checkpoint inhibitor, in patients with advanced urothelial bladder cancer. J Clin Oncol. 2016;34(26):3119–25.
19. Powles T, O'Donnell PH, Massard C, Arkenau HT, Friedlander TW, Hoimes CJ, et al. Efficacy and safety of durvalumab in locally advanced or metastatic urothelial carcinoma: updated results from a phase 1/2 open-label study. JAMA Oncol. 2017;3(9):e172411.
20. Sharma P, Retz M, Siefker-Radtke A, Baron A, Necchi A, Bedke J, et al. Nivolumab in metastatic urothelial carcinoma after platinum therapy (CheckMate 275): a multicentre, single-arm, phase 2 trial. Lancet Oncol. 2017;18(3):312–22.
21. Apolo AB, Infante JR, Balmanoukian A, Patel MR, Wang D, Kelly K, et al. Avelumab, an anti-programmed death-ligand 1 antibody, in patients with refractory metastatic urothelial carcinoma: results from a multicenter, phase Ib study. J Clin Oncol. 2017;35(19):2117–24.
22. Patel MR, Ellerton J, Infante JR, Agrawal M, Gordon M, Aljumaily R, et al. Avelumab in metastatic urothelial carcinoma after platinum failure (JAVELIN Solid Tumor): pooled results from two expansion cohorts of an open-label, phase 1 trial. Lancet Oncol. 2018;19(1):51–64.
23. Powles T, Duran I, van der Heijden MS, Loriot Y, Vogelzang NJ, De Giorgi U, et al. Atezolizumab versus chemotherapy in patients with platinum-treated locally advanced or metastatic urothelial carcinoma (IMvigor211): a multicentre, open-label, phase 3 randomised controlled trial. Lancet. 2018;391(10122):748–57.
24. Gong J, Chehrazi-Raffle A, Reddi S, Salgia R. Development of PD-1 and PD-L1 inhibitors as a form of cancer immunotherapy: a comprehensive review of registration trials and future considerations. J Immunother Cancer. 2018;6(1):8.
25. Meng X, Huang Z, Teng F, Xing L, Yu J. Predictive biomarkers in PD-1/PD-L1 checkpoint blockade immunotherapy. Cancer Treat Rev. 2015;41(10):868–76.

26. Carosella ED, Ploussard G, LeMaoult J, Desgrandchamps F. A systematic review of immunotherapy in urologic cancer: evolving roles for targeting of CTLA-4, PD-1/PD-L1, and HLA-G. Eur Urol. 2015;68(2):267–79.
27. Puzanov I, Diab A, Abdallah K, Bingham CO 3rd, Brogdon C, Dadu R, et al. Managing toxicities associated with immune checkpoint inhibitors: consensus recommendations from the Society for Immunotherapy of Cancer (SITC) Toxicity Management Working Group. J Immunother Cancer. 2017;5(1):95.
28. Thompson JA, Schneider BJ, Brahmer J, Andrews S, Armand P, Bhatia S, et al. Management of immunotherapy-related toxicities, version 1.2019. J Natl Compr Cancer Netw. 2019;17(3):255–89.
29. Brahmer JR, Lacchetti C, Schneider BJ, Atkins MB, Brassil KJ, Caterino JM, et al. Management of immune-related adverse events in patients treated with immune checkpoint inhibitor therapy: American Society of Clinical Oncology clinical practice guideline. J Clin Oncol. 2018;36(17):1714–68.

# Chapter 18
# Novel and Experimental Strategies in the Treatment of Metastatic Urothelial Carcinoma

**Joseph K. Izes and Seungeun Oh**

## Introduction

In spite of the recent considerable increase in effective treatment options, metastatic urothelial carcinoma remains a highly morbid disease, and current available therapies produce relatively low rates of long-term durable response. The American Cancer Society estimates that in 2019, there will be 17,670 deaths from 80,470 new cases of urothelial carcinoma, making this cancer the sixth most common cause of cancer deaths [1]. Approximately 25% of newly diagnosed patients have muscle invasive bladder cancer or metastatic disease [2].

## Recent Advances

As summarized in proceeding chapters, the treatment options for first-line therapy of metastatic urothelial carcinoma continue to include platinum-based chemotherapy for patients who are eligible and immune checkpoint inhibitors for patients who are platinum ineligible or have progressed following platinum therapy. While platinum-based chemotherapy (MVAC: methotrexate, vinblastine, doxorubicin, cisplatin, or gemcitabine with cis-platinum) remains the standard therapy, up to half of

J. K. Izes (✉)
Department of Urology, Sidney Kimmel Cancer Center, Sidney Kimmel Medical College, Thomas Jefferson University/Thomas Jefferson University Hospital, Philadelphia, PA, USA
e-mail: Joseph.izes@jeffferson.edu

S. Oh
Department of Urology, Thomas Jefferson University, Philadelphia, PA, USA
e-mail: Seungeun.oh@jeferson.edu



E. J. Trabulsi et al. (eds.), *Chemotherapy and Immunotherapy in Urologic Oncology*, https://doi.org/10.1007/978-3-030-52021-2_18

patients cannot tolerate cis-platinum-based [3] regimens. Second-line chemotherapy, such as taxanes, has been utilized historically with disappointing outcomes.

More recently, treatment options have expanded dramatically. Within the past several years, immunotherapeutic antibodies directed at PD-1 and its ligand PD-L1 have become available in routine clinical settings. Immune checkpoints maintain immune tolerance against self-antigen and dampen immune response. Immune checkpoint inhibitors (ICI) overcome this downregulation of antitumor immune response effectively increasing immune response. These agents have a much more manageable safety profile than platinum-based chemotherapy and are more appropriate for elderly or infirm patients. They are far from side effect-free however, and these immunotherapies also generate immune-related adverse events that mainly involve the gut, skin, endocrine glands, liver, and lung but can potentially affect any tissue [4]. Currently, five immune checkpoint inhibitors have been approved for the second-line (cis-platinum ineligible or platinum resistant) setting. Pembrolizumab and atezolizumab are currently approved in the first-line setting for PD-L1-positive and platinum-ineligible patients.

Several trials are underway to explore combination therapy. IMvigor130 is a phase 3 trial that examines the effect of first-line atezolizumab given alone or in combination with platinum-based chemotherapy [5]. Combinations of PD-1/PD-L1 inhibitors and other immune modulators combined with antiangiogenic agents have also been proposed [6].

## Molecular Markers and Genomic and Targeted Therapy

It has long been recognized that urothelial cancers are a heterogeneous group of neoplasms that vary dramatically in aggressiveness and invasiveness. This clinical observation has recently been refined on a molecular level. Biomarker-based treatment strategies have been successfully adopted in the treatment of several malignancies, and it has long been felt that identification of molecular subtypes could facilitate more precise treatment selection, or in popular parlance "personalized medicine." The Cancer Genome Atlas Project (TCGA) has elucidated the tumor molecular biology of advanced urothelial carcinoma with identification of new mutations and identification of potentially targetable cell survival pathways.

The diversity and heterogeneity of urothelial carcinoma, which has long been well appreciated on a clinical and histologic basis (low-grade papillary tumors versus high-grade invasive tumors) is now recognized to have well-defined genomic correlates [4]. Genomic analysis of 412 patients with bladder cancer and comprehensive molecular characterization of primary bladder cancers were carried out demonstrating a high tumor mutational burden. Understanding the genomic alterations and urothelial cancer has led to the identification of novel therapeutic targets.

TCGA identified genetic drivers of muscle-invasive bladder cancer (MIBC) as well as subtypes of MIBC with distinct characteristics and therapeutic responses [7]. Historically, locally advanced and metastatic urinary tract tumors have been traditionally treated similarly based on histopathology. Such histopathologic classification was occasionally predictive of response to chemotherapy, but overall, this distinction was extremely limited. Recent advances in multi-platform high-throughput genomic profiling have allowed some amount of subclassification of metastatic tumors on a molecular basis. A molecular classification of distinct subsets within the broader classification of high-grade urothelial carcinoma (UC) has already been shown to have implications for treatment. Particular markers in the TCGA dataset correlated with a high likelihood of response to cis-platinum-based chemotherapy and immune checkpoint inhibitors [8]. Five subtypes of MIBC have been identified based on RNA expression, which correlate with outcomes and might guide treatment: basal-squamous, luminal-infiltrated, luminal and luminal-papillary, and neuronal. These subtypes each have differing genetic make-up with potential implications for treatment selection. For example, the luminal-papillary variant has been shown to exhibit overexpression of FGFR3, making this subtype a target for anti-FGFR3 tyrosine kinase inhibitors. The basal-squamous subtype shows frequent mutations in TP53 and elevated PD-L1 as well as high epithelial growth factor receptor expression and may be particularly sensitive to cis-platinum-based chemotherapy as well as PD-1 inhibitors. The luminal subtype shows high expression of human epidermal growth factor receptor to (HER-2) with a possible role of HER-2 targeting drugs and a good response to neoadjuvant chemotherapy. Neuronal subtype, the most rare, indicates exquisite sensitivity to PD 1 inhibitors [9].

## FGFR Inhibitors

TCGA identified aberrant fibroblast growth factor receptor (FGFR) with oncogenic FGFR3 fusions being seen more commonly in high-grade invasive tumors [10]. These tumors seemed to have a decreased sensitivity to immune interventions. Erdafitinib, an oral pan-FGFR-targeted agent, has recently been given accelerated FDA approval based on relevant clinical activity in metastatic UC patients whose tumors bear actionable FGFR alterations [11]. In an open label phase 2 study, an objective tumor response was seen in 40% of previously treated patients who had locally advanced unresectable or metastatic urothelial carcinoma with FGFR alterations [12, 13]. The most common adverse events were hyperphosphatemia, elevated creatinine, stomatitis, decreased appetite, nausea, and dry mouth [14].

FGFR has also been targeted with monoclonal antibodies in preliminary studies with promising initial findings [15].

## ErbB

Somatic mutations in the ErbB family of cell surface tyrosine kinase receptors (consisting of EGFR, HER2, and ErbB3/ErbB4) are frequently expressed in urothelial carcinoma and have long been thought to represent viable therapeutic targets. EGFR is the cell surface receptor for members of the epidermal growth factor family of extracellular protein. Receptor activation initiates several signal transduction cascades leading to DNA synthesis and cell proliferation. Previous studies showed that overexpression of EGFR in bladder cancer correlates with tumor grade stage and survival [16]. This is also true of HER-2 overexpression. Several trials of agents based on EGFR and HER-2 inhibition have failed to show conclusive benefit. In a phase 2 trial, afatinib, an oral irreversible inhibitor of the ErbB family, approved for the treatment of metastatic non-small cell lung cancer, demonstrated significant activity in patients with platinum refractory urothelial carcinoma with HER-2 or ErbB3 alterations [17].

## *Antibody-Drug Conjugates*

Antibody-drug conjugates (ADC) targeting specific cell surface antigens represent an attractive therapeutic strategy for chemotherapy refractory tumors as the ADC has the potential to deliver a significant proportion of the potent drug to the tumor cells rather than to normal cells [18]. Enfortumab vedotin (EV) selectively targets cells expressing Nectin-4 by delivering a potent microtubule-disrupting agent. Almost all metastatic urothelial carcinoma tumors express Nectin-4, a cell adhesion molecule that is highly expressed in multiple cancers. A breakthrough therapy designation has been granted by the FDA for patients with locally advanced or metastatic urothelial carcinoma who previously received immune checkpoint therapy [19]. A phase 1 study demonstrated an objective response rate of 41%. A phase 1 trial combining EV with atezolizumab or pembrolizumab is underway.

## *Angiogenesis Inhibitors*

Angiogenesis is necessary for the growth, invasion, and metastasis of solid tumors. Vascular endothelial growth factor (VEGF) levels appear to be prognostic for outcomes in bladder cancer, and preclinical evaluation of angiogenesis inhibition has appeared to demonstrate anticancer activity [20]. Vascular endothelial growth factor receptors 1 and 2 and their ligands are important mediators of tumor angiogenesis and contribute to the pathogenesis and progression of urothelial carcinoma. Many trials with antiangiogenic therapies have showed modest, if any benefit. These include single-agent sorafenib, pazopanib, and sunitinib.

More recently, bevacizumab, a monoclonal antibody directed against circulating VEGF, has shown clinical activity in a phase 2 trial of gemcitabine and cis-platinum and bevacizumab as first-line therapy for metastatic urothelial cancer. This study demonstrated an overall response rate (ORR) of 72% and an encouraging overall survival (OS) of 19.1 months [21]. A recent randomized double-blind phase 3 trial of ramucirumab plus docetaxel versus placebo plus docetaxel was performed in patients with platinum refractory urothelial carcinoma, some of whom received

PD-1 immune checkpoint inhibitors. Progression-free survival benefit, 4.1 months versus 2.8 months, was noted as was median overall survival, 9.4 months versus 7.9 months [22].

## Conclusions

While patients with advanced urothelial carcinoma are faced with a rapidly progressive disease with a narrow window for therapeutic intervention, there has been substantial progress over a relatively short period of time in the number of clinically available effective treatments. In addition to progress in immunotherapy, targeted therapies for patients with appropriate biomarkers and combinations of new therapies are extremely promising. Novel FGFR inhibitors, progress in the application of angiogenesis inhibitors, combined immunotherapy regimens, and antibody-drug conjugates offer new options to patients who otherwise would have extremely short survival following progression after first-line therapy.

**Clinical Pearls**

- First-line therapy continues to be cisplatin-based chemotherapy regimens in the treatment of metastatic urothelial carcinoma; however, up to half of patients cannot tolerate or are ineligible for cisplatin-based treatments.
- Immunotherapeutic agents directed at PD-1 and PD-L1 have shown a more manageable safety profile and effective outcomes.
- Atezolizumab and pembrolizumab have been approved as second-line therapy.
- The Cancer Genome Atlas Project (TCGA) has helped to identify new mutations and potentially targetable cell survival pathways.
- FGFR VEGF-targeted therapies and antibody-drug conjugates have shown improved outcomes in patients less responsive to immune interventions.

## Bibliography


1. Cokkinides V, Albano J, Samuels A, Ward ME. American Cancer Society: cancer facts and figures. Atlanta: American Cancer Society; 2005.
2. Antoni S, Ferlay J, Soerjomataram I, Znaor A, Jemal A, Bray F. Bladder cancer incidence and mortality: a global overview and recent trends. Eur Urol. 2017;71(1):96–108. https://doi.org/10.1016/j.eururo.2016.06.010.
3. Galsky MD, Hahn NM, Rosenberg J, et al. Treatment of patients with metastatic urothelial cancer "unfit" for Cisplatin-based chemotherapy. J Clin Oncol. 2011;29(17):2432–8. https://doi.org/10.1200/JCO.2011.34.8433.
4. Michot JM, Bigenwald C, Champiat S, et al. Immune-related adverse events with immune checkpoint blockade: a comprehensive review. Eur J Cancer. 2016;54:139–48. https://doi.org/10.1016/j.ejca.2015.11.016.

5. Galsky MD, Grande E, Davis ID, et al. IMvigor130: a randomized, phase III study evaluating first-line (1L) atezolizumab (atezo) as monotherapy and in combination with platinum-based chemotherapy (chemo) in patients (pts) with locally advanced or metastatic urothelial carcinoma (mUC). J Clin Oncol. 2018;36(15_suppl):TPS4589-TPS4589. https://doi.org/10.1200/JCO.2018.36.15_suppl.TPS4589.
6. Nadal R, Bellmunt J. Management of metastatic bladder cancer. Cancer Treat Rev. 2019;76:10–21. https://doi.org/10.1016/j.ctrv.2019.04.002.
7. Sanli O, Dobruch J, Knowles MA, et al. Bladder cancer. Nat Rev Dis Primers. 2017;3:17022. https://doi.org/10.1038/nrdp.2017.22.
8. Robertson AG, Kim J, Al-Ahmadie H, et al. Comprehensive molecular characterization of muscle-invasive bladder cancer. Cell. 2017;171(3):540–556.e25. https://doi.org/10.1016/j.cell.2017.09.007.
9. Alessandrino F, Ghaith O, Williams K, Sonpavde GP, Silverman SG, Shinagare AB. Advanced urothelial cancer: a radiology update. Abdom Radiol (NY). 2019;44(12):3858–73. https://doi.org/10.1007/s00261-019-02148-3.
10. Roskoski R. The role of fibroblast growth factor receptor (FGFR) protein-tyrosine kinase inhibitors in the treatment of cancers including those of the urinary bladder. Pharmacol Res. 2019;151:104567. https://doi.org/10.1016/j.phrs.2019.104567.
11. Montazeri K, Bellmunt J. Erdafitinib for the treatment of metastatic bladder cancer. Expert Rev Clin Pharmacol. 2020;13(1):1–6. https://doi.org/10.1080/17512433.2020.1702025.
12. Loriot Y, Necchi A, Park SH, et al. Erdafitinib in locally advanced or metastatic urothelial carcinoma. N Engl J Med. 2019;381(4):338–48. https://doi.org/10.1056/NEJMoa1817323.
13. Siefker-Radtke AO, Necchi A, Park SH, et al. First results from the primary analysis population of the phase 2 study of erdafitinib (ERDA; JNJ-42756493) in patients (pts) with metastatic or unresectable urothelial carcinoma (mUC) and FGFR alterations (FGFRalt). J Clin Oncol. 2018;36(15_suppl):4503. https://doi.org/10.1200/JCO.2018.36.15_suppl.4503.
14. Nishina T, Takahashi S, Iwasawa R, Noguchi H, Aoki M, Doi T. Safety, pharmacokinetic, and pharmacodynamics of erdafitinib, a pan-fibroblast growth factor receptor (FGFR) tyrosine kinase inhibitor, in patients with advanced or refractory solid tumors. Investig New Drugs. 2017;36(3):1–11. https://doi.org/10.1007/s10637-017-0514-4.
15. Bellmunt J, Picus J, Kohli M, Arriaga YE, Milowsky MI. FIERCE-21: phase 1b/2 study of docetaxel+ b-701, a selective inhibitor of FGFR3, in relapsed or refractory (R/R) metastatic urothelial carcinoma (mUCC). J Clin Oncol. 2018;36(15_suppl):4534.
16. Chiyomaru T, Seki N, Inoguchi S, et al. Dual regulation of receptor tyrosine kinase genes EGFR and c-Met by the tumor-suppressive microRNA-23b/27b cluster in bladder cancer. Int J Oncol. 2015;46(2):487–96. https://doi.org/10.3892/ijo.2014.2752.
17. Choudhury NJ, Campanile A, Antic T, et al. Afatinib activity in platinum-refractory metastatic urothelial carcinoma in patients with ERBB alterations. J Clin Oncol. 2016;34(18):2165–71. https://doi.org/10.1200/JCO.2015.66.3047.
18. Faltas B, Goldenberg DM, Ocean AJ, et al. Sacituzumab Govitecan, a novel antibody--drug conjugate, in patients with metastatic platinum-resistant urothelial carcinoma. Clin Genitourin Cancer. 2016;14(1):e75–9. https://doi.org/10.1016/j.clgc.2015.10.002.
19. Rosenberg JE, Heath EI, O'Donnell PH, et al. EV-201 study: a single-arm, open-label, multicenter study of enfortumab vedotin for treatment of patients with locally advanced or metastatic urothelial cancer who previously received immune checkpoint inhibitor therapy. J Clin Oncol. 2018;36(15_suppl):TPS4590-TPS4590. https://doi.org/10.1200/JCO.2018.36.15_suppl.TPS4590.
20. Elfiky AA, Rosenberg JE. Targeting angiogenesis in bladder cancer. Curr Oncol Rep. 2009;11(3):244–9.
21. Hahn NM, Stadler WM, Zon RT, et al. Phase II trial of cisplatin, gemcitabine, and bevacizumab as first-line therapy for metastatic urothelial carcinoma: Hoosier Oncology Group GU 04-75. J Clin Oncol. 2011;29(12):1525–30. https://doi.org/10.1200/JCO.2010.31.6067.
22. Petrylak DP, de Wit R, Chi KN, et al. Ramucirumab plus docetaxel versus placebo plus docetaxel in patients with locally advanced or metastatic urothelial carcinoma after platinum-based therapy (RANGE): a randomised, double-blind, phase 3 trial. Lancet. 2017;390(10109):2266–77. https://doi.org/10.1016/S0140-6736(17)32365-6.

# Chapter 19
# Upper Tract Urothelial Carcinoma

**Anne E. Lizardi-Calvaresi, Demetrius Bagley, and Katherine Smentkowski**

## Introduction

The urothelium is the epithelial lining of the urethra, bladder, ureters, and renal pelvis of the kidneys. Upper tract urothelial carcinoma (UTUC) is defined as cancer that develops in the lining of the upper portion of the urinary tract, which extends from the distal ureter proximally to the renal pelvis [1, 2]. UTUC may also be referred to as cancer of the upper urinary tract, renal pelvis cancer, ureteral cancer, or cancer in the lining of the kidney. Historically, UTUC was called transitional cell carcinoma.

### *Occurrence*

Upper tract urothelial carcinoma is rare, accounting for only 5–10% of all urinary tract cancers, including bladder cancer [1]. There are approximately two to three cases per 100,000 persons. Approximately 75% of cases present in men. Major risk includes increased age, with most cases presenting in the seventh to ninth decades of life [1, 3].

A. E. Lizardi-Calvaresi (✉)
Sidney Kimmel Medical College at Thomas Jefferson University, Philadelphia, PA, USA
e-mail: Anne.Calvaresi@jefferson.edu

D. Bagley
Department of Urology, Thomas Jefferson University, Philadelphia, PA, USA

K. Smentkowski
Department of Urology, Thomas Jefferson University Hospital, Philadelphia, PA, USA



E. J. Trabulsi et al. (eds.), *Chemotherapy and Immunotherapy in Urologic Oncology*, https://doi.org/10.1007/978-3-030-52021-2_19

## *Relation to Bladder Cancer*

Many instances of UTUC are multifocal (approximately 30%), meaning identified in several areas. They may be detected simultaneously with the presence of a bladder urothelial carcinoma or in patients who were previously treated for a diagnosis of urothelial carcinoma of the bladder (3–5%). The risk of developing a bladder urothelial carcinoma is near 15–50% following treatment for an upper tract urothelial carcinoma [1, 3].

## *Etiology*

There are several modifiable risk factors directly related to the development of UTUC. The most common is cigarette smoking or exposure to secondhand smoke. Environmental exposures including certain chemicals such as petroleum, coal, asphalt, tar, aniline dyes, beta-naphthylamine, and benzidine also increase the risk of developing UTUC. Hereditary cases are relatively uncommon but present in some instances of genetic instability or genetic mutations. The most well-known genetic risk factor is microsatellite instability as a result of Lynch syndrome, also known as hereditary nonpolyposis colorectal cancer (HNPCC) [1, 3, 4].

## Presentation

UTUC usually presents with very few, if any, symptoms. The most common presenting symptom is painless gross hematuria or microscopic hematuria. This is present in approximately 75% of cases. Obstruction or hydronephrosis may be present, either with or without flank pain or dull ache. More acute pain or renal colic usually presents in patients with the passage of clot or with severe obstruction of the renal collecting system or ureter. Nearly 15% of patients present asymptomatically and are diagnosed with an incidental finding on radiographic imaging. Patients with advanced disease may present with bone or back pain, flank or abdominal pain, flank or an abdominal mass, or weight loss [1, 3, 4].

## Diagnosis

***Imaging*** Once upper tract malignancy is suspected, it must be confirmed before definitive treatment and therapy. Computed tomography urogram (CTU) is a cornerstone of diagnosis, with the highest diagnostic accuracy of current imaging modalities. A recent meta-analysis reported a sensitivity of 88–100% and a specificity of 93–100% in the detection of UTUC using CTU; furthermore, lesions as small as 5 mm may be detected [5, 6]. For these reasons, CTU has replaced older techniques such as intravenous pyelogram (IVP).

Patient factors such as renal insufficiency or a significant iodinated contrast allergy may preclude CTU. In these cases, it is necessary to obtain alternative means of imaging. Depending on the contraindication, a retrograde pyelogram (RPG) or magnetic resonance urography (MRU) may be used to screen for filling defects. These imaging modalities are already indicated in the workup of asymptomatic microscopic hematuria, according to the American Urological Association (AUA) guidelines, and therefore may be obtained during initial presentation [7]. MRU has a slightly decreased sensitivity of 63–75% depending on the size of the lesion, while RPG only has 53–71% sensitivity for detecting upper tract malignancies [8–10].

***Biomarkers*** The use of biomarkers in the diagnosis of upper tract urothelial carcinoma is limited. When cytology is positive in the absence of bladder or prostatic carcinoma in situ or other malignancy, it may be suggestive of UTUC [8]. For that reason, voided urine cytology is generally performed as part of the workup but is notoriously worse at detection than when used for bladder malignancy, with sensitivities of 50–59% for UTUC [8, 11]. European guidelines for UTUC recommend that cytology should be obtained via ureteral catheterization. Unfortunately, meta-analysis reports a similarly poor sensitivity of 53.1% for selective urine cytology [12]. Also similar to bladder cancer detection, cytology performs poorly in the setting of low-grade tumors. High-grade UTUC has a slightly better sensitivity of 69.9% on similar meta-analysis, compared to 45.6 for low-grade UTUC [12].

Adjuvant urinary markers for the detection of UTUC are few. Fluorescence in situ hybridization (FISH) testing, which detects abnormalities in chromosomes 3, 7, 17, and 9p21, is used in bladder cancer detection but has been disappointing in its application to UTUC. Efforts have been made to apply FISH to voided UTUC cytology specimens with inconsistent results – reported sensitivity and specificity vary widely at 54–76.7% and 78–94.7%, respectively [13, 14]. Other urinary biomarkers based on gene mutation and DNA methylation have been described but are not part of routine practice.

***Cystoscopy and Ureteroscopy*** When UTUC is suspected, cystoscopy should always be performed to rule out a concomitant bladder tumor [8]. Synchronous bladder and upper tract tumors have been reported in 17% of patients [15]. Histological biopsy of upper tract tumors is notoriously difficult due to small sample sizes obtained with available biopsy techniques. Despite this, ureteroscopy and subsequent biopsy are recommended in cases where further information would impact treatment decisions [8]. There were early concerns that pyelovenous backflow could increase rates of tumor seeding and metastatic disease, but this has since been disproved [16].

To perform ureteroscopy, a "no-touch" technique with cytological, rather than histological, processing of specimens has allowed for accurate determination of tumor grading to guide further treatment decisions. This technique begins with cystoscopy, followed by semirigid ureteroscopy of the ureter suspected to harbor tumor. Once the extent of the semirigid ureteroscope is reached, a wire is passed to that level of the ureter. The flexible ureteroscope is then advanced over the wire under direct vision, and the remainder of the collecting system is examined. This allows for examination of the entire ureter and renal pelvis with minimal manipulation [13]. Enhanced techniques used for bladder cancer detection, such as blue light cystoscopy and narrow-band imaging, are not routinely employed for detecting upper tract lesions. Preliminary data, however, reports a promising 22.7% increase in tumor detection rate when narrow-band imaging is used [18].

When a suspected tumor is encountered, cytological washings are taken from this area, and the area is biopsied. The biopsy may be performed using a variety of techniques. Biopsy forceps are often utilized, but a flat wire basket may obtain superior results when the tumor is larger or amenable to biopsy in this manner [19]. Due to the small size of ureteroscopically obtained specimens, diagnostic accuracy presents a challenge. The ability to accurately stage tumors in a manner similar to bladder cancer specimens is often impossible. For these reasons, grade, rather than stage, is used to guide treatment decisions as ureteroscopic biopsy can determine tumor grade in the majority of cases [8]. Even when relying on grade, the specimens obtained can be nondiagnostic due to destruction during processing. To overcome this, specimens can be sent for cytological processing, rather than traditional hematoxylin and eosin staining. Larger specimens can then be prepared using a cell block technique. This has increased diagnostic accuracy from 42.9% to 97.2% [20].

***Workup*** Once UTUC is highly suspected or diagnosed, evaluation of renal function and metastatic disease must be completed. National Comprehensive Cancer Network (NCCN) guidelines advocate a laboratory workup including complete blood count (CBC), chemistry profile, and renal function tests. If CTU was not obtained in the initial workup, it should be completed for staging, along with a chest x-ray. A nuclear renal medicine scan to assess for split function may be performed according to clinician discretion, and a bone scan should be obtained if the patient complains of any symptoms suggestive of bone metastasis [21].

Family history should also be assessed at this time if not obtained in original consultation to screen for hereditary nonpolyposis colorectal carcinoma (Lynch syndrome) [8, 21]. Hereditary UTUC comprises 10–20% of cases and should be suspected if the patient is less than 60 years of age and has (1) a personal history of HNPCC-spectrum cancer or (2) a first-degree relative <50 years of age with HNPCC-spectrum cancer or (3) two first-degree relatives with HNPCC-spectrum cancer. If the patient fits these criteria, they should be referred for germ-line DNA sequencing and undergo clinical evaluation for other HNPCC as well as familial genetic counseling [8].

## Treatment and Follow-Up

***Initial management*** Stage is the greatest predictor of tumor survival and recurrence [22]. However, due to the aforementioned difficulties in clinical staging, grade is the cornerstone of decision-making algorithms for treatment. Radical nephroureterectomy is considered the gold standard for treatment. However, the development of improved endoscopic technologies and the desire for renal sparing surgery have expanded treatment options for this disease.

***Low Grade*** When low-grade disease is present, endoscopic renal sparing management with laser tumor ablation can be considered rather than surgical removal. This is an option for both tumors within the renal pelvis, as well as those within the ureter [20]. However, not all patients with low-grade disease are candidates for endoscopic ablation, and current European Association of Urology (EAU) guidelines further stratify patients into low-risk and high-risk UTUC. Low-risk UTUC dictates tumors must be unifocal, should be less than 2 cm, and should not have invasive aspects on cross-sectional imaging in addition to being determined as low risk. Additionally, some authors advocate that a low-risk patient should not be a current smoker and must be reliable in their ability to follow up for surveillance [23]. When these criteria are not met, the patient with low-grade disease must be considered for similar treatment (i.e., surgical excision) as those who present with high-grade disease.

***High Grade*** The mainstay of treatment for high-grade disease is surgical excision with nephroureterectomy and bladder cuff excision. Alternatively, a distal ureterectomy and reimplantation may be considered if the tumor is isolated to the distal ureter. Regional lymphadenectomy should also be performed at the time of surgery [21].

***Endoscopic Management*** The role of endoscopic management in UTUC is well established. While nephroureterectomy with bladder cuff has been the described the "gold standard" for treatment of UTUC, the use of endoscopy for ablative treatment has gained popularity for its ability to preserve renal function while addressing cancer control. In addition to its indication for unifocal low-grade disease as described above, other patients may be considered for endoscopic management in select situations. These include patients with a solitary kidney, bilateral disease (with or without concurrent hereditary risk factors such as HNPCC), chronic kidney disease (CKD), or inability to tolerate radical surgery [24]. Although no level 1 evidence exists, the response of low-grade disease to endoscopic management has been described as excellent, with 5-year disease-specific survival rates of 86.4–100%. As expected, high-grade disease-specific survival rates are less reassuring at 47.3–63%. Renal preservation rates range from 64% to 82.5%, with 36% of cases ultimately requiring nephroureterectomy [24].

***Ureteroscopy*** When a lesion is encountered ureteroscopically, it can be treated using a variety of methods. Ureteroscopy with laser ablation is the mainstay of endoscopic therapy. Laser ablation is most frequently used in the form of holmium:yttrium aluminum garnet (Ho:YAG), neodymium:yttrium aluminum garnet (Nd: YAG), or thulium (TL) laser energy [25, 26]. Each laser varies in its coagulative ability and depth of penetration and therefore has different indications depending on exact tumor location and characteristics. In addition to laser ablation, other methods have been described including manual debulking with forceps or basket and electrofulguration/resection.

***Percutaneous Ablation*** Percutaneous nephroscopy with subsequent ablation or resection has been described for large (>2 cm) or multifocal tumors of the renal pelvis, as well as lower pole tumors that are difficult or impossible to reach ureteroscopically [24]. However, the efficacy and long-term outcomes of this method are difficult to assess, as there is limited evidence. In a systematic review article encompassing 11 percutaneous studies, only one patient out of 236 was noted to have tumor tract seeding. However, this remains a known risk of percutaneous approach, with other limited accounts of tumor seeding noted in case reports [27, 28].

***Surgical Management*** As previously described, radical nephroureterectomy is the gold standard for treatment and the recommended treatment for all high-grade or high-risk disease. In select cases, a distal high-grade tumor may be treated with distal ureterectomy and reimplantation [8, 21].

***Nephroureterectomy*** Classic radical nephroureterectomy involves removal of the kidney, ureter, intramural tunnel, and ureteral orifice with a surrounding bladder cuff. Inclusion of the bladder cuff is critical, as ureteral stump recurrences have been quoted at 30–64% [29]. Nephroureterectomy may be performed via an open, laparoscopic, or robotic approach. Retrospective analysis suggests similar cancer mortality and recurrence rates between open and laparoscopic nephroureterectomy [8, 30]. Therefore, the approach may be determined based on patient/tumor characteristics and surgeon experience. Following surgery, the administration of a single dose of intravesical chemotherapy within 72 hours has been shown to decrease intravesical recurrence rates [8].

***Neoadjuvant/Adjuvant Therapy*** The use of neoadjuvant cisplatin-based chemotherapy prior to radical cystectomy is level 1 evidence in the treatment of muscle-invasive bladder cancer [21, 31]. Therefore, there has been much interest in extrapolating its use to upper tract urothelial carcinoma treatment. Furthermore, as cisplatin-based chemotherapy requires intact renal function, it is ideal to administer before surgical removal of the kidney. Despite this, objective evidence supporting its use preoperatively is still limited. In patients who did not receive neoadjuvant chemotherapy and who maintain adequate renal function following nephroureterectomy, adjuvant chemotherapy has shown overall survival benefit, including in patients with pT3/4 and N+ disease [8].

***Follow-Up*** Following treatment, patients with UTUC must be monitored closely for recurrence. Based on EUA and NCCN guidelines, patients who undergo nephron-sparing surgery (i.e., endoscopic management) should have cystoscopy with cytology every 3 months and ureteroscopy every 3–6 months for the first 1–2 years. This should be performed along with cross-sectional imaging, ideally CTU. After the first 1–2 years, surveillance can then proceed yearly for >5 years [8, 21]. Following nephroureterectomy, cystoscopy with cytology is advocated every 3 months for the first year with cross-sectional imaging every 6–12 months, depending on the pathological stage. After the first year, surveillance may be spaced out to at least annually but should proceed out to greater than 5 years [8, 21].

**Clinical Pearls**

- Upper tract urothelial carcinoma is relatively rare but should be considered in patients who present with gross hematuria.
- The standard of care for high-grade upper tract urothelial carcinoma is a radical nephroureterectomy.
- Consideration of neoadjuvant treatment should be considered in this population.

## References


1. Bagley DH, Tanimoto R, Healy KA. Upper tract urothelial carcinoma: ureteroscopic biopsy and specimen preparation. In: Upper urinary tract urothelial carcinoma. 1st ed. Switzerland: Springer; 2015.
2. Munoz JJ, Ellison LM. Upper tract urothelial neoplasms: incidence and survival during the last 2 decades. J Urol. 2000;164(5):1523–5.
3. Flanigan RC. Urothelial tumors of the upper urinary tract. In: Campbell-Walsh urology. 9th ed. Philadelphia: Saunders Elsevier; 2007.
4. Azemar MD, Comperate E, Richard F, Cussenot O, Roupret M. Bladder recurrence after surgery for upper urinary tract urothelial cell carcinoma: frequency, risk factors, and surveillance. Urol Oncol. 2011;29(2):130–6.
5. Chlapoutakis K, Theocharopoulos N, Yarmentitis S, et al. Performance of computed tomographic urography in diagnosis of upper urinary tract urothelial carcinoma, in patients presenting with hematuria: systematic review and meta-analysis. Eur J Radiol. 2010;73:334–8.
6. Cacili EM, Cohan RH, Inampudi P, et al. MDCT urography of upper tract urothelial neoplasms. Am J Roentgenol. 2005;184:1873–81.
7. Davis R, Jones JS, Barocas DA, et al. Diagnosis, evaluation and follow-up of asymptomatic microhematuria (AMH) in adults: AUA guideline. J Urol. 2012;188:2473–81.
8. Roupret M, Babjuk M, Comperat E, et al. European Association of Urology Guidelines on upper urinary tract urothelial carcinoma: 2017 update. Eur Urol. 2018;73:111–22.
9. Lee KS, Zeikus E, DeWolf WC, et al. MR urography versus retrograde pyelography/ureteroscopy for the exclusion of upper urinary tract malignancy. Clin Radiol. 2010;65:185–92.
10. Chen GL, El-Gabry E, Bagley DL. Surveillance of upper urinary tract transitional cell carcinoma: the role of ureteroscopy, retrograde pyelography, cytology and urinalysis. J Urol. 2000;164:1901–4.

11. Miyake M, Owari T, Hori S, et al. Emerging biomarkers for the diagnosis and monitoring of urothelial carcinoma. Res Rep Urol. 2018;10:251–61.
12. Potretzke AM, Knight BA, Vetter JM, et al. Diagnostic utility of selective upper tract urinary cytology: a systematic review and meta-analysis of the literature. Urology. 2016;96:35–43.
13. Sokolova IA, Halling KC, Jenkins RB, et al. The development of a multitarget, multicolor florescence in situ hybridization assay for the detection of urothelial carcinoma in urine. J Mol Diagn. 2000;2:116–23.
14. Johannas JR, Nelson E, Bibbo M. Voided urine fluorescence in situ hybridization testing for upper tract urothelial carcinoma surveillance. J Urol. 2010;184:879–82.
15. Cosentino M, Palou J, Gaya JM, et al. Upper urinary tract urothelial cell carcinoma: location as a predictive factor for concomitant bladder carcinoma. World J Urol. 2013;31:14–5.
16. Hendin BN, Streem SB, Levin HS, et al. Impact of diagnostic ureteroscopy on long term survival in patients with upper tract transitional cell carcinoma. J Urol. 1999;161:783–5.
17. Tawfiek E, Bibbo M, Bagley D. Ureteroscopic biopsy: technique and specimen preparation. Urology. 1997;50:117–9.
18. Traxer O, Geavlete B, de Medina SG, et al. Narrow-band imaging digital flexible ureteroscopy in detection of upper urinary tract transitional-cell carcinoma: initial experience. J Endourol. 2011;25:19–23.
19. Kleinmann N, Healy KA, Hubosky SG, et al. Ureteroscopic biopsy of upper tract urothelial carcinoma: comparison of basket and forceps. J Endourol. 2013;27:1450–4.
20. Keeley FX, Kulp DA, Bibbo M, et al. Diagnostic accuracy of ureteroscopic biopsy in upper tract transitional cell carcinoma. J Urol. 1997;157:33–7.
21. National Comprehensive Cancer Network. Bladder cancer (Version 1.2020). https://www.nccn.org/professionals/physician_gls/pdf/bladder.pdf. Accessed 6 Dec 2019.
22. Png KS, Lim EK, Chong KT, et al. Prognostic factors for upper tract transitional cell carcinoma; a retrospective review of 66 patients. Asian J Surg. 2008;31:20–4.
23. Seisen T, Colin P, Roupret M. Risk-adapted strategy for the kidney-sparing management of upper tract tumors. Nat Rev Urol. 2015;12:155–66.
24. Verges DP, Lallas CD, Hubosky SG, et al. Endoscopic treatment of upper tract urothelial carcinoma. Curr Urol Rep. 2017;18:31.
25. Park BH, Jeon SS. Endoscopic management of upper urinary tract urothelial carcinoma. Korean J Urol. 2013;54:426–32.
26. Musi G, Mistretta FA, Marenghi C, et al. Thulium laser treatment of upper urinary tract carcinoma; a multi-institutional analysis of surgical and oncological outcomes. J Endourol. 2018;32:257–63.
27. Cutress ML, Stewart GD, Zakikhani P, et al. Ureteroscopic and percutaneous management of upper tract urothelial carcinoma (UTUC): systematic review. BJU Int. 2011;110:614–28.
28. Rouprêt M, Traxer O, Tligui M, et al. Upper urinary tract transitional cell carcinoma: recurrence rate after percutaneous endoscopic resection. Eur Urol. 2007;51:709–13.
29. Srirangam SJ, Cleynenbreugel B, Poppel H. Laparoscopic nephroureterectomy: the distal ureteral dilemma. Adv Urol. 2009;2009:316807.
30. Capitanio U, Shariat SF, Isbarn H, et al. Comparison of oncologic outcomes for open and laparoscopic nephroureterectomy: a multi-institutional analysis of 1249 cases. Eur Urol. 2009;56:1–9.3.
31. Grossman HB, Natale RB, Tangen CM, et al. Neoadjuvant chemotherapy plus cystectomy compared with cystectomy alone for locally advanced bladder cancer. N Engl J Med. 2003;349:859–66.

# Part III
# Kidney Cancer

# Chapter 20
# Kidney Cancer and Its Treatment

**Elena Dreyzin and Alexander Kutikov**

## Chapter Content

**Initial Visit** A smiling young man gets up to shake my hand when I enter the exam room. As he sits down, his wife reassuringly pats him on the back. They appear calm and pleasant, but I sense the familiar tension as they gaze at the stack of papers in my hands. Meet KC, a 42-year-old man who immigrated to the United States from Africa 10 years ago. He works as a driver, prides himself on being a family man, and enjoys bike riding with his wife along the Schuylkill River in Philadelphia. Though sickle cell trait positive, KC has always been generally healthy and fit. He thus saw no need to contact a medical professional when the annual screening urine test performed during a work physical exam revealed microhematuria for 3 years in a row. Finally, a hematuria workup was performed, and a computed tomography (CT) scan showed a 5.0-cm enhancing lesion on the left kidney. KC feels "fine" and has never actually seen blood in his urine. KC does not know a lot about his grandparents' medical history; his mom died young of breast cancer and dad is back home battling kidney failure. While I perform the initial physical exam and record medical history, the urologic oncologist is reviewing scans and labs, consulting with radiology, and finalizing a treatment plan. KC is at the very beginning of his cancer journey.

**Type of Kidney Tumors** Tumors of the kidney can either stem from the renal parenchyma, which are known as renal cell carcinomas, or arise from the inner lining of the urothelium that covers the kidney's collecting system. The latter are known as urothelial carcinomas and are biologically very similar to bladder cancer. This chapter will focus on renal cell carcinomas.

E. Dreyzin (✉) · A. Kutikov
Department of Surgical Oncology, Fox Chase Cancer Center, Philadelphia, PA, USA
e-mail: Elena.Dreyzin@fccc.edu; Alexander.Kutikov@fccc.edu



E. J. Trabulsi et al. (eds.), *Chemotherapy and Immunotherapy in Urologic Oncology*, https://doi.org/10.1007/978-3-030-52021-2_20

**Overview of RCC** Renal cell carcinomas (RCCs) originate from the renal cortex and represent approximately 80–85% of all malignant kidney masses. The most common type of RCC is clear cell carcinoma (75–85%) followed by papillary (10–15%) and chromophobe (5–10%). It is important to remember that benign oncocytoma may mimic malignant renal cell carcinoma and is harbored by up to 30% of patients who undergo renal surgery in the United States [1]. Smoking, persistent hypertension, diabetes mellitus (DM), obesity, acquired cystic disease of the kidney, von Hippel-Lindau syndrome, and exposure to toxic elements such as cadmium, asbestos, and petroleum are among the risk factors for kidney malignancy. Sickle cell trait is a risk factor for medullary RCC.

**Imaging Studies** Many early kidney neoplasms are discovered incidentally when scans are done for other reasons. The classic triad of RCC – flank pain, hematuria, and a palpable renal mass – is now a rare form of presentation and strongly suggests advanced disease. To fully characterize a renal mass, cross-sectional imaging with and without contrast is necessary to determine whether the lesion is enhancing. Lesion enhancement indicates blood flow and thus confirms neoplasia. Renal ultrasound can also be used to differentiate between a non-hyperdense cyst and a solid tumor. On images, benign cysts are "anechoic" with a strong posterior wall echo indicating good transmission through a fluid-filled sac; a solid mass will show echo within it. It is important to remember that hyperdense cysts (those cysts that are filled with blood or protein) are largely indistinguishable from renal masses on ultrasound. Since most common sites of metastases are lungs and intra-abdominal sites such as lymph nodes, bone, and liver, guidelines advocate for appropriate staging with a CT of chest. Nuclear bone scans and brain magnetic resonance imaging (MRI) are reserved for patients with very high-risk localized disease. MRI with gadolinium is excellent at delineating renal vein and vena cava tumor invasion if present. FDG-PET (fluorodeoxyglucose-positron emission tomography) scans have a very limited role in RCC evaluation, since test characteristics of this modality in patients with RCC are poor.

**Renal Biopsy** Is kidney biopsy useful for the diagnosis of renal cancer? Absolutely, but arguably not for all patients. At our center, patients who would receive surgery regardless of biopsy results (e.g., young and non-comorbid patients with worrisome masses) proceed directly to treatment. Meanwhile, other patients who are ideal active surveillance candidates also do not undergo a procedure that would not change the treatment strategy. Otherwise, we believe renal biopsy can help calibrate treatment strategy and avoid overtreatment of benign masses [2]. Indeed, recent data suggest that up to 30% of renal tumors that are resected in the United States are benign [3].

**Staging** Treatment for RCC spans active surveillance, focal ablation, partial and radical nephrectomy, targeted therapy, immunotherapy, and radiation in select cases. TNM Staging System universally classifies the extent of tumor spread and assists in treatment decision-making: T, tumor size; N, regional lymph node involvement; and

M, distant metastasis involvement [4]. For example, T1aN0M0 is a person with a small <4 cm tumor in greatest dimension without regional nodes or distant metastasis. This combination describes a patient ideally suited for active surveillance (AS) route, a person with small asymptomatic lesion demonstrating slow growth (< 0.5 cm/year). AS is not for everyone. While some patients are comfortable with frequent visits and imaging, others prefer to surgically remove even the smallest mass. AS is well suited for the elderly and those with significant comorbidities (other cancers, advanced cardiovascular disease, poorly controlled diabetes, hypercoagulation syndromes, etc.). Active surveillance is safe; data suggests a very low metastatic rate only in tumors that show rapid growth kinetics [5]. Most current AS guidelines dictate a thorough H&P with CT of abdomen/MRI, CT of chest, and BMP every 6 months for the first year and then annually for 5 years. During that time, renal ultrasound (RUS) may be substituted for CT abdomen/MRI. Physician extenders can handle most AS patients and refer back to the attending physician if the tumor exhibits rapid growth, there are changes in lab work, or any other evidence of disease progression is noted.

**Ablation and Cryotherapy** Goals of treatment always need to be identified and discussed with the patient and family. It is especially relevant when patient transitions from active surveillance to active treatment (e.g., surgery). While surgery is the gold standard, percutaneous cryotherapy ("freezing") and radiofrequency ablation ("heating") are reasonable options, especially for elderly patients with appropriate masses for whom risks of surgery are not trivial. Laparoscopic ablation was performed in the past but has fallen out of favor with the advent of expertise in minimally invasive partial nephrectomy. Percutaneous ablation procedures, also known as focal therapy, avoid general anesthesia and invasive dissection. Of note, AS should still be considered as the primary treatment approach in that population [6]. Another goal of renal tumor therapy is kidney tissue preservation, which focal therapy generally can achieve successfully. Many centers with deep minimally invasive partial nephrectomy expertise and strong active surveillance programs use ablation therapy quite sparingly.

**Partial Versus Radical Nephrectomy: RENAL Score** Indications for surgical management of RCC are based on the disease stage and the extent of the disease. Location of the lesion, presence of bilateral tumors, compromised renal function (chronic kidney disease and/or solitary kidney status), and history of a genetic syndrome (von Hippel-Lindau disease) all influence the decision to proceed and how to best calibrate type/extent of surgery. The radical nephrectomy (RN) involves ligation of the renal vasculature and removal of the kidney and the Gerota's fascia (a fibrous tissue encapsulating the kidneys). Historically, the adrenal gland was routinely resected along with the kidney, but in current practice, the adrenal is removed only if it radiographically appears abnormal. RN is now the procedure of choice in a resectable primary tumor and a concurrent single metastatic lesion into adrenal gland, renal vein, or perinephric fat, and in these cases, the complete resection may be curative. However, when adrenal gland is not affected by metastasis, it should be surgically spared as the incidence of adrenal metastasis is not typical. Decision between partial and radical nephrectomy is complex; however, RN is generally preferred in cases where tumors are ≥7 cm and/or are endophytic (less than 40% extending off the surface of the kidney) and centrally located. While patients with cancers localized to the kidney have an excellent 5-year survival rate, 80–90%, they are also at risk for loss of renal function [7]. As such, patient's age and preoperative renal function must be integrated into the decision between radical and partial nephrectomy. Even though open surgery was the traditional surgical approach for RN, most kidneys can now be resected employing minimally invasive techniques.

Partial nephrectomy (PN), unlike RN, affords maximum renal tissue preservation while generally providing excellent cancer control. Absolute indications for this operation include solitary kidney, bilateral masses, and those with risk for chronic renal disease who cannot undergo RN without risking dialysis. While the benefits and minimal risks of PN are evident in small and peripherally located tumors, anatomically complex masses may expose patient to perioperative and potential oncologic risks that would have been avoided if RN were performed. These risks become especially burdensome on the comorbid and elderly population [8]. Thus, surgeons often debate how far to push relative indications of PN. In order to better communicate kidney tumor anatomic complexity and meaningfully compare surgical results, several renal surgery risk scoring systems have been published. The RENAL nephrometry system was proposed in 2009 and provides a measurable and reproducible method to categorize renal masses according to their anatomic relationship to the kidney's anatomy. Using axial cuts of CT or MRI scans, providers can quantify anatomic complexity of the renal mass in the following manner:

1. *R*adius: a diameter of <4 (one point), 4–7 (two points), and >7 cm (three points).
2. *E*xophytic/endophytic: ≥50% exophytic (one point), <50% exophytic (two points), and entirely endophytic (three points).
3. *N*earness to collecting system or sinus: the closer the tumor to the system, the more risks associated with PN (one to three points).
4. *A*nterior/posterior tumor (a or p assignment).
5. *L*ocation relative to polar lines (one to three points with central tumors being a score of three). Details to the scoring system can be found at http://www.nephrometry.com.

The RENAL scoring system and those like it have been shown to correlate to critical decision-making for patients with renal mass. For those seeing patients with kidney tumors, it is important to understand the variables that are communicated by such scoring systems [9].

In addition to age and comorbidity status, key clinical factors affecting the RN vs PN decision are dependence on anticoagulation and antiplatelet agents, history of complications at previous surgeries, impaired renal function (diabetes mellitus, chronic kidney disease, morbid obesity, etc.), tumor size, surgeon skill/confidence level, and, of course, patient preference/comfort level. Radical nephrectomy is considered in the case of centrally positioned tumors and in extension of tumor into lymph nodes, renal vein or inferior vena cava, or ipsilateral adrenal gland. The benefits and risks of both partial and radical nephrectomies must be well considered prior to making a treatment decision. Despite advanced modern surgical techniques, many patients present to medical attention with existing metastases or recur after treatment of localized disease. Recent revolutionary advances in the field of medical oncology offer many novel options for such patients.

**Radiation (XRT)** Although RCC has been described as a radioresistant tumor, XRT is often used to selectively treat metastatic lesions. It is also helpful in painful bone metastases, cancer progression into the brain, and recurrences in the renal bed [10].

**Chemotherapy** Cytotoxic chemotherapy largely does not have a role in kidney cancer treatment except for the use of gemcitabine/cisplatin in patients with collecting duct RCC, an extremely rare type of non-clear cell RCC that biologically resembles urothelial carcinoma [11].

**Antiangiogenic Therapy** Antiangiogenic therapy works by inhibiting the growth of new blood vessels to the tumor. Most commonly used agents are sunitinib, pazopanib, axitinib, and cabozantinib. These agents target the vascular endothelial growth factor (VEGF) pathway. The therapy can prolong survival in metastatic clear cell RCC and is now being used in combination with immunotherapy.

**Immunotherapy** Immunotherapy is the golden child of medical oncology and is a relatively novel approach to metastatic cancer. Instead of attacking the tumor directly, these agents harness the body's own immune system to respond to the cancer. While the human body likely constantly develops cancer, the immune system destroys these cells, preventing tumor formation. Occasionally, cancer cells escape and multiply using a network of supporting cells that protect it. Antigen-presenting cells (APCs) are the "look-out" entities that circulate in the body seeking potential oncologic developments, and T cells are the "army" of the immune system. Upon encountering a suspicious activity in the body, the APCs send a signal to a T cell soldier to multiply and attack the cancer. Since nonstop flow of T cells can be damaging to healthy cells, a checkpoint protein mechanism (PD-1) is set up to stop T cell multiplication just as the right number of these cells has been produced. Some tumors manage to shut off the T cell multiplication too early in the immune process. Therefore, the checkpoint inhibitor drugs, the most common type of immunotherapy, prevent T cells from being switched off and allow the immune system to safely destroy cancerous sites. Immunotherapy has now been approved to treat multiple cancers including bladder cancer, head and neck cancer, Hodgkin's lymphoma, non-small cell lung cancer, melanoma, and kidney cancer. PD-1 inhibitors such as pembrolizumab (Keytruda) and nivolumab (Opdivo) are most commonly used in RCC [12]. Although objective responses can be seen in a large proportion of patients, immunotherapy side effects need to be kept top of mind. These include thyroiditis, pneumonitis, adrenal insufficiency/hypotension, cardiac arrhythmias, neuro- and liver toxicity, and dermatologic complications. Vigilance must be high in patients receiving these therapies, since delay in diagnosis can result in death. For instance, patients on immunotherapy presenting with symptoms of pneumonia need to be started on steroid therapy to stem what can be a rapidly evolving immunotherapy-induced pneumonitis. Indeed, some patients are placed on long-term steroid courses or required to discontinue immunotherapy completely due to toxicity.

**Screening of General Population** To a patient and family, a diagnosis of renal cancer is emotionally and physically challenging. A provider then may logically contemplate whether universal screening renal ultrasounds (much like mammogram at 40 and colonoscopy at 50) have merit. Renal cell carcinoma though has a low prevalence in general population; therefore, screening *everyone* is not recommended at this time in order to avoid financial stress and unnecessary anxiety to a patient. Indeed, many subclinical lesions that never need treatment are likely to be uncovered, resulting in overdiagnosis and overtreatment. Those with inherited conditions such as von Hippel-Lindau syndrome and tuberous sclerosis, younger patients with end-stage renal disease, those with family history of RCC, and those with prior kidney irradiation should be carefully monitored with periodic imaging.

What about patient KC whom we met in the beginning of the chapter? Staging workup was ordered after the first visit, and KC was free from metastasis. His 5-cm renal was of intermediate complexity based on the RENAL nephrometry scoring system. A robotic partial nephrectomy was successfully performed, and pathology revealed a 5-cm grade-3 clear-cell renal cell carcinoma. KC will have close follow-up with urologic oncology. At each visit, we will order restaging imaging and blood work. Follow-up is a long road ahead, but for now, the patient and his family exhale a cautious sigh of relief. So do I.

**Pearls for the Advanced Practice Practitioner**

- Kidney mass is often discovered incidentally. Not all lesions are cancer and not every tumor needs invasive treatment.
- Kidney cancer risk factors: smoking, hypertension, obesity, acquired cystic disease of the kidney, exposure to toxins (cadmium, asbestos, petroleum), genetic factors, sickle cell trait, DM, and polycystic kidney disease.
- Kidney lesion biopsy can help patients avoid invasive treatment of a benign renal mass.
- Refer to a genetic counselor if multiple family members are involved and younger at the time of diagnosis (40 or below) and if bilateral tumors or known inherited syndromes are present.
- Use NCCN guidelines: user-friendly format; registration is free for APCs (NCCN.org).

## References


1. Ljungberg B, Campbell SC, Choi HY, Cho HY, Jacqmin D, Lee JE, Weikert S, Kiemeney LA. The epidemiology of renal cell carcinoma. Eur Urol. 2011;60(4):615–21.
2. Kutikov A, et al. Renal mass biopsy: always, sometimes, or never? Eur Urol. 2016;70(3):403–6.
3. Kim JH, Li S, Khandwala Y, Chung KJ, Park HK, Chung BI. Association of prevalence of benign pathologic findings after partial nephrectomy with preoperative imaging patterns in the United States from 2007 to 2014. JAMA Surg. 2019;154(3):225–31.
4. Rini BI, McKiernan JM, Chang SS, et al. Kidney. In: Amin MB, editor. AJCC cancer staging manual. 8th ed. New York: Springer; 2017. p. 739.
5. Ristau BT, et al. Active surveillance for small renal masses: when less is more. Eur Urol Focus. 2016;2(6):660–8.
6. Ginzburg S, et al. Focal ablation therapy for renal cancer in the era of active surveillance and minimally invasive partial nephrectomy. Nat Rev Urol. 2017;14:669–82.
7. Colombo JR Jr, Haber GP, Jelovsek JE, Lane B, Novick AC, Gill IS. Seven years after laparoscopic radical nephrectomy: oncologic and renal functional outcomes. Urology. 2008;71(6):1149.
8. Kim SP, et al. Collaborative review of risk benefit trade-offs between partial and radical nephrectomy in the management of anatomically complex renal masses. Eur Urol. 2017;72(1):64–75. https://doi.org/10.1016/j.eururo.2016.11.038.
9. Kutikov A, Uzzo RG. The R.E.N.A.L. nephrometry score: a comprehensive standardized system for quantitating renal tumor size, location and depth. J Urol. 2009;182(3):844–53. https://doi.org/10.1016/j.juro.2009.05.035.
10. Kjaer M, Frederiksen PL, Engelholm SA. Postoperative radiotherapy in stage II and III renal adenocarcinoma. A randomized trial by the Copenhagen Renal Cancer Study Group. Int J Radiat Oncol Biol Phys. 1987;13(5):665.
11. Oudard S, etal. GETUG (Groupe d'Etudes des Tumeurs Uro-Génitales). Prospective multicenter phase II study of gemcitabine plus platinum salt for metastatic collecting duct carcinoma: results of a GETUG (Groupe d'Etudes des Tumeurs Uro-Génitales) study. J Urol. 2007;177(5):1698.
12. McDermott DF, Lee JL, Szczylik C, et al. Pembrolizumab monotherapy as first-line therapy in advanced clear cell renal cell carcinoma: results from cohort A of KEYNOTE-427. J Clin Oncol. 2018;36S:ASCO #4500.

# Chapter 21
# Targeted Therapies for Treatment of Metastatic Renal Cell Carcinoma

**Jessica Matande and Adam C. Reese**

## Introduction

In the United States, renal cell carcinoma (RCC) is the seventh most common cancer in men and the ninth most common cancer in women, with over 60,000 new diagnoses annually [1]. Furthermore, the incidence of RCC has increased over the past several decades, largely due to the widespread adoption of cross-sectional imaging resulting in a higher incidence of incidentally detected renal masses. Unfortunately, despite the enhanced detection of these early-stage lesions, approximately 20–30% of patients with kidney cancer have metastatic disease at diagnosis [2]. Prognosis in such patients is poor, with 5-year survival rates of roughly 26% [3].

Several centers have identified prognostic criteria to characterize disease risk among patients with metastatic RCC. One of the most widely employed prognostication systems is that developed by Memorial Sloan Kettering Cancer Center (MSKCC), which stratifies patients with advanced or metastatic renal cell carcinoma into favorable, intermediate, or poor risk categories based on the presence or absence of five risk criteria (Fig. 21.1) [4]. Figure 21.2 elucidates the Karnofsky performance score used in the MSKCC system. The MSKCC system is useful in predicting patient prognosis, ranging from a median survival of only 4 months for those with poor risk disease to 20 months for those with favorable disease. Furthermore, this categorization helps clinicians delineate treatment protocols, as recommended management strategies often differ by disease risk.

This chapter discusses the various targeted therapies used to manage metastatic renal cell carcinoma (metastatic RCC). Several of these agents are currently considered first-line treatment for favorable risk metastatic RCC by the National Comprehensive Cancer Network (NCCN). Immunotherapies, which will be

J. Matande (✉) · A. C. Reese
Department of Urologic Oncology, Temple University Hospital, Philadelphia, PA, USA
e-mail: jessica.matande@tuhs.temple.edu



E. J. Trabulsi et al. (eds.), *Chemotherapy and Immunotherapy in Urologic Oncology*, https://doi.org/10.1007/978-3-030-52021-2_21

**MSKCC (Memorial Sloan Kettering Cancer center) Risk Classification**

**Poor Prognostic Features**

Lactate dehydrogenase level >1.5 times upper limit of normal
Hemoglobin level < lower limit of normal
Corrected serum calcium level >10 mg/dl
Absence of prior nephrectomy
Karnofsky performance score 80 or less
2 or more sites of organ metastasis

**MSKCC Risk Classification (Includes the First Five Poor prognostic Features)**

Poor risk (3 or more of 5 factors)
Intermediate risk (1 or 2 of 5 factors)

**Fig. 21.1** Memorial Sloan Kettering Cancer Center risk classification [4]

| Score (category) | Karnofsky |
|---|---|
| 100 | Normal; no complaints; no evidence of disease. |
| 90 | Able to carry on normal activity; minor signs or symptoms. |
| 80 | Normal activity with effort; some signs or symptoms of disease. |
| 70 | Care for self; unable to carry on normal activity or to do active work. |
| 60 | Requires occasional assistance but is able to care for most of his needs. |
| 50 | Requires considerable assistance and frequent medical care. |
| 40 | Disabled; requires special care and assistance. |
| 30 | Severely disabled; hospitalization necessary; active supportive treatment is necessary. |
| 20 | Very sick; hospitalization necessary; active supportive treatment is necessary. |
| 10 | Moribund; fatal processes progressing rapidly. |
| 0 | Dead. |

**Fig. 21.2** Karnofsky performance status scale definition rating (%) criteria [5]

discussed in a separate chapter, are now often considered preferred initial management for patients with intermediate/poor risk disease, although targeted therapies may be beneficial in these patients as well.

Targeted therapies for metastatic RCC were initially discovered through the characterization of molecular pathways resulting in hereditary kidney cancer syndromes. One of the best characterized hereditary RCC syndromes is von Hippel-Lindau (VHL) syndrome, an autosomal dominant syndrome resulting in various malignancies that can manifest in the retina, central nervous system, and kidneys [6]. Patients with VHL syndrome inherit one mutated *VHL* allele, and the second allele undergoes somatic mutation or deletion in order to promote the oncologic process, which follows the "two-hit hypothesis" model [6]. VHL is a tumor suppressor gene and encodes the VHL protein which is involved in growth factor signaling and cell division. Mutations of the *VHL* gene disrupt this signaling pathway, thereby promoting tumor development. As such, patients with germline *VHL* mutation, resulting in VHL disease, are prone to early-onset, multifocal, and bilateral clear cell RCC.

Interestingly, aberrations of the VHL gene also appear to play a role in sporadic (non-syndromic) RCC. Somatic mutations of the *VHL* gene have been found in roughly 60% of patients with sporadic clear cell renal cell carcinomas [6]. Thus, aberrations in this VHL signaling pathway appear to promote carcinogenesis in both syndromic and sporadic cases of clear cell RCC.

The *VHL* gene was first identified in 1993, and a more detailed characterization of the *VHL* signaling pathway followed in subsequent years, ushering in the discovery of targeted therapy [3]. Manipulating various aspects of the *VHL* molecular signaling pathway allowed for the development of targeted therapies that revolutionized the treatment of metastatic RCC and have since been incorporated into standard treatment paradigms for advanced kidney cancers. These targeted therapies include tyrosine kinase inhibitors (TKI), vascular endothelial growth factor (VEGF) inhibitors, and mammalian target of rapamycin (mTOR) inhibitors. Each of these agents works at a different stage of the oncologic process, exhibiting antitumor effects through inhibition of tumor angiogenesis and cell proliferation (see Fig. 21.3).

It is important to note that aberrations in the *VHL* signaling pathway typically result in clear cell RCC, as opposed to other histologic subtypes such as papillary or chromophobe RCC. Since tumors with these non-clear cell histologies likely develop through distinct molecular pathways, conventional targeted therapies are typically not as effective in managing metastatic non-clear cell RCC. Therefore, it is important to obtain tissue for histologic evaluation, as treatment recommendations often differ for clear cell RCC versus other histologies. For patients with newly diagnosed metastatic RCC, tissue sampling can be performed via biopsy of the kidney or through cytoreductive nephrectomy if otherwise indicated. NCCN guidelines recommend performing tissue sampling of some form to confirm diagnosis of RCC and also to determine histology in order to guide patient management [7].

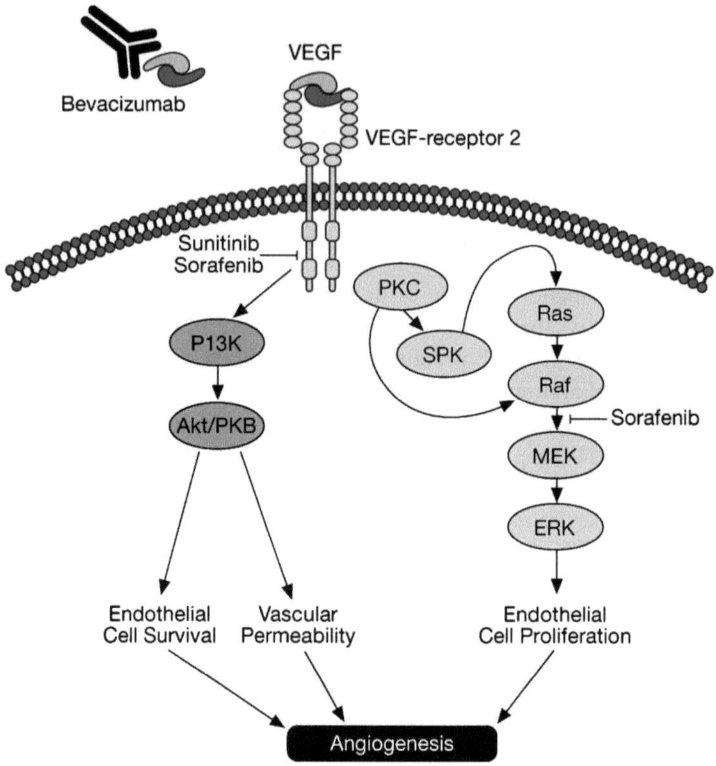


**Fig. 21.3** Targeted therapy pathways [1]

## Tyrosine Kinase Inhibitors

Tyrosine kinase inhibitors (TKIs) are currently considered first-line therapy for favorable risk metastatic clear cell RCC. The medications in this treatment category include sunitinib, pazopanib, sorafenib, cabozantinib, and axitinib. TKI's mechanism of action is through competitive inhibition of ATP at the catalytic binding site of tyrosine kinase. Tyrosine kinase is essentially an "on" or "off" switch for many cellular functions, including cell growth and division.

Tyrosine kinase inhibitors were first introduced as treatment options for RCC in 2005 with the development of oral sorafenib. Sorafenib is a small molecule that inhibits several tyrosine kinases [8]. At the time TKIs were being developed, cytokine therapies such as interferon-α-2a and interleukin 2 were first-line therapy for advanced RCC, albeit with relatively low tumor response rates and poor patient tolerability due to adverse effects. A randomized phase II trial published in 2009 was performed to test the efficacy and safety of sorafenib against cytokine-directed therapy with interferon-α [9]. This study demonstrated no difference in progression-free survival (PFS); however, patients receiving sorafenib showed greater tumor regression, better quality of life, and improved tolerability compared to those receiving interferon-α [9]. Due to development of multiple alternative options and lack of recent use of sorafenib as first-line therapy in this category, the NCCN no longer recommends it as first-line treatment for these patients. The results of the TARGET trial, testing this medication against placebo in patients with disease progression after prior cytokine therapy, relegated sorafenib to an acceptable choice as a subsequent therapy option for patients failing cytokine therapies [10]. However, due to its relative affordability as well as acceptable clinical efficacy and safety profile, it is an appropriate option for first-line treatment in settings where cost is a concern [9].

Sorafenib is an oral medication that comes as 200-mg tablets. It is dosed 400 mg (two tablets) orally twice daily without food [11].

Sunitinib, an agent that targets multiple tyrosine kinases, was approved by the FDA for treatment of metastatic RCC in 2006. An initial phase III trial comparing sunitinib to interferon-α demonstrated superiority of sunitinib in treatment efficacy, with an improvement in median progression-free survival of 6 months, as well as superior patient tolerability [12]. A subsequent update of this trial reported improved overall survival rates in patients managed with sunitinib [13]. Based on these data, sunitinib is now considered a preferred initial therapy for patients with favorable risk metastatic clear cell RCC.

Sunitinib has also shown efficacy, primarily in data from phase II clinical trials, in the management of patients with non-clear cell histologies including papillary and chromophobe RCC [14, 15]. Nonetheless, outcomes in this population are poor compared to patients with metastatic clear cell RCC, underscoring a need for better systemic therapies in patients with non-clear cell histology.

Sunitinib comes in capsule formation and is usually prescribed to be taken 50 mg orally once daily, with or without food. It is taken for 4 weeks followed by a drug holiday for 2 weeks [16, 17].

Pazopanib is another targeted therapy currently considered to be first line for the management of favorable risk metastatic clear cell RCC. Pazopanib functions as an antiangiogenic agent targeting several intracellular receptors. Pazopanib was initially compared to placebo in a trial of 435 patients with advanced or metastatic RCC, including patients who were treatment naive as well as those previously treated with cytokine therapy [18]. Pazopanib resulted in improved progression-free survival and tumor response rates in both groups of patients. The COMPARZ trial was subsequently performed as a head-to-head study comparing pazopanib and sunitinib. The final results demonstrated similar efficacy in terms of overall survival, but differences in adverse effects between these agents [12]. The later PISCES trial supported results of COMPARZ trial but suggested that pazopanib was better tolerated by patients, with less fatigue and less changes in food taste. Based on these data, both pazopanib and sunitinib are considered acceptable first-line therapies for metastatic clear cell RCC [19].

Pazopanib comes in tablet formation and is prescribed 800 mg orally once daily without food. It should be given at least 1 hour before or 2 hours after a meal following the standard TKI dosage cycle discussed above. Pazopanib comes in 200- and 400-mg tablets [20].

Cabozantinib is a small molecule inhibitor of several tyrosine kinases. This agent has shown efficacy in the initial management of patients with intermediate or poor risk disease, as well as among patients progressing after prior targeted therapy. The CABOSUN trial compared cabozantinib to sunitinib in patients with newly diagnosed intermediate or poor risk metastatic RCC and found an increase in progression-free survival and significantly higher objective response rates compared to sunitinib [21]. As such, it is considered to be a first-line therapy for patients with poor- and intermediate-risk metastatic clear cell RCC. Cabozantinib has also shown to be effective in the managing patients with disease progression after prior TKI-directed therapy. The METEOR trial compared cabozantinib to everolimus in such patients and found increased overall survival, delayed disease progression, and improved object response rates in the cabozantinib group [22]. As such, cabozantinib is considered a preferred option for managing patients with recurrent disease after failing prior targeted therapy.

Cabozantinib is prescribed 60 mg orally daily without food [23].

Axitinib is a selective, second-generation inhibitor of VEGFR-1, VEGFR-2, and VEGFR-3. This agent was previously used predominantly as second-line treatment. More recently, however, it has shown efficacy as initial therapy. As initial therapy, axitinib has demonstrated improved objective response rates compared to placebo and a similar efficacy and safety profile when compared to sunitinib [24, 25]. Based on these results, axitinib is now considered a first-line treatment option for patients with favorable risk metastatic clear cell RCC [24].

Axitinib comes in tablet formation, and it is typically dosed as 5 mg orally twice daily with or without food [26].

The most commonly reported side effects of these treatments listed during their clinical trials and per manufacturer guidelines are reviewed in the table below [16, 20, 21, 23]. You will see that many of these treatments have similar side effect profiles. In a later section, breakdown of how to monitor and manage the side effects will be reviewed in detail. Distinct from the other TKIs, pazopanib has the potential for grade 3 hepatotoxicity. It is critical to monitor liver function before and during treatment with all TKIs, as they can all affect liver function, and in particular with pazopanib treatment [27]. Despite this extensive list, TKIs generally appear to be well tolerated [28].

**TKI side effect comparison**

| | Pazopanib | Sunitinib | Axitinib | Sorafenib | Cabozantinib |
|---|---|---|---|---|---|
| Hepatotoxicity (+++ = grade 3 toxicity) | +++ | + | + | + | + |
| Diarrhea | + | + | + | + | + |
| Hypertension | + | + | + | + | + |
| Hair color changes | + | + | | | |
| Nausea/vomiting | + | + | + | | + |
| Anorexia | + | | | | |
| Fatigue | + | + | + | + | + |
| Weakness | + | | + | | |
| Abdominal pain | + | | | | |

| | Pazopanib | Sunitinib | Axitinib | Sorafenib | Cabozantinib |
|---|---|---|---|---|---|
| Headache | + | | | | |
| Hematologic abnormalities | + | + | + | | + |
| Hand-foot syndrome | | + | | + | + |
| Weight loss | | | + | | + |
| Decreased appetite | | | + | | + |
| Thyroid dysfunction | | + | + | + | |
| Congestive heart failure | + | + | | | |
| QTc prolongation | + | | | | |
| Rash | | | | + | |
| Alopecia | | | | + | |
| Fistula or GI perforation | | | + | | + |
| Stomatitis | | + | + | | |

Per manufacturer guidelines, a complete blood count (CBC), thyroid-stimulating hormone (TSH), and liver function tests (LFTs) should be performed before treatment to establish a baseline. CBC should be repeated on day 1 of each subsequent treatment cycle, or every 6 weeks [16, 17]. TSH should be repeated on day 1 of each cycle for 4 cycles and then every 3 months thereafter, with particular attention for patients taking sorafenib, axitinib, or sunitinib. A baseline comprehensive metabolic panel (CMP) and urinalysis (UA) should be collected and repeated every 6 weeks to monitor renal function. For patients on pazopanib, it is recommended that LFTs are rechecked at weeks 3, 5, 7, and 9 and then months 3 and 4 and periodically or as needed thereafter [20]. Pazopanib also carries a risk of QTc prolongation. It should be used with caution in patients who take antiarrhythmics or other medications that can also cause this side effect. Baseline and periodic electrocardiogram is recommended [20].

Patients are generally expected to continue the treatment regimen until disease progression is noted or they experience unacceptable toxicity. The toxicities are medication and dosage dependent as discussed above. In regard to TKIs as a whole, the major concern is for hepatotoxicity, particularly with pazopanib. It can be evaluated and monitored using the National Cancer Institute's Common Toxicity Criteria, which are broken down by body part affected or symptoms experienced. This helps define when to alter dosages, put the patient on a drug holiday, or discontinue the treatment altogether. For dose modifications, the respective medication's manufacturer guidelines should be referenced.

The NCCN guidelines for RCC state patients undergoing treatment for advanced RCC should be reevaluated in the office and have follow-up imaging every 6–16 weeks. Repeat chest, abdominal, and pelvic imaging with CT or MRI should be ordered and compared to baseline imaging. Imaging of the spine or full body bone scans can be ordered if and when clinically indicated [7]. Radiographic evidence of disease progression typically indicates a change in treatment is needed. These guidelines should be followed for all targeted therapy treatments.

A difficulty in assessing treatment success versus failure with TKI agents is that these therapies, when effective, often result in central necrosis of the tumor while the overall size of the tumor remains stable. Response Evaluation Criteria in Solid Tumors

(RECIST) have classically been used to determine radiographic response to therapy and are the most widely accepted method to objectively assess treatment response in metastatic RCC. This system notes the size of metastatic lesion and assesses treatment response by measuring changes in the size of these lesions on serial imaging [29]. Because this system is based on the size of metastatic lesions, it can give a potentially false impression of treatment failure if the lesions do not obviously shrink in size but rather are experiencing central necrosis, as often is the case with TKIs.

## Anti-vascular Endothelial Growth Factor (VEGF) Antibodies

Vascular endothelial growth factor (VEGF) is a member of the platelet-derived growth factor (PDGF) family of growth factors. Signaling via VEGF results in angiogenesis and cell division and has been implicated in carcinogenesis of tumors in multiple organs. VEGF signaling plays a role in the VHL pathway described above (Fig. 21.1), whereby VHL gene inactivation leads to VEGF overexpression, which can promote RCC development. Inhibitors of the VEGF receptor have demonstrated efficacy in the treatment of metastatic RCC.

Bevacizumab is an anti-VEGF antibody that interferes with the VEGF signaling pathway and is used to treat several types of cancers including colorectal and lung cancers, as well as RCC. In the management of RCC, bevacizumab is typically paired with interferon-α. This treatment was FDA approved in 2009, based on results from two large trials comparing bevacizumab plus interferon-α to interferon-α alone, showing an increase in progression-free survival and a nonsignificant trend toward improved overall survival in the bevacizumab group, albeit with increased toxicity [30, 31].

Bevacizumab is dosed 10 mg/kg every 2 weeks with interferon-α, and it is administered as an intravenous infusion. The first dose is recommended to be infused over 19 minutes. If that is well tolerated, the second dose can be infused over 60 minutes, and subsequent doses can be infused over 30 minutes thereafter. Due to its potential effects on wound healing, patients should wait at least 28 days after surgery (such as cytoreductive nephrectomy) or until the surgical wound is fully healed to initiate treatment with bevacizumab [32].

The most common side effects of bevacizumab are hypertension, proteinuria, fatigue, headache, and bleeding. Other manufacturer warnings include bowel perforation or fistula formation, arterial and venous thromboembolic events, posterior reversible encephalopathy syndrome, infusion reaction, embryo-fetal toxicity, ovarian failure, and congestive heart failure. Side effects attributed to interferon include fatigue, neutropenia, fever, and depression. Bevacizumab's bleeding risk carries a black box warning. Women of child-bearing age should be advised of the potential risk of ovarian failure and potential risk to a fetus and therefore should be encouraged to use reliable contraception [33].

Patients using bevacizumab should have a full blood panel to establish baseline values prior to treatment. Blood pressure monitoring and UA should be repeated every 2 weeks, so this can be done at each infusion appointment [32]. As with previous treatments, these patients should also be reevaluated with full blood panel and imaging every 6–16 weeks [7]. Treatment should be altered or discontinued if patients develop concerning toxicities – particularly with hemorrhage in this treatment class. Treatment should be discontinued if there is evidence of disease progression.

## Mammalian Target of Rapamycin (mTOR)

The mammalian target of rapamycin (mTOR) is a catalytic subunit of two protein kinase complexes and plays an important part in cell growth and proliferation/regulation. The mTORC1 site signal is switched on by several oncogenic pathways and is overactive in an estimated 70% of all human tumors. It drives many anabolic pathways in the cell and also suppresses important catabolic processes – most importantly autophagy.

Inhibitors of mTOR signaling have shown efficacy in the management of metastatic RCC. The first agent found to inhibit mTOR was rapamycin, which was originally developed as an immunosuppressant to prevent solid organ rejection after transplantation. Rapamycin inhibits only some of the functions of mTORC1 and is cystostatic rather than cytotoxic, so it can cause promotion of other tumorigenic events. Because mTOR signaling is essential for normal cell viability, inhibiting it can cause unavoidable damage to healthy tissue [34].

Two analogs of rapamycin, everolimus and temsirolimus, are used to treat metastatic RCC. Temsirolimus was FDA approved for advanced RCC in 2007 and has since expanded its use to several other cancers. The ARCC trial was a phase III, multicenter, randomized, open-label study of patients with metastatic RCC who were treatment naive and were categorized as poor risk group [22]. The study patients received interferon-α alone, temsirolimus alone, or a combination of temsirolimus and interferon-α. The end results demonstrated that temsirolimus alone produced improved overall survival (OS) compared to the other two treatment groups. Thus, temsirolimus is considered a first-line treatment for patients with poor risk metastatic RCC, but it is not typically used for those with favorable risk disease.

Temsirolimus has also shown benefit as a second-line agent in patients progressing after prior targeted therapy. The INTORSECT trial compared temsirolimus to sorafenib in patients who were previously treated with sunitinib as first-line therapy [25]. The results of this trial showed a benefit of temsirolimus in patients who had received less than 180 days of sunitinib therapy prior to progression. Thus, it was concluded that temsirolimus could be considered as second-line therapy in patients with an abbreviated response to first-line TKI treatment [35].

Temsirolimus is administered as a 25-mg intravenous infusion over a 30–60-minute period once a week [36].

Everolimus is an mTOR inhibitor that was originally approved for second- and third-line therapy in patients with advanced RCC who progressed after initial TKI therapy. This recommendation was based on data from the RECORD-1 phase III trial comparing everolimus to placebo in patients who experienced disease progression on sunitinib or sorafenib [37]. Everolimus treatment resulted in improved progression-free survival of about 2 months compared to placebo. However, the subsequent METEOR and CheckMate 025 trials comparing VEGF medications to everolimus demonstrated VEGF superiority, thereby relegating mTOR inhibitors to third-line treatment [22, 38].

Everolimus is orally administered 10 mg once daily [17].

The RECORD-3 trial was recently performed to determine the optimal sequencing of TKIs vs mTOR inhibitors in the initial management of metastatic RCC. This study compared sunitinib followed by everolimus after treatment failure to the opposite order of medications. Results showing the superiority of initial treatment with sunitinib suggest that TKIs, as opposed to mTOR inhibitors, should remain the initial therapy of choice in most patients.

The most common side effects of mTOR inhibitors include stomatitis, fatigue, hyperglycemia, hyperlipidemia, rash, diarrhea, anorexia, and nausea [39]. For everolimus specifically, noninfectious pneumonitis is a less common but concerning side effect. Noninfectious pneumonitis can be detected clinically or with chest x-ray if necessary [17]. Manufacturer warnings include monitoring for infection, severe hypersensitivity reactions, angioedema, renal failure, impaired wound healing, myelosuppression, and embryo-fetal toxicity [17]. Based on the severity of the side effect, treatment should be temporarily withheld or permanently discontinued.

Patients taking these medications should avoid live vaccines, and it is recommended they receive complete childhood vaccinations prior to starting treatment [39]. Female patients who could become pregnant should be advised of potential risk to a fetus and use reliable contraception [36]. Patients taking an angiotensin-converting enzyme (ACE) inhibitor in addition to this treatment are at increased risk of developing angioedema, and if they do experience this side effect, the mTOR should be permanently discontinued [17].

Prior to starting treatment with an mTOR inhibitor, baseline labs including CBC, basic metabolic panel (BMP), serum glucose, and lipid panel should be checked. These labs should be rechecked every 2 weeks for the first three cycles and then every 4 weeks thereafter [40]. As discussed with previous treatments, these patients should also be reevaluated with imaging every 6–16 weeks [7].

## Summary of TKIs in Managing Metastatic Renal Cell Carcinoma

Over the past decade, the development of targeted therapies and immuno-oncology agents has revolutionized the treatment of patients with metastatic RCC. These therapies, however, are in their infancy, and so we have much to learn about how they can best be deployed to optimize patient outcomes. Clearly, certain agents are preferred over others as first-line versus second-line therapy, to treat clear cell versus non-clear cell histology, and for favorable versus intermediate or poor risk disease. Figures 21.4 and 21.5 summarize the current recommendations from the National Comprehensive Cancer Network (NCCN) regarding preferred management strategies in each of these settings. However, as novel agents are developed and additional research is published, these recommendations are likely to change. It is therefore of paramount importance that the provider remains up to date on the current literature to allow for delivery of the best possible treatment regimen to patients with metastatic RCC.

NCCN National Comprehensive Cancer Network®

**NCCN Guidelines Version 2.2019**
**Kidney Cancer**

NCCN Guidelines Index
Table of Contents
Discussion

| RELAPSE OR STAGE IV: FIRST-LINE THERAPY FOR CLEAR CELL HISTOLOGY | | | |
|---|---|---|---|
| | **Preferred regimens** | **Other recommended regimens** | **Useful under certain circumstances** |
| **Favorable risk**[j] | • Pazopanib (category 1)<br>• Sunitinib (category 1) | • Ipilimumab + nivolumab<br>• Cabozantinib (category 2B) | • Active surveillance[k]<br>• Axitinib (category 2B)<br>• Bevacizumab + interferon alfa-2b (category 1)<br>• High-dose IL-2[l] |
| **Poor/ intermediate risk**[j] | • Ipilimumab + nivolumab (category 1)<br>• Cabozantinib | • Pazopanib (category 1)<br>• Sunitinib (category 1) | • Axitinib (category 2B)<br>• Bevacizumab + interferon alfa-2b (category 1)<br>• High-dose IL-2[l]<br>• Temsirolimus (category 1)[m] |

| RELAPSE OR STAGE IV: SUBSEQUENT THERAPY FOR CLEAR CELL HISTOLOGY[n] | | |
|---|---|---|
| **Preferred regimens** | **Other recommended regimens** | **Useful under certain circumstances** |
| • Cabozantinib (category 1)<br>• Nivolumab (category 1)<br>• Ipilimumab + nivolumab | • Axitinib (category 1)<br>• Lenvatinib + everolimus (category 1)<br>• Everolimus<br>• Pazopanib<br>• Sunitinib | • Bevacizumab (category 2B)<br>• Sorafenib (category 2B)<br>• High-dose IL-2 for selected patients[l] (category 2B)<br>• Temsirolimus (category 2B)[m] |

[j] See Risk Models to Direct Treatment (IMDC criteria) (KID-C).
[k] Rini BI, Dorff TB, Elson P, et al. Active surveillance in metastatic renal-cell carcinoma: a prospective, phase 2 trial. Lancet Oncol 2016;17:1317-1324.
[l] Patients with excellent performance status and normal organ function.
[m] See Risk Models to Direct Treatment (Predictors of Short Survival Used to Select Patients for Temsirolimus) (KID-C).
[n] In clear cell and non-clear cell RCC with predominant sarcomatoid features, gemcitabine + doxorubicin (category 2B) and gemcitabine + sunitinib (category 2B) have shown benefit.

**Note: All recommendations are category 2A unless otherwise indicated.**
**Clinical Trials: NCCN believes that the best management of any patient with cancer is in a clinical trial. Participation in clinical trials is especially encouraged.**

 KID-4

**Fig. 21.4** NCCN guidelines for relapse or stage IV disease – clear cell renal cell carcinoma



NCCN National Comprehensive Cancer Network®

**NCCN Guidelines Version 2.2019**
**Kidney Cancer**

NCCN Guidelines Index
Table of Contents
Discussion

| RELAPSE OR STAGE IV: SYSTEMIC THERAPY NON-CLEAR CELL HISTOLOGY[n,o] | | |
|---|---|---|
| **Preferred regimens** | **Other recommended regimens** | **Useful under certain circumstances** |
| • Clinical trial<br>• Sunitinib | • Cabozantinib<br>• Everolimus | • Axitinib<br>• Bevacizumab<br>• Erlotinib<br>• Lenvatinib + everolimus<br>• Nivolumab<br>• Pazopanib<br>• Bevacizumab + erlotinib for selected patients with advanced papillary RCC including HLRCC<br>• Bevacizumab + everolimus<br>• Temsirolimus (category 1 for poor-prognosis risk group;[m] category 2A for other risk groups) |

**HLRCC: Hereditary leiomyomatosis and renal cell cancer**

[m] See Risk Models to Direct Treatment (Predictors of Short Survival Used to Select Patients for Temsirolimus) (KID-C).
[n] In clear cell and non-clear cell RCC with predominant sarcomatoid features, gemcitabine + doxorubicin (category 2B) and gemcitabine + sunitinib (category 2B) have shown benefit.
[o] For collecting duct or medullary subtypes, partial responses have been observed with cytotoxic chemotherapy (carboplatin + gemcitabine, carboplatin + paclitaxel, or cisplatin + gemcitabine) and other platinum-based chemotherapies currently used for urothelial carcinomas.

**Note: All recommendations are category 2A unless otherwise indicated.**
**Clinical Trials: NCCN believes that the best management of any patient with cancer is in a clinical trial. Participation in clinical trials is especially encouraged.**

 KID-5

**Fig. 21.5** NCCN guidelines for relapse or stage IV disease – non-clear cell renal cell carcinoma

## Management of Treatment Side Effects

It is important to help patients manage their symptoms in order to optimize their health, ability to continue tolerating treatment, and overall sense of well-being. Patients should generally be encouraged to eat well, stay hydrated, walk or perform light exercise if they are able, and attempt to maintain normal routines with work and social life.

There are several more specific side effects that may require management, which can include reassurance, lifestyle modifications, or medical therapy. These are reviewed here and also included below in a reference table.

***GI Complaints*** Patients with diarrhea should be encouraged to try probiotics/yogurt, eat low fiber foods, have small but frequent meals, avoid spicy and fatty foods, and avoid caffeine and fruit. Over-the-counter medications, such as loperamide, can be used as needed. For complaints of stomatitis, similar recommendations are made but also include frequent mouth rinses, use of a straw to drink liquids, and consumption of soft foods. "Magic mouthwash," which can include various combinations of viscous lidocaine 2%, Mylanta, nystatin, hydrocortisone, tetracycline, and diphenhydramine, can be useful. Patients are instructed to swish the solution in their mouth and then spit it out and can repeat this every 4 hours as needed. They should avoid drinking and eating afterward for about 30 minutes to ensure the medication stays on the affected area. For anorexia, patients should be encouraged to try and eat several small meals a day, find snacks they can enjoy that are also nutritious, add gravy, butter, or cheese for added protein and calories, and drink fluids between meals instead of filling up on them while eating. For nausea and vomiting, ondansetron sublingual dissolving tablets and other anti-nausea medications can be helpful. If patients are bothered by certain food smells, it might be helpful to consume them at room temperature or cold. If they are too tired to cook, friends or family may be able to help prepare food. If they have trouble tasting food, you can suggest adding herbs and condiments. Getting a registered dietician involved can be very beneficial. Patients with abdominal pain and dyspepsia should be encouraged to eat slowly, remain upright after meals, and avoid heavy meals, coffee, and alcohol. Over-the-counter treatments such as antacid tablets or bismuth subsalicylate can be used short term and as needed. Patients should be monitored for bowel perforation or fistula formation throughout treatment with cabozantinib and axitinib. If the patient develops signs or symptoms of either complication, obtain abdominal imaging and consider admission for surgical evaluation and management [26].

***Dermatologic Complaints*** Patients with hand-foot syndrome, also known as palmar-plantar erythrodysesthesia, should be advised to wear loose fitting cotton clothes, use sunscreen, clean their hands and feet with warm water daily, and apply creams often and liberally. For patients with rash, determine whether it is due to an allergic reaction, dermatitis, dry skin, or other cause. Avoid exposure to allergens. Additionally, they may also benefit from short-term use of topical corticosteroid cream or emollients.

***Hypertension*** Blood pressure should be monitored at each visit. Treat hypertension with appropriate antihypertensives as needed. If hypertension persists despite medical therapy, adjust TKI medication dosage or discontinue TKI treatment [26].

***Congestive Heart Failure*** Monitor patients for signs and symptoms throughout treatment. If symptoms arise, treat the condition and evaluate for the need to alter or discontinue use of the offending TKI [26].

***Thyroid Dysfunction*** Monitor TSH for the respective medication as suggested previously. Treat hyper- or hypothyroidism when indicated to maintain euthyroid levels [26].

***Fatigue*** Fatigue is arguably one of the most common cancer-related symptoms. It can be a result of the disease itself or a side effect of treatment. It is difficult to quantify and surprisingly underdiagnosed. The National Cancer Institute's Common Toxicity Criteria that were discussed previously also have a grading scale for fatigue. Classifying the severity of a patient's fatigue will help determine the best way to address it. The NCCN discusses four interventions for fatigue. The first should be approached with every patient, and it involves general counseling of the patient and their family members regarding the expected effects of their treatment. The second intervention centers around teaching general strategies for managing fatigue such as self-monitoring, energy conservation, and diversions to keep patients occupied and their attention focused on other things. The third intervention is more complex and involves nonpharmacologic treatments such as exercise, referral to rehabilitation services, psychosocial treatments, support groups, and nutrition consultation. The fourth intervention involves treatment with medication that can include psychostimulants, treatment for anemia, and sleep medication. It is important to listen to your patient and not to dismiss their complaints. Fatigue, though seemingly ubiquitous and insurmountable, can be managed [3].

| Side effect | Lifestyle management options | Medical management options |
|---|---|---|
| Diarrhea | Do: probiotics, yogurt, low fiber foods; eat small, frequent meals<br>Don't: spicy foods, fatty foods, caffeine, and fruit | Loperamide |
| Stomatitis | See above | "Magic mouthwash" |
| Anorexia | Do: several small meals a day, find enjoyable and nutritious snacks; add gravy, butter, or cheese; drink fluids between meals; ask friends/family to prepare meals; add herbs and condiments for flavor; consult registered dietician, consume foods at room temperature or cold to avoid bothersome food odors | |
| Abdominal pain and dyspepsia | Do: eat slowly; stay upright after meals; avoid heavy meals, coffee, and alcohol | Antacid tablets<br>Bismuth subsalicylate |

| Side effect | Lifestyle management options | Medical management options |
|---|---|---|
| Palmar-plantar erythrodysesthesia (hand-foot syndrome) | Do: wear loose fitting cotton clothes, use sunscreen, clean hands and feet with warm water daily, apply creams often and liberally | Short-term use of topical corticosteroid creams |
| Hypertension | Do: diet modification (particularly salt intake) if indicated | Antihypertensive medication as indicated<br>Adjust TKI therapy dose or discontinue if HTN persists despite medical therapy |
| Fistula or bowel perforation | | Monitor for symptoms throughout treatment<br>Obtain abdominal imaging when clinically indicated<br>Admit for surgical evaluation/intervention prn |
| Nausea/vomiting | Do: avoid triggers if possible | Ondansetron<br>Hydration assistance (PO or IV prn) |
| Thyroid dysfunction | | Monitor TSH<br>Treat hyper- or hypothyroidism as indicated to maintain euthyroid levels |
| Rash | Do: identify the cause: allergic reaction, dermatitis, or dry skin; avoid allergens; wear loose fitting cotton clothes; use sunscreen; clean hands and feet with warm water daily; apply creams often and liberally | Corticosteroid cream – short-term use only |

**Pearls for the Advanced Practice Provider**

- Refer to NCCN Kidney Cancer guidelines as needed.
- Manufacturer guidelines are helpful references for questions regarding administration of each medication and management of side effects.
- Follow the guidelines discussed regarding when to order follow-up labs and imaging, in addition to obtaining a thorough history and physical, to ensure the patient is tolerating treatment and responding as expected.
- Refer to the suggested management for side effects in order to help patients maintain or improve their quality of life during treatment and avoid the early termination of treatment due to adverse effects.

## References

1. Linehan WM, Bratslavsky G, Pinto PA, Schmidt LS, Neckers L, Bottaro DP, et al. Molecular diagnosis and therapy of kidney cancer. Annu Rev Med. 2010;61:329–43. https://doi.org/10.1146/annurev.med.042808.171650.
2. Janzen NK, Kim HL, Figlin RA, Belldegrun AS. Surveillance after radical or partial nephrectomy for localized renal cell carcinoma and management of recurrent disease. Urol Clin North Am. 2003;30(4):843–52.
3. Latif F, Tory K, Gnarra J, Yao M, Duh FM, Orcutt ML, et al. Identification of the von Hippel-Lindau disease tumor suppressor gene. Science. 1993;260(5112):1317–20.
4. Mekhail TM, Abou-Jawde RM, Boumerhi G, Malhi S, Wood L, Elson P, et al. Validation and extension of the Memorial Sloan-Kettering prognostic factors model for survival in patients with previously untreated metastatic renal cell carcinoma. J Clin Oncol. 2005;23(4):832–41. https://doi.org/10.1200/JCO.2005.05.179.
5. Schag CC, Heinrich RL, Ganz PA. Karnofsky performance status revisited: reliability, validity, and guidelines. J Clin Oncol. 1984;2(3):187–93. https://doi.org/10.1200/JCO.1984.2.3.187.
6. Cohen HT, McGovern FJ. Renal cell carcinoma. N Engl J Med. 2005;353:2477–90.
7. Practice guidelines in oncology: kidney cancer. [database on the Internet] Version 2.2019. Accessed. https://www.nccn.org/professionals/physician_gls/pdf/kidney.pdf.
8. Awada A, Hendlisz A, Gil T, Bartholomeus S, Mano M, de Valeriola D, et al. Phase I safety and pharmacokinetics of BAY 43-9006 administered for 21 days on/7 days off in patients with advanced, refractory solid tumours. Br J Cancer. 2005;92(10):1855–61. https://doi.org/10.1038/sj.bjc.6602584.
9. Escudier B, Szczylik C, Hutson TE, Demkow T, Staehler M, Rolland F, et al. Randomized phase II trial of first-line treatment with sorafenib versus interferon Alfa-2a in patients with metastatic renal cell carcinoma. J Clin Oncol. 2009;27(8):1280–9. https://doi.org/10.1200/JCO.2008.19.3342.
10. Escudier B, Eisen T, Stadler WM, Szczylik C, Oudard S, Staehler M, et al. Sorafenib for treatment of renal cell carcinoma: final efficacy and safety results of the phase III treatment approaches in renal cancer global evaluation trial. J Clin Oncol. 2009;27(20):3312–8. https://doi.org/10.1200/JCO.2008.19.5511.
11. Bayer. Nexavar (sorafenib). Prescribing information. 2005.
12. Motzer RJ, McCann L, Deen K. Pazopanib versus sunitinib in renal cancer. N Engl J Med. 2013;369(20):1970. https://doi.org/10.1056/NEJMc1311795.
13. Motzer RJ, Hutson TE, McCann L, Deen K, Choueiri TK. Overall survival in renal-cell carcinoma with pazopanib versus sunitinib. N Engl J Med. 2014;370(18):1769–70. https://doi.org/10.1056/NEJMc1400731.
14. Choueiri TK, Plantade A, Elson P, Negrier S, Ravaud A, Oudard S, et al. Efficacy of sunitinib and sorafenib in metastatic papillary and chromophobe renal cell carcinoma. J Clin Oncol. 2008;26(1):127–31. https://doi.org/10.1200/JCO.2007.13.3223.
15. Lee JL, Ahn JH, Lim HY, Park SH, Lee SH, Kim TM, et al. Multicenter phase II study of sunitinib in patients with non-clear cell renal cell carcinoma. Ann Oncol. 2012;23(8):2108–14. https://doi.org/10.1093/annonc/mdr586.
16. Ltd. P. Sutent (sunitinib malate). Highlights of prescribing information. 2006.
17. Novartis. Afinitor (everolimus). Highlights of prescribing information. 2009.
18. Sternberg CN, Davis ID, Mardiak J, Szczylik C, Lee E, Wagstaff J, et al. Pazopanib in locally advanced or metastatic renal cell carcinoma: results of a randomized phase III trial. J Clin Oncol. 2010;28(6):1061–8. https://doi.org/10.1200/JCO.2009.23.9764.
19. Escudier B, Porta C, Bono P, Powles T, Eisen T, Sternberg CN, et al. Randomized, controlled, double-blind, cross-over trial assessing treatment preference for pazopanib versus sunitinib in patients with metastatic renal cell carcinoma: PISCES Study. J Clin Oncol. 2014;32(14):1412–8. https://doi.org/10.1200/JCO.2013.50.8267.
20. GlaxoSmithKline. Votrient (pazopanib). Summary of product characteristics. 2009.

21. Choueiri TK, Halabi S, Sanford BL, Hahn O, Michaelson MD, Walsh MK, et al. Cabozantinib versus Sunitinib as initial targeted therapy for patients with metastatic renal cell carcinoma of poor or intermediate risk: the Alliance A031203 CABOSUN trial. J Clin Oncol. 2017;35(6):591–7. https://doi.org/10.1200/JCO.2016.70.7398.
22. Choueiri TK, Escudier B, Powles T, Tannir NM, Mainwaring PN, Rini BI, et al. Cabozantinib versus everolimus in advanced renal cell carcinoma (METEOR): final results from a randomised, open-label, phase 3 trial. Lancet Oncol. 2016;17(7):917–27. https://doi.org/10.1016/S1470-2045(16)30107-3.
23. Exelexis. Cabometyx (cabozantinib). Highlights of prescribing information. 2012.
24. Rini BI, Melichar B, Ueda T, Grünwald V, Fishman MN, Arranz JA, et al. Axitinib with or without dose titration for first-line metastatic renal-cell carcinoma: a randomised double-blind phase 2 trial. Lancet Oncol. 2013;14(12):1233–42. https://doi.org/10.1016/S1470-2045(13)70464-9.
25. Hutson TE, Lesovoy V, Al-Shukri S, Stus VP, Lipatov ON, Bair AH, et al. Axitinib versus sorafenib as first-line therapy in patients with metastatic renal-cell carcinoma: a randomised open-label phase 3 trial. Lancet Oncol. 2013;14(13):1287–94. https://doi.org/10.1016/S1470-2045(13)70465-0.
26. Pfizer. Inlyta (axitinib). Highlights of prescribing information. 2012.
27. Sternberg CN, Hawkins RE, Wagstaff J, Salman P, Mardiak J, Barrios CH, et al. A randomised, double-blind phase III study of pazopanib in patients with advanced and/or metastatic renal cell carcinoma: final overall survival results and safety update. Eur J Cancer. 2013;49(6):1287–96. https://doi.org/10.1016/j.ejca.2012.12.010.
28. Hartmann JT, Haap M, Kopp HG, Lipp HP. Tyrosine kinase inhibitors - a review on pharmacology, metabolism and side effects. Curr Drug Metab. 2009;10(5):470–81.
29. Krajewski KM, Nishino M, Ramaiya NH, Choueiri TK. RECIST 1.1 compared with RECIST 1.0 in patients with advanced renal cell carcinoma receiving vascular endothelial growth factor-targeted therapy. AJR Am J Roentgenol. 2015;204(3):W282–8. https://doi.org/10.2214/AJR.14.13236.
30. Rini BI, Halabi S, Rosenberg JE, Stadler WM, Vaena DA, Archer L, et al. Phase III trial of bevacizumab plus interferon alfa versus interferon alfa monotherapy in patients with metastatic renal cell carcinoma: final results of CALGB 90206. J Clin Oncol. 2010;28(13):2137–43. https://doi.org/10.1200/JCO.2009.26.5561.
31. Rini BI, Escudier B, Tomczak P, Kaprin A, Szczylik C, Hutson TE, et al. Comparative effectiveness of axitinib versus sorafenib in advanced renal cell carcinoma (AXIS): a randomised phase 3 trial. Lancet. 2011;378(9807):1931–9. https://doi.org/10.1016/S0140-6736(11)61613-9.
32. Genentech. Avastin (bevacizumab). Highlights of prescribing information. 2004.
33. Harshman LC, Srinivas S. The bevacizumab experience in advanced renal cell carcinoma. Onco Targets Ther. 2010;3:179–89.
34. Xie J, Wang X, Proud CG. mTOR inhibitors in cancer therapy. F1000Res. 2016;5 https://doi.org/10.12688/f1000research.9207.1.
35. Hwang C, Heath EI. The judgment of Paris: treatment dilemmas in advanced renal cell carcinoma. J Clin Oncol. 2014;32(8):729–34. https://doi.org/10.1200/JCO.2013.53.6029.
36. Pfizer. Torisel (temsirolimus). Highlights of prescribing information. 2007.
37. Motzer RJ, Escudier B, Oudard S, Hutson TE, Porta C, Bracarda S, et al. Efficacy of everolimus in advanced renal cell carcinoma: a double-blind, randomised, placebo-controlled phase III trial. Lancet. 2008;372(9637):449–56. https://doi.org/10.1016/S0140-6736(08)61039-9.
38. Escudier B, Sharma P, McDermott DF, George S, Hammers HJ, Srinivas S, et al. CheckMate 025 randomized phase 3 study: outcomes by key baseline factors and prior therapy for Nivolumab versus Everolimus in advanced renal cell carcinoma. Eur Urol. 2017;72(6):962–71. https://doi.org/10.1016/j.eururo.2017.02.010.
39. Buti S, Leonetti A, Dallatomasina A, Bersanelli M. Everolimus in the management of metastatic renal cell carcinoma: an evidence-based review of its place in therapy. Core Evid. 2016;11:23–36. https://doi.org/10.2147/CE.S98687.
40. George S, Bukowski R. Role of everolimus in the treatment of renal cell carcinoma. Therapeutics and Clinical Risk Management. 2009;5:699–706.

# Chapter 22
# Immune Therapies for Metastatic Kidney Cancer

**Kassem S. Faraj, Thai H. Ho, Mark D. Tyson, and Erik P. Castle**

## Background

One of the earliest reports demonstrating the potential application of immunomodulation for tumor regression was when administration of interleukin-2 (IL-2) led to a reduction of tumor burden in a patient with melanoma in 1984 [1]. This has since led to significant interest in the field of immunology and its role in managing various malignancies. The earliest studies evaluating the efficacy of immune system modulation in cancer demonstrated responses in advanced melanoma, lung cancer, colorectal cancer, bladder cancer, and renal cell carcinoma (RCC). The specific modulators that have been studied and used for therapy in advanced RCC include drugs involved in the pathways of IL-2, interferon alfa, cytotoxic T-lymphocyte antigen-4 (CTLA-4), and programmed cell death protein-1 (PD-1). This chapter will discuss the clinical use of agents that modulate the above pathways.

## Interleukin-2

Interleukin-2 is a cytokine created by antigen-stimulated CD4 cells, CD8 cells, natural killers cells, and activated dendritic cells during the immune response. In early in vitro studies, this cytokine was found to be a potent stimulator of the immune system, facilitating and inducing various components of the immune

K. S. Faraj (✉) · M. D. Tyson · E. P. Castle
Department of Urology, Mayo Clinic, Phoenix, AZ, USA
e-mail: faraj.kassem@mayo.edu; Tyson.mark@mayo.edu; castle.erik@mayo.edu

T. H. Ho
Department of Hematology and Oncology, Mayo Clinic, Phoenix, AZ, USA
e-mail: ho.thai@mayo.edu



E. J. Trabulsi et al. (eds.), *Chemotherapy and Immunotherapy in Urologic Oncology*, https://doi.org/10.1007/978-3-030-52021-2_22

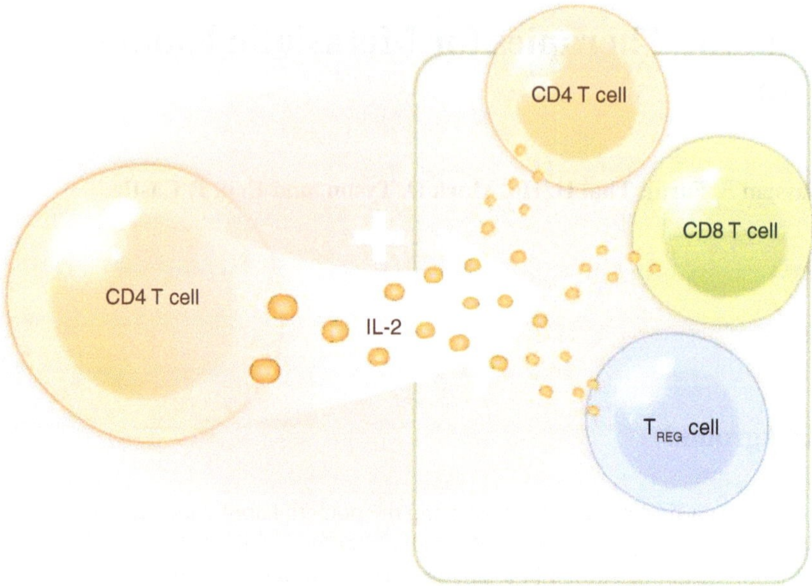


**Fig. 22.1** Interleukin-2 release from CD4 cell permitting activation of various T cells

system (Fig. 22.1) [2]. Specifically, studies in mice found that administration of IL-2 permits the induction of T-helper cells, cytotoxic T cells, and antibody production [3].

One the earliest studies in humans that evaluated the effect of IL-2 on cancer was published by Lotze et al. This study involved ten patients with melanoma, colon cancer, and ovarian cancer. Patients were administered intravenously or intraperitoneally with high-dose IL-2 (30,000 U/kg) three times a day. Half of the melanoma patients exhibited an objective response that was sustained up to 6 months after conclusion of therapy. This study discussed that at the time of preparation of the manuscript, one patient with metastatic renal cell carcinoma (RCC) with pulmonary metastasis demonstrated a complete response with IL-2 [4]. One report by Rosenberg et al. in 1989 described the use of IL-2 in 652 cancer patients. IL-2 was administered alone or in conjunction with various adjunctive immunomodulators, cytokines, monoclonal antibodies, or chemotherapeutic agents [5]. The report revealed that objective regression was appreciated in 20–35% of patients and was durable. As a result of the encouraging potential effectiveness of this therapy, numerous trials at that time were performed [4, 6–9]. Metastatic RCC was one of the cancers that was found to be favorably responsive to this treatment.

A study in 1994 that enrolled 283 consecutive patients with both metastatic melanoma and RCC evaluated its efficacy in oncological outcomes. Seven percent of the RCC patients experienced complete regression, and 13% experienced partial regression [10]. At a 4-year update, the study reported a 19% overall response rate and 9% complete response rate in the metastatic RCC patients. As result of the encouraging data, the US Food and Drug Administration (FDA) approved the use of high-dose IL-2 for patients with metastatic renal cell carcinoma. Further studies confirmed both the efficacy and durability of this treatment. One study that reviewed seven phase 2 clinical trials involved 255 patients with metastatic renal cell carcinoma and reported objective response rates of 15% of patients, with 7% complete responses and 8% partial responses. The responses were durable in many patients, as some experienced complete and partial responses for up to 80 and 131 months, respectively [11]. Although early studies suggested that administration of lymphokine-activated killer (LAK) cells with IL-2 facilitated tumor regression, this was found to be an ineffective adjunct to the IL-2 regimens in patients with metastatic RCC [6].

IL-2 was one of the first-line therapies for metastatic RCC for years but was not without its risks. Its use had been associated with significant toxicity and costs and its limitation to only be used at specialized centers. The toxicity of IL-2 was recognized in early studies, as Margolin et al. reported on toxicities in 93 patients who received high-dose IL-2 [12]. The most frequent toxicities observed were a capillary leak syndrome, which resulted in significant fluid shifts, hypotension, and vasopressor support. Nearly all patients experienced hepatic and kidney dysfunction. These adverse effects were found to be highly dose dependent and reversible after stopping treatment [7].

In an attempt to reduce the incidence and severity of adverse events, various therapy modifications were attempted. Reduced doses of IL-2 were studied in comparison to the standard high-dose regimen and were found to be less clinically active than the higher dose [13]. High-dose IL-2 was also compared to a combination of subcutaneous IL-2 with interferon in metastatic RCC, and the high-dose IL-2 was superior in regards to response rate. This study also suggested that patients with liver or bone metastasis may specially benefit from the high-dose regimen [14]. It was maintained as one of the first-line treatments for patients with metastatic RCC until recent years, when some of the less toxic, more efficacious therapies were described. Some of these therapies will be discussed later in this chapter.

## *Dose*

The therapeutic dose and regimen of IL-2 varies in the literature. It has been found to be effective when used via an intravenous or subcutaneous route. The intravenous cycle typically consists of administration of a range of doses ($7 \times 10^4$ to $18 \times 10^6$ U/kg). Various treatment regimens have been described using the intravenous route. One of the examples of an effective regimen described using an induction cycle of $18 \times 10^6$ IU/m$^2$ body surface area per day for 5 days for two courses, separated by at least 6 days. This is followed by a maintenance cycle consisting of one 5-day course of treatment. It was recommended that patients undergo two induction cycles and two maintenance cycles, with each cycle separated by 3 weeks of no therapy [15]. Additional effective regimens have been described in the literature [9, 13, 16, 17].

The subcutaneous regimen also varies. Some have described daily treatments (Monday–Friday) for a given cycle, usually involving 250,000 U/kg/dose in the first week and then 125,000 U/kg/dose in subsequent weeks [13]. Another report that combined the subcutaneous route with interferon described using an initial dose of $5 \times 10^6$ every 8 hours for the first day, followed by daily treatments (Monday–Friday) for 4 weeks for each 6-week cycle [14].

### *Adverse Events*

High-dose IL-2 is associated with many adverse events. Some are discussed above, but to summarize, patients can experience a range of adverse effects. Some of the low-grade complications include nausea, diarrhea, mild hematologic toxicities, elevation in liver enzymes, fevers, chills, fatigue, and rash. The high-grade complications can be related to a capillary leak syndrome that can result in significant vasodilation, severe fluid overload, and hypotension. Other side effects include confusion, depressed level of consciousness, renal dysfunction leading to oliguria, neurotoxicities, and cardiac toxicities. Patients can also experience severe infections due to neutrophil dysfunction [9, 16]. Patients commonly require intensive care unit admission and vasopressor support [16].

## Interferon Alfa-2a

Interferon alfa-2a (IFN $\alpha$2a) is a protein with immunomodulatory effects, including tumor regression. It is thought to increase the expression of HLA molecules, as well as facilitate activation of CD8 cells, which can have cytotoxic effects on tumor cells (Fig. 22.2) [18]. In some of the earliest reports, this drug was found to be effective as an antitumor agent in malignancies such as Kaposi's sarcoma, hairy cell leukemia, and cutaneous T-cell lymphoma [19]. As a result, it was eventually studied in metastatic RCC.

In a retrospective study by Quesada et al., 19 patients with metastatic RCC were given $3 \times 10^6$ units of daily IFN $\alpha$2a or doses of $18 \times 10^6$ or $36 \times 10^6$ units twice weekly. Twenty-six percent of patients showed a partial response, 10.5% experienced an objective minor response, 16% of patients experienced mixed effects (i.e., progression in some sites and regression in other sites), 10.5% had disease stabilization, and 37% progressed [20]. In a prospective study that looked at various doses of IFN $\alpha$2a in 159 patients with metastatic RCC, a 10% overall response rate was observed, and median overall survival was 11.4 months, with only 3% of patients

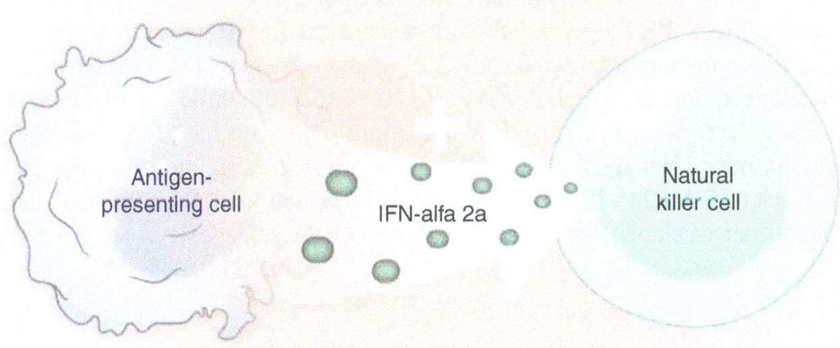


**Fig. 22.2** IFN-alfa-2a release from antigen-presenting cells leading to activation of natural killer cell

being alive at 5 years or more [21]. A later randomized trial that looked at IL-2, IFN α2a, or both in patients with metastatic RCC revealed response rates of 6.5%, 7.5%, and 18.6% for the three groups, respectively. Event-free survival rates were 15%, 12%, and 20%, respectively. The combination group experienced a greater incidence of adverse events. Overall survival was similar in the three groups [15]. The overall median survival between the three groups was 12, 13, and 17 months, respectively. These differences were not statistically significant. Several other studies revealed similar survival benefit with interferon monotherapy [22, 23]. As a result of its efficacy, though limited in nature, it was considered one of the first-line therapeutic options in patients with metastatic RCC.

IFN α2a was commonly used until it was found to be inferior to some of the newer agents that were introduced for metastatic RCC around 10 years ago. In a multicenter, phase 3, randomized trial of 626 patients with previously untreated, poor prognostic metastatic RCC, patients were stratified to receive the mTOR (mammalian target of rapamycin) kinase inhibitor (temsirolimus), IFN α2a, or combination therapy. The patients who received temsirolimus alone had a significantly longer overall survival compared to the other two groups. Median overall survival times were 10.9, 7.3, and 8.4 months, respectively. Fewer patient experienced adverse events in the temsirolimus group than the interferon group. As newer agents such as mTOR inhibitors and checkpoint inhibitors became better understood and studied more, the use of both interferon and IL-2 significantly decreased due to decreased comparative efficacy and/or increased toxicity.

### *Dose*

There are various doses and regimens that have been described for IFN α2a use in metastatic RCC. One of the regimens described for IFN α2a has been a subcutaneous route of $18 \times 10^6$ IU per day three times a week for 10 weeks as an induction treatment and then an additional 13 weeks as maintenance [15]. Another regimen includes subcutaneous injection of $5 \times 10^6$ IU of IFN α2a three times per week for 4 weeks as a 6-week cycle, with a maximum of six cycles [14]. The Medical Research Council Renal Cancer Collaborators described a regimen that consisted of a first week of IFN α2a with three treatments of 5, 5, and $\times 10^6$ IU, followed by three treatments per week of $10 \times 10^6$ IU, for a total of 12 weeks [23].

### *Adverse Events*

Some of the side effects that have been described for interferon treatment include lack of appetite, anorexia, fatigue, nausea, dry mouth, shivering, heartburn, and hepatotoxicity [21, 23, 24].

## Immunomodulators and Checkpoint Inhibitors

### *Mechanism and Biology*

There are various factors that regulate T-cell homeostasis in the immune system. For a T cell to be activated, the T-cell receptor must bind the antigen of interest. This interaction alone is insufficient to activate a T cell. As a result, if only this interaction occurs, without an additional costimulatory stimulus, the T cells will become unresponsive (i.e., anergy) [25]. A second signal is required to permit T-cell activation (i.e., costimulation). This second signal typically involves the protein CD28, which is on the T cells. Upon stimulation by ligands on antigen-presenting cells (B7-1 or B7-2), activation of the T cell ensues [26]. Cytotoxic T-lymphocyte antigen-4 (CTLA-4) is a protein that is a competitive inhibitor for B7-1/B7-2 that has a much greater affinity for these proteins than CD28. This protein functions as an inhibitor for T-cell activation [25, 26]. Consequently, increased activity of CTLA-4 can result in T-cell inhibition.

Another important pathway involves programmed cell death protein (PD-1) and the related ligand (PD-L1). PD-L1 is expressed by the various tumor cells and helps facilitate continued growth of the tumor cells by negatively regulating the immune system. When PD-L1 on tumor cells binds PD-1 on T cells, there is an inhibition of cytokine release and cytotoxic activity of antitumor T cells, permitting tumor growth [27]. Therapies involved in the above pathways (Table 22.1) will be discussed below in the form of CTLA-4 and PD-1 inhibitors.

**Table 22.1** Key trials involving checkpoint inhibitors in metastatic renal cell carcinoma

| Drug | Trial | Agents | Patients | PFS, mo | *P* | OS, mo | *P* | ORR (%) |
|---|---|---|---|---|---|---|---|---|
| PD-1 inhibitors | | | | | | | | |
| Nivolumab | CheckMate 025 | Nivolumab vs everolimus | 821 | 4.6 vs 4.4 | 0.11 | 25.0 vs 19.6 | 0.002 | 25.0 vs 5.0 |
| | CheckMate 214 | Nivolumab + ipilimumab vs sunitinib | 1096 | 11.6 vs 8.4 | 0.03 | NR vs 26.0 | <0.001 | 42.0 vs 27.0 |
| | NCT03141177 | Nivolumab + cabozantinib vs sunitinib (ongoing) | 630 | N/A | N/A | N/A | N/A | N/A |
| Pembrolizumab | KEYNOTE-427 | Pembrolizumab | 110 | 8.7 | NR | NR | NR | 33.6 |
| | NCT02501096 | Lenvatinib + pembrolizumab | 30 | 13.8 | NR | NR | NR | 63.3 |
| | NCT02133742 | Pembrolizumab + axitinib | 52 | 20.9 | N/A | Not reached | N/A | 73.0 |
| | NCT02853331 | Pembrolizumab + axitinib vs sunitinib (ongoing) | 862 | N/A | N/A | N/A | N/A | N/A |
| | NCT02811861 | Pembrolizumab + lenvatinib vs Everolimus +lenvatinib vs sunitinib (ongoing) | 1050 | N/A | N/A | N/A | N/A | N/A |
| PD-L1 inhibitors | | | | | | | | |
| Atezolizumab | IMmotion151[a] | Atezolizumab + bevacizumab vs sunitinib | 915 | 11.2 vs 8.4 | 0.002 | NR | NR | 37.0 vs 33.0 |
| Durvalumab | NCT03308396 | Durvalumab + guadecitabine (ongoing) | 58 | N/A | N/A | N/A | N/A | N/A |
| Avelumab | JAVELIN Renal 101 | Avelumab + axitinib vs sunitinib | 888 | 13.8 vs 7.2 | <0.001 | NR | NR | 55.2 vs 25.5 |
| CTLA-4 inhibitors | | | | | | | | |
| Ipilimumab | Yang et al | Ipilimumab 3 mg/kg followed by 1 mg/kg vs 3 mg/kg | 21 | NR | NR | NR | NR | 4.8 vs 12.5 PR |
| | CheckMate 214 (see above) | | | | | | | |
| Tremelimumab | NCT00372853[b] | Dose escalation of tremelimumab + sunitinib | 28 | NR | N/A | NR | NA | 43% PR |

Abbreviations: *ORR* objective response rate, *PR* partial response, *OS* overall survival, *PFS* progression-free survival, *NR* not reported, *N/A* not applicable, *mo* months

[a]IMmotion151 primarily evaluated PFS in PD-L1+ patients. Secondary endpoints were PFS in ITT patient, ORR, and DOR. This table reports the results of the ITT analysis that included the entire cohort of the study

[b]NCT00372853 led to grade 3 or 4 adverse events in 61% of patients

## *Cytotoxic T-lymphocyte Antigen-4*

One of the early reports that studied the antitumor effects of inhibiting CTLA-4 involved a study in mice that were injected with transfected tumor cells. These mice were then treated with anti-CTLA-4 or anti-CD28. Mice injected with anti-CTLA-4 exhibited inhibited tumor growth as compared with the anti-CD28-treated mice and the controls. The study concluded that removing inhibitory signals in the costimulatory pathway can enhance antitumor immunity (Fig. 22.3a and b) [28]. As a result of the encouraging preclinical studies, this therapy was investigated in clinical trials.

Ipilimumab is a CTLA-4 antibody that was found to be initially effective in achieving durable tumor regression in patients with melanoma [29]. Because RCC has previously been found to be immunoresponsive, a phase II trial was performed to evaluate the efficacy of ipilimumab in metastatic RCC. The trial consisted of 61 patients with metastatic RCC who were given two different regimens of ipilimumab. One group received 3 mg/kg for the first treatment followed by 1 mg/kg every 3 weeks, while the other received 3 mg/kg every 3 weeks. Partial responses were experienced 5/40 (12.5%) and 1/21 (4.8%) of the high- and low-dose groups, respectively [30]. The higher-dose cohort experienced a greater incidence of high-grade adverse reactions compared to the lower-dose group (42.5% vs 14%, respectively). Interestingly, in the aforementioned study, the incidence of autoimmune adverse events was associated positively with tumor regression. Despite the encouraging data related to tumor regression, the high adverse effect profile was concerning. As a result, the lower dose was used in trials as an adjunctive therapy option and will be discussed more in the section on PD-1 inhibition [31].

### *Dose*

Two doses have been described for ipilimumab monotherapy in the use of metastatic RCC, 3 mg/kg and 1 mg/kg, as described in the previous section [30]. In modern studies, it is most effectively used as an adjunctive regimen. When used with nivolumab, it can be given at a dose of 1 mg/kg every 3 weeks for four doses during the induction regimen of therapy [32].

### *Toxicity*

Some of the toxicities experienced by patients receiving ipilimumab therapy include autoimmune toxicity (enteritis, hypophysitis), adrenal insufficiency, gastrointestinal toxicity, colonic perforation, diarrhea, or aseptic meningitis [30].

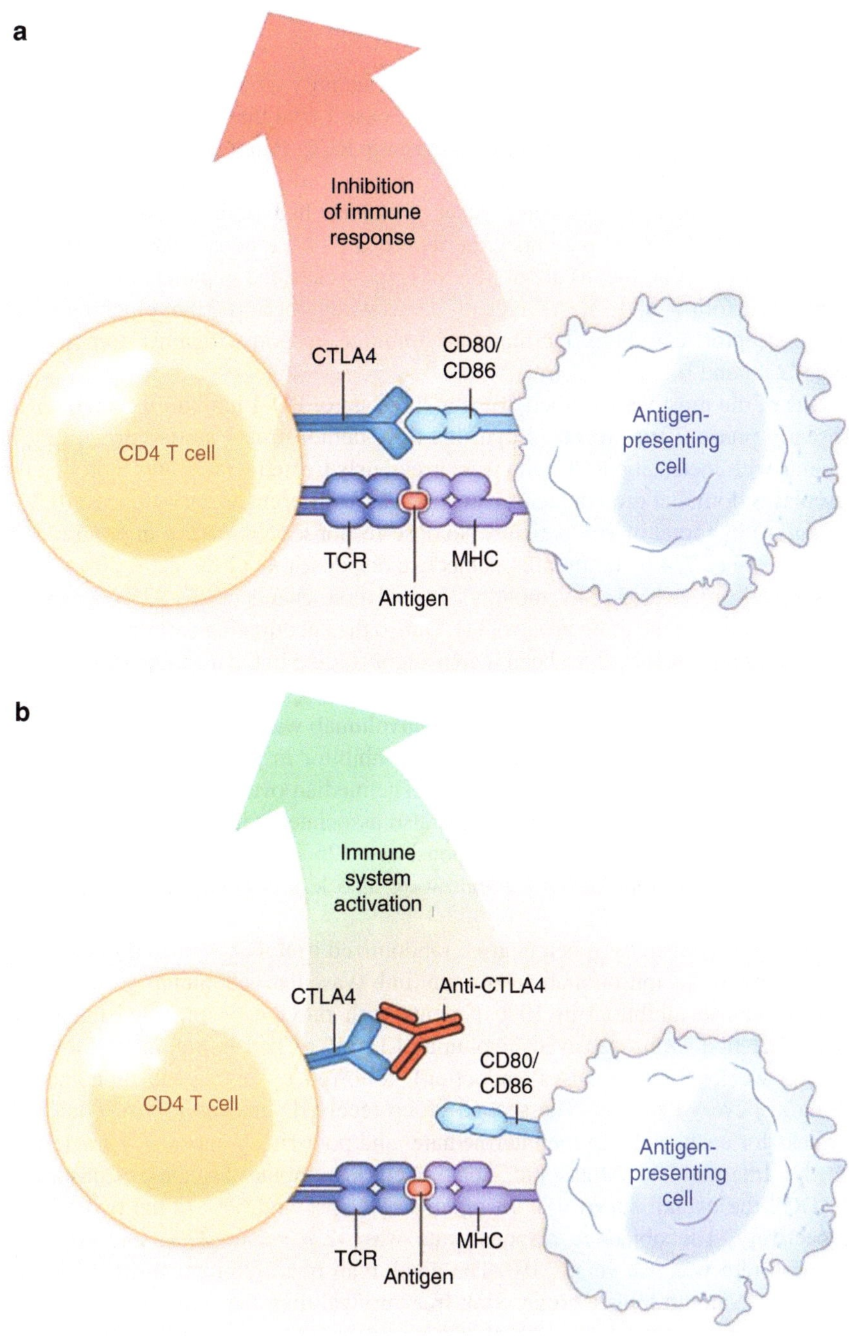


**Fig. 22.3** (**a**) Binding of CTLA4 to CD80/CD86 leads to inhibition of immune response. (**b**) Binding of anti CTLA4 molecule to CTLA4 leads to activation of immune response

## *Programmed Cell Death Protein-1*

An early study that evaluated the safety and activity of anti-PD-1 antibodies in patients with advanced malignancies was a phase 1 trial that included 296 patients with various malignancies, including metastatic RCC. Patients in each malignancy cohort were stratified into three groups that received different doses of the antibody (1, 3, 10 mg/kg). Fourteen percent of patients had grade 3 or higher adverse events. Metastatic RCC patients experienced a 27% response rate with therapy. Responses were durable, as about 65% of responses lasted in patients with greater than 1-year follow-up [33]. As a result, it was widely believed that blocking of the PD-1 receptor can help facilitate an immune response against tumor cells (Fig. 22.4a and b).

One of the most well-studied drugs in the class of PD-1 inhibitors is nivolumab. An early phase 2 trial revealed that this drug demonstrated antitumor activity in patients with metastatic RCC who were previously treated with agents targeting the vascular endothelial growth factor pathway. Three different doses were used (0.3, 2, 10 mg/kg) in a total of 168 patients. No dose-response relationship in progression-free survival (2.7, 4.0, 4.2 months), objective response rate (20%, 22%, 20%), overall survival (18.2, 25.5, 24.7 months), and adverse events (24%, 22%, 35%) was observed between the three groups [34]. Due to the encouraging antitumor activities of PD-1 inhibitors, they have been increasingly studied in the management of metastatic RCC.

In a randomized study of 821 patients, nivolumab was compared to everolimus, a mammalian target of rapamycin (mTOR) inhibitor in patients who were previously treated with antiangiogenic therapy. The median overall survival was 25 and 20 months, respectively. Nivolumab was also associated with a lower risk of death (HR 0.73) and a greater objective response rate (25% vs 5%), when compared to everolimus. High-grade adverse events were also less common in the nivolumab cohort (19% vs 37%) [35].

Another recent study was a phase 3 randomized trial that evaluated the efficacy of nivolumab plus ipilimumab versus sunitinib (vascular endothelial growth factor tyrosine kinase inhibitor) in 1096 patients with previously untreated metastatic RCC. The first group received nivolumab (3 mg/kg) and ipilimumab (1 mg/kg) every 3 weeks for four doses (induction), followed by nivolumab monotherapy (3 mg/kg) every 2 weeks. The second group received sunitinib (50 mg) daily for 4 weeks for each cycle. In the intermediate- and poor-risk groups, as characterized by the International Metastatic Renal Cell Carcinoma Database Consortium (IMDC), the overall survival at 18 months was 75% and 60% in the two groups, respectively. The objective response rate was 42% versus 27%, and complete response rate was 9% versus 1%. The nivolumab plus ipilimumab group experienced a 3.2-month longer progression-free survival than the sunitinib cohort. The overall adverse event rates were high in both groups (93% and 97%), with a grade 3 or 4 event occurring in 46% and 63% of patients, respectively [32].

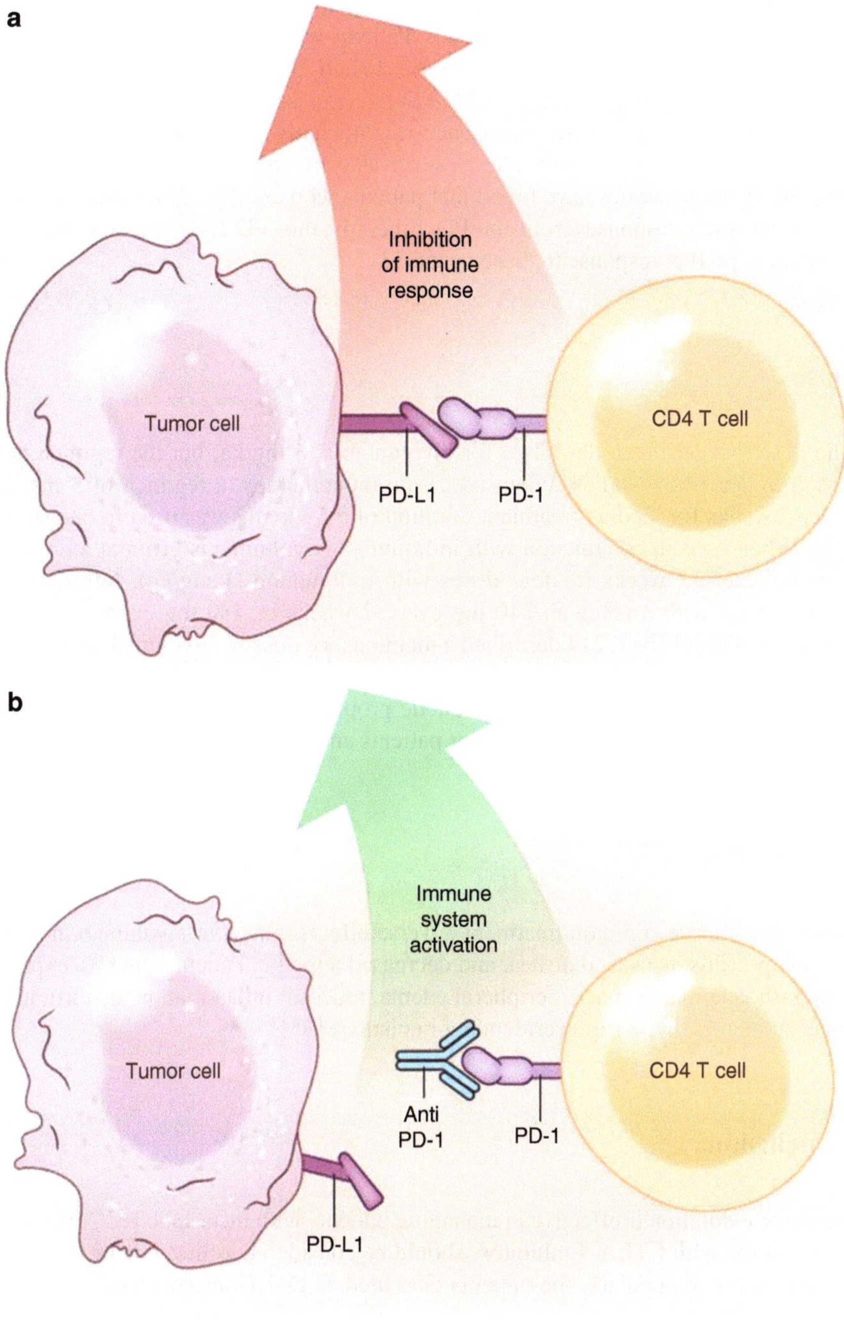


**Fig. 22.4** (**a**) Binding of PD-1 and PD-L1 leads to inhibition of immune response. (**b**) Binding of anti PD-1 molecule to PD-1 leads to activation of immune response

An aspect that can be related to the PD-1 inhibitor therapy effectiveness is the extent of PD-L1 expression on tumor cells. Patients who have tumors that are PD-L1 negative may potentially have poor responses to anti PD-1 therapy [33]. When comparing tumors that have >1% vs <1% PD-L1 expression in patients undergoing anti-PD1 therapy, the former experiences significantly better objective response, progression-free survival, and overall survival compared with the latter. On the other hand, some studies have found that patients who are PD-L1 negative can still exhibit favorable responses from anti PD-1 therapy; thus PD-L1 expression may not adequately predict response to these agents [32].

### *Dose*

The dose that has been described for nivolumab is 3 mg/kg, but the regimen has varied in described studies. When used as a monotherapy, a regimen of 3 mg/kg every 2 weeks for median treatment duration of 5.5 months was used in one study [35]. When used in conjunction with ipilimumab, nivolumab is given at a dose of 3 mg/kg every 3 weeks for four doses with ipilimumab (1 mg/kg), followed by monotherapy with nivolumab 240 mg every 2 weeks or 480 mg every 4 weeks. Though CHECKMATE 214 described a maintenance dose of Nivolumab at 3mg/kg every 2 weeks, the flat dosage is approved by the FDA in this setting. Both dosages have demonstrated similar pharmacokinetic properties, with the flat dosage potentially providing a convenient option for patients and physicians.

### *Adverse Events*

Some of the more common treatment adverse effects related to nivolumab include fatigue, pruritus, nausea, diarrhea, and decreased appetite. Patients can also experience rash, anemia, dyspnea, peripheral edema, mucosal inflammation, distortion of taste, stomatitis, hypertriglyceridemia, or epistaxis [35].

## Conclusions

Immunomodulation is effective in managing patients with metastatic RCC. PD-1 in combination with CTLA-4 inhibitors should be considered as first-line therapies in these patients, particularly the patients classified as IMDC intermediate/poor risk. IL-2 and IFN α2a are historic options that are increasingly being replaced by checkpoint inhibitors. Additional studies with novel checkpoint inhibitors as well as novel regimens and combinations are needed to further increase the armamentarium for the treatment of patients with metastatic renal cell carcinoma.

**Clinical Pearls**

- Immunomodulation can be very effective in the metastatic renal cell cancer patient.
- Historically, IL-2 was used for metastatic renal cell cancer but is associated with significant toxicity, cost, and limitations.
- Interferon alfa-2a has been used for metastatic renal cell cancer but is viewed as inferior to some of the newer agents.
- PD-1 inhibitors and CTLA-4 inhibitors have shown improved outcomes and fewer adverse events in this patient population and should be considered as first-line treatments.

# References

1. Rosenberg SA, Lotze MT, Muul LM, Leitman S, Chang AE, Ettinghausen SE, et al. Observations on the systemic administration of autologous lymphokine-activated killer cells and recombinant interleukin-2 to patients with metastatic cancer. New Engl J Med. 1985;313(23):1485–92, Rosenberg SA. IL-2: The first effective immunotherapy for human cancer. J Immunol. 2014;192(12):5451–8.
2. Rosenberg SA, Grimm EA, McGrogan M, Doyle M, Kawasaki E, Koths K, et al. Biological activity of recombinant human interleukin-2 produced in Escherichia coli. Science. 1984;223(4643):1412–4.
3. Farrar WL, Johnson HM, Farrar JJ. Regulation of the production of immune interferon and cytotoxic T lymphocytes by interleukin 2. J Immunol. 1981;126(3):1120–5.
4. Lotze MT, Chang AE, Seipp CA, Simpson C, Vetto JT, Rosenberg SA. High-dose recombinant Interleukin-2 in the treatment of patients with disseminated cancer – responses, treatment-related morbidity, and histologic-findings. JAMA J Am Med Assoc. 1986;256(22):3117–24.
5. Rosenberg SA, Lotze MT, Yang JC, Aebersold PM, Linehan WM, Seipp CA, et al. Experience with the use of high-dose Interleukin-2 in the treatment of 652 cancer-patients. Ann Surg. 1989;210(4):474–85.
6. Rosenberg SA. Prospective randomized trial of high-dose interleukin-2 alone or in conjunction with lymphokine-activated killer-cells for the treatment of patients with advanced cancer (Vol 85, Pg 622, 1993). J Natl Cancer Inst. 1993;85(13):1091.
7. Rosenberg SA, Lotze MT, Muul LM, Chang AE, Avis FP, Leitman S, et al. A progress report on the treatment of 157 patients with advanced cancer using lymphokine-activated killer-cells and interleukin-2 or high-dose interleukin-2 alone. New Engl J Med. 1987;316(15):889–97.
8. Law TM, Motzer RJ, Mazumdar M, Sell KW, Walther PJ, O'Connell M, et al. Phase III randomized trial of interleukin-2 with or without lymphokine-activated killer cells in the treatment of patients with advanced renal cell carcinoma. Cancer. 1995;76(5):824–32.
9. Klapper JA, Downey SG, Smith FO, Yang JC, Hughes MS, Kammula US, et al. High-dose interleukin-2 for the treatment of metastatic renal cell carcinoma – a retrospective analysis of response and survival in patients treated in the Surgery Branch at the National Cancer Institute between 1986 and 2006. Cancer. 2008;113(2):293–301.
10. Rosenberg SA, Yang JC, Topalian SL, Schwartzentruber DJ, Weber JS, Parkinson DR, et al. Treatment of 283 consecutive patients with metastatic melanoma or renal-cell cancer using high-dose bolus interleukin-2. JAMA J Am Med Assoc. 1994;271(12):907–13.

11. Fisher RI, Rosenberg SA, Fyfe G. Long-term survival update for high-dose recombinant interleukin-2 in patients with renal cell carcinoma. Cancer J Sci Am. 2000;6:S55–S7.
12. Margolin KA, Rayner AA, Hawkins MJ, Atkins MB, Dutcher JP, Fisher RI, et al. Interleukin-2 and lymphokine-activated killer cell therapy of solid tumors – analysis of toxicity and management guidelines. J Clin Oncol. 1989;7(4):486–98.
13. Yang JC, Sherry RM, Steinberg SM, Topalian SL, Schwartzentruber DJ, Hwu P, et al. Randomized study of high-dose and low-dose interleukin-2 in patients with metastatic renal cancer. J Clin Oncol. 2003;21(16):3127–32.
14. McDermott DF, Regan MM, Clark JI, Flaherty LE, Weiss GR, Logan TF, et al. Randomized phase III trial of high-dose interleukin-2 versus subcutaneous interleukin-2 and interferon in patients with metastatic renal cell carcinoma. J Clin Oncol. 2005;23(1):133–41.
15. Negrier S, Escudier B, Lasset C, Douillard JY, Savary J, Chevreau C, et al. Recombinant human interleukin-2, recombinant human interferon alfa-2a, or both in metastatic renal-cell carcinoma. New Engl J Med. 1998;338(18):1272–8.
16. Allard CB, Gelpi-Hammerschmidt F, Harshman LC, Choueiri TK, Faiena I, Modi P, et al. Contemporary trends in high-dose interleukin-2 use for metastatic renal cell carcinoma in the United States. Urol Oncol. 2015;33(11):496 e11–6.
17. Fyfe G, Fisher RI, Rosenberg SA, Sznol M, Parkinson DR, Louie AC. Results of treatment of 255 patients with metastatic renal cell carcinoma who received high-dose recombinant interleukin-2 therapy. J Clin Oncol. 1995;13(3):688–96.
18. Hiroishi K, Tuting T, Lotze MT. IFN-alpha-expressing tumor cells enhance generation and promote survival of tumor-specific CTLs. J Immunol. 2000;164(2):567–72.
19. Krown SE, Real FX, Cunningham-Rundles S, Myskowski PL, Koziner B, Fein S, et al. Preliminary observations on the effect of recombinant leukocyte A interferon in homosexual men with Kaposi's sarcoma. N Engl J Med. 1983;308(18):1071–6, Golomb HM, Jacobs A, Fefer A, Ozer H, Thompson J, Portlock C, et al. Alpha-2 interferon therapy of hairy-cell leukemia: a multicenter study of 64 patients. J Clin Oncol. 1986;4(6):900–5, Foon KA, Sherwin SA, Abrams PG, Longo DL, Fer MF, Stevenson HC, et al. Treatment of advanced non-Hodgkin's lymphoma with recombinant leukocyte A interferon. N Engl J Med. 1984;311(18):1148–52.
20. Quesada JR, Swanson DA, Trindade A, Gutterman JU. Renal cell carcinoma: antitumor effects of leukocyte interferon. Cancer Res. 1983;43(2):940–7.
21. Minasian LM, Motzer RJ, Gluck L, Mazumdar M, Vlamis V, Krown SE. Interferon alfa-2a in advanced renal cell carcinoma: treatment results and survival in 159 patients with long-term follow-up. J Clin Oncol. 1993;11(7):1368–75.
22. Motzer RJ, Bacik J, Murphy BA, Russo P, Mazumdar M. Interferon-alfa as a comparative treatment for clinical trials of new therapies against advanced renal cell carcinoma. J Clin Oncol. 2002;20(1):289–96, Flanigan RC, Salmon SE, Blumenstein BA, Bearman SI, Roy V, McGrath PC, et al. Nephrectomy followed by interferon alfa-2b compared with interferon alfa-2b alone for metastatic renal-cell cancer. New Engl J Med. 2001;345(23):1655–9.
23. Medical Research Council Renal Cancer Collaborators. Interferon-alpha and survival in metastatic renal carcinoma: early results of a randomised controlled trial. Lancet. 1999;353(9146):14–7.
24. Quesada JR, Rios A, Swanson D, Trown P, Gutterman JU. Antitumor activity of recombinant-derived interferon alpha in metastatic renal cell carcinoma. J Clin Oncol. 1985;3(11):1522–8.
25. Chambers CA, Kuhns MS, Egen JG, Allison JP. CTLA-4-mediated inhibition in regulation of T cell responses: mechanisms and manipulation in tumor immunotherapy. Annu Rev Immunol. 2001;19:565–94.
26. Wolchok JD, Saenger Y. The mechanism of anti-CTLA-4 activity and the negative regulation of T-cell activation. Oncologist. 2008;13(Suppl 4):2–9.
27. Choueiri TK, Motzer RJ. Systemic therapy for metastatic renal-cell carcinoma. N Engl J Med. 2017;376(4):354–66.
28. Leach DR, Krummel MF, Allison JP. Enhancement of antitumor immunity by CTLA-4 blockade. Science. 1996;271(5256):1734–6.

29. Phan GQ, Yang JC, Sherry RM, Hwu P, Topalian SL, Schwartzentruber DJ, et al. Cancer regression and autoimmunity induced by cytotoxic T lymphocyte-associated antigen 4 blockade in patients with metastatic melanoma. Proc Natl Acad Sci U S A. 2003;100(14):8372–7.
30. Yang JC, Hughes M, Kammula U, Royal R, Sherry RM, Topalian SL, et al. Ipilimumab (anti-CTLA4 antibody) causes regression of metastatic renal cell cancer associated with enteritis and hypophysitis. J Immunother. 2007;30(8):825–30.
31. Hammers HJ, Plimack ER, Infante JR, Rini BI, McDermott DF, Lewis LD, et al. Safety and efficacy of nivolumab in combination with ipilimumab in metastatic renal cell carcinoma: the CheckMate 016 study. J Clin Oncol. 2017;35(34):3851–8.
32. Motzer RJ, Tannir NM, McDermott DF, Frontera OA, Melichar B, Choueiri TK, et al. Nivolumab plus ipilimumab versus sunitinib in advanced renal-cell carcinoma. New Engl J Med. 2018;378(14):1277–90.
33. Topalian SL, Hodi FS, Brahmer JR, Gettinger SN, Smith DC, McDermott DF, et al. Safety, activity, and immune correlates of anti-PD-1 antibody in cancer. New Engl J Med. 2012;366(26):2443–54.
34. Motzer RJ, Rini BI, McDermott DF, Redman BG, Kuzel TM, Harrison MR, et al. Nivolumab for metastatic renal cell carcinoma: results of a randomized phase II trial. J Clin Oncol. 2015;33(13):1430–7.
35. Motzer RJ, Escudier B, McDermott DF, George S, Hammers HJ, Srinivas S, et al. Nivolumab versus everolimus in advanced renal-cell carcinoma. New Engl J Med. 2015;373(19):1803–13.

# Chapter 23
# Novel Therapies for Renal Cell Carcinoma

**Brooke Zilinskas**

Despite the increased use of imaging modalities throughout medicine, and the overall increase in diagnosis of renal cell carcinoma (RCC), almost one third of patients with RCC will have metastasis at the time of their diagnosis. Furthermore, in patients diagnosed with organ-confined RCC, metastatic disease will develop 20–40% of the time [1]. Metastatic RCC has an extremely poor prognosis with 10-year survival rates less than 5% [2]. However, in the past decade, there have been some "novel" therapies in the treatment of metastatic RCC that show promise. A quick Internet search through the National Institutes of Health will show many ongoing clinical trials in all phases. Some novel agents and some older agents, being used in these trials, may offer more hope to our patients presenting with or progressing to metastasis. In this chapter, we will discuss some of the novel agents that have changed current treatment guidelines and show promise in these clinical trials. It is also noteworthy to mention that the current landscape of treatment for metastatic RCC is changing so rapidly, with the publication of new data from clinical trials of all phases, that by the time of this publication, there will surely be new data released and potentially updated guidelines. The best way for the practitioner to stay current in the treatment of metastatic RCC is to review published literature and trusted guidelines regularly.

## Nivolumab

Nivolumab is a novel agent that interferes with the inhibition of the body's immune system response. After shrinking tumors in mouse models, it has been used on a wide variety of cancers. Melanoma, non-small cell lung cancer, hepatocellular

B. Zilinskas (✉)
Department of Urology, UT Southwestern Medical Center, Dallas, TX, USA
e-mail: brooke.zilinskas@utsouthwestern.edu; vitaly.margulis@utsouthwestern.edu

 
E. J. Trabulsi et al. (eds.), *Chemotherapy and Immunotherapy in Urologic Oncology*, https://doi.org/10.1007/978-3-030-52021-2_23

carcinoma, and renal cell carcinoma are only a few of the cancers that have been targeted with this agent [3].

At a cellular level, nivolumab interferes with the programmed death receptor-1 (PD-1), which is partly responsible for tumor-induced immune suppression. Nivolumab allows the body to mount an immune response and fight the cancer cells. It is given intravenously every 2 or 3 weeks depending on study protocol and guidelines. Adverse reactions include adrenocortical insufficiency, aplastic anemia, colitis, diabetes, encephalopathy, hand and foot syndrome, and other inflammatory- or immune-mediated conditions. High-dose corticosteroids may be necessary if an immune-mediated response occurs during treatment [3].

Checkmate-214, a randomized phase III clinical trial, paired ipilimumab and nivolumab (IN arm) versus sunitinib in the treatment of patients with metastatic RCC. The findings of Checkmate-214 showed a statistically significant survival curve, and longer remission periods, in patients receiving the IN arm versus those receiving sunitinib. These findings have already led to a 2018 update of the European Association of Urology (EAU) guidelines for the treatment of first-line metastatic clear cell RCC [4–6].

It is important to mention that in the Checkmate-214 trial, patients were stratified into favorable-, intermediate-, and poor-risk groups based on the International Metastatic Renal Cell Carcinoma Database Consortium (IMDC) risk model. This model takes into account Karnofsky performance status, time from diagnosis to treatment, and lab findings. It has been tested and validated and is a recurring theme in metastatic RCC research [6, 7]. Checkmate-214 showed a statistical significance in disease-free progression in the IN arm versus sunitinib in patients with intermediate or poor risk. However, this benefit was not seen in the favorable-risk group, and therefore sunitinib remains the treatment of choice for those patients as per the EAU guidelines.

## Ipilimumab

Ipilimumab is not actually a novel therapy, but its use in the Checkpoint-214 trial with nivolumab made this agent resurface in the treatment of metastatic RCC. Ipilimumab is a monoclonal antibody that binds to the cytotoxic T-lymphocyte antigen 4 (CTLA-4). By binding to this antigen, it is believed that antitumor T cells are increased allowing the body to mount an immune response [8]. This agent was originally researched and used in clinical trials more than a decade ago, but the side effects including enterocolitis, hepatitis, and neuropathy which can even be fatal limited ipilimumab use as a single agent. It is indicated as first-line treatment in patients with intermediate or poor risk in combination with nivolumab per the European Association of Urology's 2018 guidelines [8]. It is given as an infusion every 3 weeks for up to four cycles [8].

## Cabozantinib

Cabozantinib is classified as a tyrosine kinase inhibitor. It broadly inhibits these receptors including VEGFR, MET, and AXL [4]. Targeting the VEGF receptor is not novel, but cabozantinib's ability to more broadly affect tyrosine kinase via multiple receptor targets led researchers to suspect that less resistance would occur in patients on this medication. In the CABOSUN trial, patients were given cabozantinib versus the gold standard sunitinib. All patients in this study were intermediate or poor risk based on IMDC classification. The primary endpoint was met, showing that patients in the cabozantinib arm had a statistically significant progression-free survival over the sunitinib arm. These results were upheld (though were a bit less impressive) after independent radiology interpretation of progression-free survival on imaging [4, 9]. Side effects of cabozantinib include fatigue and diarrhea, hypertension, and thrombocytopenia.

## Other Novel Agents

With the positive results from the Checkmate-214 and CABOSUN trials, it is reasonable to consider treatments combining agents that target the PD-1 receptor with those interrupting the VEGF pathway. There are clinical trials involving these types of agents versus sunitinib currently underway, such as the IMmotion-151 trial. IMmotion-151 looks at bevacizumab (a VEGF inhibitor) with atezolizumab (a PD-L1 monoclonal antibody) versus sunitinib. This study is unique as participants were required to have a tissue biopsy which was evaluated for PD-L1 expression, and this, as well as risk score and presence of liver metastasis, was included in the stratification of patients. The study is ongoing, but some of the data that has been released shows statistically significant progression-free survival for patients in the PD-L1 subset. This drug regimen appears to be well tolerated by patients, but until the data has been completely collected, analyzed, and released, as well as independent review of the radiographic data, it is too soon to implement into clinical guidelines [10].

Axitinib is an oral agent indicated in the treatment of metastatic RCC after progression of disease is documented on an IV first-line agent. It is an oral kinase inhibitor that slows and inhibits tumor growth. It is given twice daily in various doses depending on tolerability, not to exceed 20 mg per day. It can be used as monotherapy or in combination with avelumab (a PD-L1 monoclonal antibody). Serious side effects can include blood clots, hemorrhage, hepatotoxicity, and fistulas. There is a current clinical trial (JAVELIN-101) which looks at axitinib/avelumab versus sunitinib that may expand treatment options as results become available and are independently validated [11].

## Tumor and Biomarkers

Currently, there are no standard and validated biomarkers to aid in the treatment of renal cell carcinoma. Finding one or more of these biomarkers is likely at the top of every researcher's wish list. The closest tool available now is the IMDC risk stratification model which would group intermediate- and poor-risk patients into receiving nivolumab and ipilimumab while good-risk patients would continue to receive sunitinib, as the EAU guidelines have recommended [6].

While the IMmotion-151 trial did subdivide patients based on the expression of their PD-L1 activity, this needs to be repeated and validated by other researchers. If these biomarkers, or tumor markers, could be identified in chemo-naive patients or even earlier at the time of initial cancer diagnosis, then opportunities for neoadjuvant or early adjuvant chemotherapy after partial or radical nephrectomy increase. Patients could benefit from better efficacy and potentially fewer side effects with tailored or personalized chemotherapy at the first sign of metastasis or even salvage chemotherapy. This advancement would hopefully allow overall survival rates for metastatic RCC to improve.

## Conclusion

The past decade has been busy for the treatment of advanced RCC. Clinical trials have led to a change in the first line of treatment for intermediate- and poor-risk patients, and ongoing trials may show this benefit for patients with less toxicity. Agents targeting programmed cell death and the VEGF pathway have shown benefit independently, and ongoing research is pairing these agents together. Biomarkers are the future of cancer care, and while some studies have tried to stratify patients to determine tailored chemotherapy, and others have run testing on PD-L1 tumor cell expression, further research needs to show that this is a reproducible finding and should be included in daily cancer care at academic and private centers alike. It is difficult to stay updated on what is new in the treatment of metastatic RCC with all the data being released, but it is comforting that in the next decade, we may have more options to offer to our patients who find themselves in the position of needing this treatment.

**Clinical Pearls**

- The current landscape of treatment for metastatic RCC is so rapidly changing that a practitioner must stay abreast of all current literature and clinical trials.
- The new checkpoint inhibitor immunotherapy agents that are approved for the treatment of mRCC include nivolumab (anti-PD-1) and ipilimumab (anti-CTLA-4).
- Cabozantinib is a tyrosine kinase inhibitor with activity against VEGFR, MET, and AXL that is approved for patients with intermediate- or poor-risk disease based on IMDC classification.
- Combination therapy with targeted and immunotherapeutic agents is actively being investigated for patients with mRCC.
- Biomarkers should help in future individualization of care for mRCC.

## References

1. Srinivasan R, Marston Linehan W. Treatment of advanced renal cell carcinoma. In: Campbell-Walsh Urology, vol. 63. Philadelphia, PA : Elsevier; 2020. p. 1500–1518.e5.
2. Motzer RJ, Mazumdar M, Bacik J, et al. Survival and prognostic stratification of 670 patients with advanced renal cell carcinoma. J Clin Oncol. 1999;17:2530–40.
3. McDermott DF, Atkins MB. PD-1 as a potential target in cancer therapy. Cancer Med. 2013;2(5):662–73.
4. Salgia NJ, Dara Y, Bergerot P, et al. Curr Treat Options Oncol. 2019;20:41. https://doi-org.foyer.swmed.edu/10.1007/s11864-019-0638-1.
5. Motzer RJ, Tannir NM, McDermott DF, Aren Frontera O, Melichar B, Choueiri TK, et al. Nivolumab plus ipilimumab versus sunitinib in advanced renal-cell carcinoma. N Engl J Med. 2018;378(14):1277–90.
6. Powles T, et al. Updated European Association of Urology Guidelines: recommendations for the treatment of first-line metastatic clear cell renal cancer. Eur Urol. 2018;73(3):311–5.
7. Heng DYC, Xie W, Regan MM, et al. External validation and comparison with other models of the International Metastatic Renal- Cell Carcinoma Database Consortium prognostic model: a population-based study. Lancet Oncol. 2013;14:141–8.
8. Yervoy (ipilimumab) injection for intravenous use (prescribing information). Princeton: Bristol-Myers Squibb; 2017.
9. Choueiri TK, et al. Cabozantinib versus sunitinib as initial therapy for metastatic renal cell carcinoma of intermediate or poor risk (Alliance A031203 CABOSUN randomised trial): progression-free survival by independent review and overall survival update. Eur J Cancer. 2018;94:115–25.
10. Motzer RJ, et al. IMmotion151: a randomized phase iii study of atezolizumab plus bevacizumab vs sunitinib in untreated metastatic Renal Cell Carcinoma (mRCC). J Clin Oncol. 2018;36(6_suppl):578.
11. Motzer RJ, Penkov K, Haanen JBAG, Rini BI, Albiges L, Campbell MT, et al. LBA6_PRJAVELIN renal 101: a randomized, phase III study of avelumab + axitinib vs sunitinib as first-line treatment of advanced renal cell carcinoma (aRCC). Ann Oncol. 2018;29(suppl_8):mdy424.036.

# Part IV
# Other Malignancies

# Chapter 24
# Testicular Cancer

Kara R. Cossis, Tara Mahan, Sara Dennin Johney, and Benjamin Lowentritt

## Signs and Symptoms

Testicular cancer is usually first discovered via a palpable mass noted within the testes. The testicle may also appear enlarged or edematous. In addition, a sensation of achiness or fullness within the scrotum or lower abdomen may occur [1]. Lymphadenopathy may also be present particularly in the supraclavicular nodes. A retroperitoneal mass, venous thrombus, or pulmonary embolism may also present clinically [33]. Breast growth or soreness and precocious puberty may be noted due to the secretion of hormones from the tumor. It is also possible to be asymptomatic. When the disease has progressed, there may be systemic symptoms such as a lower back pain, shortness of breath, chest pain, cough, abdominal pain, headaches, or confusion [1].

K. R. Cossis (✉) · T. Mahan · S. Dennin Johney · B. Lowentritt
Chesapeake Urology, Owings Mills, MD, USA
e-mail: kcossis@chesuro.com; tmahan@chesuro.com; sjohney@chesuro.com; blowentritt@uniteduro.com



E. J. Trabulsi et al. (eds.), *Chemotherapy and Immunotherapy in Urologic Oncology*, https://doi.org/10.1007/978-3-030-52021-2_24

## Epidemiology

Testicular cancer is the most common malignancy affecting young adult males with ages 15–34; however, it accounts for only 1–2% of cancers in the male population [32]. There are a few well-established and well-studied risk factors for the disease, but in general, the etiology of testicular cancer remains unknown. Epidemiologic studies estimate 72,000 newly diagnosed testicular cancers annually with an average of 9000 associated deaths each year [19, 31].

According to the National Institutes of Health, the incidence of testicular cancer has risen in the American male population from 3.35 cases/100,000 men between 1973 and 1978 to 4.48 cases per 100,000 men from 1994 to 1998 [20].

The factors responsible for increased incidence in recent years remain unclear.

## Risk Factors

Known risk factors for testicular cancer may predispose males to the development of carcinoma in situ and invasive testicular cancer. These include cryptorchidism, personal or family history of testicular cancer, testicular dysgenesis, Klinefelter syndrome, infertility, and HIV infection. Some other risk factors have been suggested and studied, but no substantial findings have been supportive to prove a direct relationship.

### *Cryptorchidism*

Cryptorchidism is defined as the failure of one of the testicle or both of the testes to descend into the scrotum during early development. Testicular malposition alone does not explain the increased risk of testicular cancer; however, incidences of testicular neoplasms have been observed to be higher in this population. Prophylactic orchiectomy is recommended for the undescended testicle still present within the abdomen. Approximately 10% of testicular tumors occur in malpositioned testicles, where 20% of the testicular tumors are found in the contralateral descended testicle [21]. In cases of inguinal cryptorchidism, these are less likely to result in malignancy, and surgery can be delayed.

### *Personal History*

A small percent of men with testicular cancer will be diagnosed with a second testicular malignancy in their lifetime. The US National Cancer Institute reports a 0.6% risk of contralateral cancer at the time of diagnosis and a 15-year risk of 1.9% [22].

## Family History

Of those diagnosed with testicular cancer, 1–3% have an affected family member also diagnosed with the disease. While this is a small percent, it statistically suggests a hereditary component [23]. The contribution of family history in testicular cancer in case-controlled studies has been observed and demonstrates a six to ten times greater risk in direct male relatives, primarily in brothers or sons [24].

## Testicular Dysgenesis

The testicular dysgenesis syndrome (TDS) refers to a spectrum of reproductive disorders that originate in male fetal life. It is thought to be a result of disturbed gonadal development in the embryo. Theory suggests it to be a combination of genetic factors, environment, and lifestyle. TDS includes cryptorchidism and hypospadias in newborn boys and testicular cancer and infertility in adult males. There is a range of phenotypes from mild/most common form in which impaired spermatogenesis is the only symptom to severe cases in which the patient may develop testicular cancer [38].

TDS can occur as a result of abnormal Leydig cell function. Testosterone, which is produced by Leydig cells, is required for normal testis descent, urethral meatus formation, and spermatogenesis.

A careful estimate of the frequency of medium severity TDS in Denmark is ~5%, based on the knowledge of the current frequencies of testicular cancer and cryptorchidism. The prevalence of TDS has not been established worldwide [34, 35].

## Klinefelter Syndrome

Klinefelter syndrome is a rare chromosomal condition in which the male karyotype contains an extra X chromosome. This aneuploidy is the most common condition associated with hypogonadism and infertility. These symptoms can vary in intensity and may include undescended testes or hypospadias. Again, an undescended testicle is correlated with an increased risk of testicular cancer [39].

## HIV

The rate of testicular seminomas has seen a modest rise in the HIV-positive infected male population. The incidence increase ratio is 0.7 to 1.8 when compared with the general population [25]. HIV status does not seem to impact the rate of nonseminomas diagnosed.

## *Ethnicity*

A review of 12 European countries found that the incidence of germ cell tumors was increasing; however mortality rates during the same period were declining. This suggests improvements in diagnosis and treatment [26]. Please note that the declining mortality rates are seen in white, non-Hispanic populations. There appears to be a higher risk of death from the cancer in the African-American, Native American, Filipino, Hawaiian, and Hispanic populations in the United States as compared to the white males [27]. The racial disparity is not fully understood.

It is confirmed that the increase primarily is in the white male population [27]. Testicular cancer is less common in the black male at a rate of 1 to 4. Studies between 1988 and 2001 show that testicular cancer is rising in the black male population. Incidence of testicular cancer in black men doubled between 1988 and 1992 and from 1998 to 2001 [28]. The worldwide incidence is lowest in Africa and Asia and highest in Scandinavian countries, Germany, Switzerland, and New Zealand [29].

## *In Utero*

Case-control studies suggest that exposure to estrogen-type products in utero increases the risk of testicular germ cell tumors; however studies have failed to prove a definite link [30].

While there may be an impact, the hormonal factor has not been quantified for significance [31].

## Summary

Many factors have been studied to evaluate for contribution to testicular cancer. Younger age, personal and family history of testicular germ cell tumor, cryptorchidism are consistently those with the most risk. History of vasectomy, use of marijuana, diet, exposure to estrogen in utero, and BMI may have some causal relation but no significant, quantifiable influence on risk.

## *Signs and Symptoms*

Testicular cancer is usually first discovered via a palpable mass noted within the testes. The testicle may also appear enlarged or edematous. In addition, a sensation of achiness or fullness within the scrotum or lower abdomen may be present. Breast growth or soreness and precocious puberty may be noted due to the secretion of hormones from the tumor. It is also possible to be asymptomatic. When the disease has progressed, there may be systemic symptoms such as a lower back pain, shortness of breath, chest pain, cough, abdominal pain, headaches, or confusion [1].

## Screening

Governing bodies for various leading organizations have offered screening recommendations for testicular cancer. The US Preventive Services Task Force (USPSTF) released initial recommendations in 2004 against screening adolescent or adult males for testicular cancer. This decision was justified though the relatively low incident of the condition combined with favorable outcomes from treatment even with more advanced disease progression. They state, "there is adequate evidence that the benefits of screening for testicular cancer are small to none." This was upheld in 2009 and again in 2011[17] after performing a literature review and has been maintained. This anti-screening method applies to both clinician examinations and patient self-examinations [4]. The American Academy of Family Physicians [5], the American Academy of Pediatrics [6], and the American Cancer Society [7] all support these published recommendations.

Further justification for this stems from the fact that regular testicular self-examinations have not been studied enough to determine if they reduce mortality and therefore cannot commit to specific screening recommendations [1]. As such, education on testicular cancer to adolescence and young men has been minimal at best but is virtually nonexistent as a standard of care. Further concerns have been raised regarding the increased anxiety created by emphasizing testicular self-examinations within a group already concerned about their body and who in this age group as a whole demonstrates a lack of concern for their health [12].

## Early Detection

Again, early detection allows for the best chance of overall survival. In addition, the financial cost of treating an advanced testicular cancer along with that of lost life years is significantly reduced. A study was published in the journal of *Cancer Medicine* reflecting the results of a cost-utility validation. In this study, the cost of treating advanced stage testicular tumors, both seminomas and nonseminomas, were compared to six other scenarios that involve clinical recognition and assessment of a testicular mass discovered during self-examination of which four were classified benign and two were classified as early stage malignancies. Costs were calculated using Current Procedural Terminology (CPT) codes thorough Medicare fee schedules. Medicare reimbursements were then used to estimate the national cost standard.

## Pre-diagnosis Workup

If there are concerns of a possible testicular cancer, a comprehensive history and physical exam should be conducted along with a testicular ultrasound ordered. In addition, serum tumor markers will be drawn. These markers include alpha-fetoprotein (AFP), β-human chorionic gonadotropin (β-HCG), and lactate dehydrogenase (LDH) [1]. In addition, a chemistry profile should be ordered along with a chest X-ray [32, 33].

## Tumor Markers

The tumor markers AFP, β-HCG, and LDH are often elevated if a testicular malignancy is present. Elevation of any of the tumor markers may indicate a seminoma tumor. AFP and β-HCG are more specific markers than that of LDH. AFP is secreted by nonseminomatous cells and is therefore elevated with embryonic and yolk sac tumors. The half-life is approximately 5–7 days and can be seen at any stage testicular tumor. β-HCG may be elevated in both seminomas and nonseminomas, especially choriocarcinomas. The half-life is approximately 1–3 days. This level may yield a false positive with hypogonadism, with marijuana use [32], with hyperthyroidism, and with heterophile antibodies. When the value is >1000 IU/L, it is more indicative of a nonseminoma. A level of >5000 IU/L post-orchiectomy may suggest brain metastasis, and therefore a brain MRI is advised. LDH is important in prognosis assessment and with disseminated nonseminomas helps to risk stratify first-line chemotherapy. This can also be used to monitor for possible relapse [33].

## Diagnosis

A biopsy can be performed to provide a confirmatory tissue diagnosis, but this is usually not the standard of care due to concerns of seeding the cancer and contributing to it spreading. The diagnosis is typically made from an orchiectomy specimen. When cancer is suspected, a radical orchiectomy via an inguinal approach is the preferred surgery to avoid introducing potential cancer spread to the scrotal wall and/or inguinal lymph nodes. Clinical suspicion leads to a confirmatory pathologic diagnosis after orchiectomy. Further staging tools include radiographic imaging with ultrasound, CT scan, MRI, PET scan, or bone scans.

## Post-diagnosis Workup

An abdominal/pelvic CT scan should be ordered post-diagnosis. A chest CT scan is further recommended if the CT scan is positive or if the chest X-ray is abnormal. Tumor markers should be repeated. In addition, a brain MRI and bone scan are recommended if clinically indicated or based on specific pathologic findings. Sperm banking should also be discussed with the patient [32].

## Sperm Banking

The sequela of this disease can be infertility from the tumor itself or through the subsequent treatments. Hence, these men should be counseled on banking sperm and referred to a fertility specialist should they desire offspring in the future [13]. This can occur before or after orchiectomy but needs to be done prior to chemotherapy, radiation therapy, or retroperitoneal lymph node dissection [33].

In making such preparations for family planning through freezing sperm, the cost of such preparations varies. The initial consultation process, however, is estimated to be just below $1000 with yearly storage fees somewhere between $275 and 500 per year [13]. According to the infertility resources, the average cost of a basic in vitro fertilization cycle ranges from about $12,000 to $15,000 [14].

## Tumor Types

The most common types of testicular cancer, accounting for over 90%, are germ cell tumors. Sperm production originates in these germ cells. Germ cell tumors are further classified as seminomas and nonseminomas with roughly equal rates of occurrences between these two types. A combination of both seminomas and nonseminomas, or mixed germ cell tumors, also exists but is treated as nonseminomas given how they grow and spread.

In general, seminomas are slower growing compared to nonseminomas. These seminomas are subtyped as classical or spermatocytic seminomas. Classical seminomas are by far the most common and affect men around 25–45 years of age. In contrast, spermatocytic seminomas tend to be seen in older men, usually around 65 years of age. They are also slower growing with a lower malignant risk.

Nonseminomas typically occur in the later teenage years and early 30s. This category of tumor is broken down into four subtypes: embryonal carcinoma, yolk sac carcinoma, choriocarcinomas, and teratoma. Many nonseminoma tumors occur as some combination of these four and may also have a seminoma component. An embryonal carcinoma is present about 40% of the time in combination but only 3–4% of the time in pure form. They tend to grown rapidly and often spread outside of the testicle. Yolk sac carcinoma is the most common form of testicular cancer in children, especially infants, but is rarely seen in adults. Choriocarcinoma is rare but extremely aggressive in adults. When this exists in its pure form, it rapidly spreads to distant organs including the lungs, bones, and brain. When combined with other germ cell tumors, a choriocarcinoma is somewhat less aggressive but always a concerning finding when present. Teratomas, however, usually do not exist in pure form. They are classified into three types: mature teratomas which rarely spread but have the potential to reoccur, immature teratomas which have metastatic and reoccurrence potential, and teratomas with somatic-type malignancy which are extremely rare. These have components of mature teratomas but other cells that are associated with malignancies occurring outside of the testicles such as a sarcoma or adenocarcinoma [1].

Occurring less often and a precursor to germ cell cancers, is carcinoma in situ or intratubular germ cell neoplasms. These are asymptomatic and usually diagnosed incidentally on a biopsy performed for another reason. Stromal tumors are another type of testicular malignancy that make up less than 5% of adult cases but up to 20% of childhood cases. Stromal tumors exist as two types, Leydig cell tumors and Sertoli cell tumors. In general, most Leydig and Sertoli cell tumors are benign and have a low metastatic potential. When stromal tumors are malignant, however, they often behave aggressively and respond poorly to chemotherapy or radiation therapy [1].

Certain risk factors have been identified that may increase the probability of developing testicular cancer. Cryptorchidism or history of an undescended testicle, which occurs in about 3% of the general male population, is one such risk factor. Further risk factors include a family history involving a first-degree relative, HIV or AIDS infections, and carcinoma in situ of the testes. A prior personal history of testicular cancer has also been found to lead to cancer in the contralateral testicle in 3–4% of the time. Again, age places men at a higher risk, specifically those between 20 and 34 years old. Caucasian men have been found to have four to five times the risk compared to African-American and Asian-American men. There is possible risk related to tall stature, but this has not always been consistent [1].

## *Treatment*

There are three common approaches for managing and treating testicular cancer. These include surgery, radiation, and chemotherapy. A patient's treatment team will often include a urologist, a medical oncologist, and a radiation oncologist. For patients with refractory disease, there are options for clinical trials and stem cell transplant [18]. Standard of care guidelines have been established for all disease stages and published through the NCCN. They should be closely followed to provide the best chance for cure with the least amount of side effects [33].

Treatment for testicular cancer factors in the histology and stage of the tumor. Testicular cancer has historically been considered a very curable cancer with low likelihood of relapse [18]. This is based on tumor markers post-orchiectomy along with AJCC T (tumor), N (node), and M (metastasis) staging system [33].

If the cancer is found incidentally and there are no signs of spread outside of the testicle on blood work or imaging, then surveillance without surgery may be appropriate. This is carcinoma in situ (CIS), or stage 0 testicular cancer. An orchiectomy is the treatment of choice for CIS if surveillance is not an option. Once surgery is performed, no additional treatment is needed [15].

The majority, 90–95% [18], of the testicular tumors are seminomas, nonseminomas, and mixed germ cell (mixture of seminoma and nonseminoma). Approximately 5–10% are stromal tumors.

Seminomas and nonseminomas are treated differently based on the staging. Mixed germ cell tumors are treated using the protocol for nonseminoma tumors. Adult patients have a higher incidence of seminoma, whereas prepubertal patients are more likely to have nonseminoma.

## Pure Seminomas

Since this type of tumor is rarely seen in preadolescent patients, there is currently no standard treatment of these tumors in this population [18]. All recommendations in this section are specific to the adult male.

### Stage 1A and 1B

Surgery is often the initial treatment which is a radical inguinal orchiectomy. A radical orchiectomy includes removal of the spermatic cord and testicle on the diseased side.

Following surgery, a decision on surveillance versus chemotherapy versus radiation treatment is considered. For men with pure seminoma, Stage 1A or 1B, who will be compliant with the strict and intense follow-up schedule, surveillance is the preferred option. Men with scrotal violation (i.e., scrotal orchiectomy, open testicular explorations) are not good candidates for surveillance. This is because the normal lymphatic drainage can be impacted [18].

Surveillance involves a strict protocol of frequent physical exams and blood tests to monitor lactate dehydrogenase (LDH), beta-human chorionic gonadotropin (β-HCG), and serum alpha-fetoprotein (AFP). Imaging of the chest, abdomen, and pelvis are obtained at the same frequency [17]. If any signs of spread are found, the next treatment steps are radiation and chemotherapy.

Radiation may be the next step in treatment should the patient have a history of scrotal violation, a history of prior radiation, or history of inflammatory bowel disease. Radiation treatment typically is 10–15 sessions over 2–3 weeks and targets the retroperitoneal lymph nodes using abdominal external beam radiation.

Chemotherapy, if appropriate, is carboplatin generally given over 2 cycles.

**Stage 1S** One or more tumor markers remains elevated despite radical orchiectomy [15]. At this point, the patient is appropriate for restaging and medical oncology evaluation to consider initiating chemotherapy or radiation treatment.

**Stage 2A and 2B** In this stage, surgery and radiation to the retroperitoneal and ipsilateral iliac lymph nodes of the abdomen are the treatment of choice. If chemotherapy is considered, common combinations are three rounds BEP (bleomycin, etoposide, and cisplatin) or four rounds of EP (etoposide and cisplatin) [16].

**Stage 2C or 3** Following radical orchiectomy, the chemotherapy regimen is outlined for a patient based on their risk. The goal of the chemotherapy is to reduce the size of the residual masses. Generally, no radiation is used in this stage (American Cancer Society, 2018) [15]. Patients are monitored through blood work and PET scans to observe for any relapse.

## Nonseminoma and Mixed Tumors

This class of tumors is also seen in the pediatric population. In Stages 1A and 1B, radical inguinal orchiectomy and surveillance are the treatment standard. Higher stages are treated with surgery and chemotherapy [18].

The remaining recommendations are for the adult males diagnosed with nonseminoma tumor types.

**Stage 1A** In this class of tumors, staging is what drives the treatment following the removal of the tumor via orchiectomy. Just as seminomas, the preferred option is close surveillance for compliant patients. Surgery may include nerve-sparing retroperitoneal lymph node dissection (RPLND). Relapses found during surveillance period are most often found in the first few years. These relapses are generally treated with chemotherapy.

For stage 1A and 1B, management depends on whether factors associated with an increased risk of relapse are present. These include:

- Lymphovascular invasion
- Predominance of embryonal carcinoma component
- A T3 or T4 primary tumor

Keeping these risk factors in mind, stage 1 nonseminomatous germ cell tumors can be divided into low- or high-risk categories.

- Low risk – men without any risk factors, consider active surveillance
- High risk – men with one or more risk factors, active surveillance, chemotherapy, and RPLND are options. For men who prefer to not pursue further treatment, active surveillance is reasonable. However, these men increase their risk of relapse to 40% [40].

**Stage 1S** The tumor is limited to the testis on clinical staging, but there is persistent elevation of tumor markers following orchiectomy. The presence of metastatic disease should be a concern. These patients may be appropriate for chemotherapy.

**Stage 1B** Following the orchiectomy and RPLND, chemotherapy is given if cancer is found in any of the dissected lymph nodes. Surveillance is not an option in this population.

**Stage 2A or 2B** Surgery is standard and includes nerve-sparing retroperitoneal lymph node dissection followed by chemotherapy.

**Stage 2C or 3** Surgery followed by chemotherapy, close monitoring of residual tumors by blood markers, and imaging. Any tumor remaining following chemotherapy treatment is usually removed surgically.

If cancer is found to be resistant to chemotherapy, a clinical trial, stem cell transplant, or other less conventional treatment may be recommended.

## Stromal Tumors

These tumors do not respond to chemotherapy and are treated with surgery, radical inguinal orchiectomy, and close surveillance.

### Continued Monitoring: Follow-up

Follow-up varies based on the initial treatment received.

As testicular cancer patients are generally diagnosed and treated at a young age, there are possible long-term consequences of treatment. Oncologic follow-up (with serum tumor markers, chest radiograph, and CT scan of the abdomen and pelvis as indicated) should be coordinated between the patient's providers.

Survivors should be followed at minimal annually for 5 to 10 years following their treatment. A decision to discontinue surveillance should be based on patient preference and discussion between the primary care and oncology teams [36].

The following guidelines are recommended [37]:

- Complete physical examination annually – Testicular cancer survivors should undergo a complete physical examination annually, with weight and blood pressure recorded. The examination should include a lymph node survey and examination of the contralateral testicle. Also, an examination of the skin. There should be a high index of suspicion for second cancers.
- Baseline lipid profile and counseling regarding cardiovascular risk factors.
- Renal function (serum creatinine) and serum magnesium annually (for patients who received cisplatin-based chemotherapy).
- Serial assessment of hormonal function (i.e., testosterone and luteinizing hormone levels) on a regular basis, particularly for men treated with chemotherapy or radiation therapy. There are no evidence-based guidelines to inform an optimal surveillance strategy, but consider their symptoms and test based on these.
- In addition, patients should be counseled about the importance of reporting new symptoms early.

## Cost Analysis

The cost analysis with respect to treating advanced stage testicular malignancies versus the cost for screenings or treating early stage malignancies is significant. According to the 2014 publication in *Cancer Medicine*, using Medicare reimbursement fee schedule as an estimate of national cost, the total treatment for an advanced stage seminoma on a per person basis was determined to be $48,877 and $51,592 for a nonseminoma. In contrast, the cost of an office screening is $156. This equates to 313–330 individuals being able to screened in the office for the same cost, 180–190 office visit screenings when a scrotal ultrasound is performed at $272, 79–83 office visits with serial scrotal ultrasounds and labs valued at $621, or 2–3 office visits for those who underwent surgery with a radical inguinal orchiectomy with benign pathology, the cost of which is $7686. Of those that were found to have an early stage testicular cancer, the cost of treatment and surveillance was $17,282 for a seminoma and $26,190 for a nonseminoma. Surveillance was based on 10 years of follow up from the time of diagnosis and treatment. Based on these numbers, many more clinical evaluations are able to be performed for benign disease compared to the cost of missing an advanced stage tumor. The cost-benefit ratio is approximately 2.4 to 1 for early detected testicular cancer compared to advanced stage disease. Naturally, health-care costs will only continue to increase, further inflating the above numbers.

## Patient Awareness and Education

Despite these statistics, literature suggests that men who are most likely to be affected have little knowledge of their risk for the disease and how to properly perform self-screenings. In fact, those classified within the most high-risk age group report from 0 to 31% knowledge on testicular self-examinations with performance ranging from 0 to 18%. A survey of college athletes revealed that of 87% were unaware of their risk for testicular cancer. In fact, only 9.6% had been taught on how to perform testicular self-examinations of which a little less than half or 4.8% obtained this knowledge through their physicians.

Given that this is a relatively curable condition, if detected early, patient education is key to a risk reduction of morbidity and mortality. Furthermore, early detection may allow for diagnosis at an earlier stage in the disease. This then has the potential to be managed with less toxic treatment. Unfortunately, sociocultural norms and religious beliefs exist as barriers for men in performing testicular self-examinations. An important consideration must be given to looking beyond the actual overall low prevalence of the disease itself and giving attention to the group this most affects, young men. As such the years of potential life lost (YPLL) can be significant [9]. The sequela of this disease can be infertility from the tumor itself or through the subsequent treatments. With respect to testicular cancer, men are significantly underrepresented when it comes to education, public outreach, and standard of care in disseminating this information. In fact, a study presented in the

*Archives of Medicine and Health Sciences* journal with respect to military soldiers found that military physicians taught female soldiers the importance of breast self-examinations 84% of the time but only 51% of the time to their male counterparts about testicular self-examinations [9].

**Pearls for the Advanced Practice Provider**

- Testicular cancer is the most frequently occurring cancer in young men with ages 15–34 but only represents 1–2% of all human malignancies and <1% of all male tumors.
- Screening has been recommended against by the USPSTF due to low incidence and favorable outcomes.
- Early detection allows increased overall survival and limits advanced disease progression, sequelae, and increased financial costs.
- Tumor markers, including AFP, β-HCG, and LDH, are used to diagnose, predict prognosis, and monitor response to treatment.
- Germ cell tumors are the most common type of testicular cancer, occurring 90% of the time. The germ cell tumors are further classified into seminomas and nonseminomas which occur at relatively equal rates.
- Treatment generally involves surgery with possible adjunctive chemotherapy or radiation depending on tumor classification and staging.

## References


1. American Cancer Society. Testicular cancer. [Internet]. Available from https://www.cancer.org/cancer/testicular-cancer/about/key-statistics.html.
2. Mellanby AR, Rees JB, Tripp, JH. Peer-led and adult-led school health education: a critical review of available comparative research. Health Educ Res. Oxford Academic. 1 Oct 2000. [Internet]. Available from https://academic.oup.com/her/article/15/5/533/639474.
3. Finney JW, Weist MD, Friman PC. Evaluation of two health education strategies for testicular self-examination. 27 Feb 2013. [Internet]. Available from https://onlinelibrary.wiley.com/doi/full/10.1901/jaba.1995.28-39.
4. Final recommendation statement testicular cancer: screening. Apr 2011. [Internet]. Available from https://www.uspreventiveservicestaskforce.org/Page/Document/RecommendationStatementFinal/testicular-cancer-screening.
5. American Academy of Family Physicians. Summary of recommendations for clinical preventive services. Leawood: American Academy of Family Physicians; 2010. [Internet]. Available from www.aafp.org/online/etc/medialib/aafp_org/documents/clinical/CPS/rcps08-2005.Par.0001.File.tmp/June2010.pdf.
6. American Academy of Pediatrics Committee on Practice and Ambulatory Medicine and Bright Futures Steering Committee. Recommendations for preventive pediatric health care. Pediatrics. 2007;120:1376.
7. Cancer screening guidelines | Detecting cancer early. 7 July 2017. [Internet]. Available from https://www.cancer.org/healthy/find-cancer-early/cancer-screening-guidelines/american-cancer-society-guidelines-for-the-early-detection-of-cancer.html.

8. Whol R, Kane W. Teachers' beliefs concerning teaching about testicular cancer and testicular self-examination. Mar 1997. [Internet]. Available from https://www.ncbi.nlm.nih.gov/pubmed/9071673.
9. Nwozichi CU. Effect of video-based teaching module on knowledge about testicular cancer and testicular self-examination among male undergraduate students. Arch Med Health Sci [serial online]. 2015;3:215–26. Available from http://www.amhsjournal.org/text.asp?2015/3/2/215/171909.
10. Matthews A. Self-examination should be taught to men: Advocate. 10 Mar 2016. [Internet]. Available from http://www.abc.net.au/news/2016-03-10/self-examination-education-for-men/7237238.
11. American Cancer Society recommendations for prostate cancer early detection. 14 April 2016. [Internet]. Available from https://www.cancer.org/cancer/prostate-cancer/early-detection/acs-recommendations.html.
12. Friman P C, Finney JW. Health education for testicular cancer. 1990. [Internet]. Available from http://citeseerx.ist.psu.edu/viewdoc/download?doi=10.1.1.1024.5345&rep=rep1&type=pdf.
13. Sperm storage costs. n.d.. [Internet]. Available from https://www.reprotech.com/sperm-storage-costs.html.
14. IVF costs – in vitro fertilization costs. (n.d.). [Internet]. Available from http://www.ihr.com/infertility/ivf/ivf-in-vitro-fertilization-cost.html.
15. American Cancer Society. www.cancer.org. 17 May 2018. [Internet]. Available from American Cancer Society: https://www.cancer.org/cancer/testicular-cancer/treating/by-stage.html#written_by.
16. Einhorn L. Curing metastatic testicular cancer. Proc Natl Acad Sci. 2002:4592–5.
17. Eric Leung PW. Treatment burden in stage I seminoma: a comparison of surveillance and adjuvant radiation therapy. BJU Int. 2013:1088–95.
18. Wieder JA. Pocket guide to urology. 5th ed. Oakland: J. Wieder Medical; 2014.
19. Fitzmaurice C, Global Burden of Disease Cancer Collaboration. Global, regional, and national cancer incidence, mortality, years of life lost, years lived with disability, and disability-adjusted life-years for 32 cancer groups, 1990 to 2015: a systematic analysis for the global burden of disease study. JAMA Oncol [Internet]. 2017;3(4):524–48. https://doi.org/10.1001/jamaoncol.2016.5688.
20. McGlynn KA, Devesa SA. Trends in the incidence of testicular germ cell tumors in the United States. Cancer [Internet]. 2002;97(1):63–70.
21. Batata MA, Chu FC, Hilaris BS, Whitmore WF, Golbey RB. Testicular cancer in cryptorchidism. Cancer [Internet]. 1982;49:1023–30. https://doi.org/10.1002/1097-0142(19820301)49:5<1023::AID-CNCR2820490528>3.0.CO;2-M.
22. Kier MG, Hansen MK, Lauritsen J, et al. Second malignant neoplasms and cause of death in patients with germ cell cancer: a Danish Nationwide Cohort Study. JAMA Oncol [Internet]. 2016;2(12):1624–7. https://doi.org/10.1001/jamaoncol.2016.3651.
23. Dong C, Lönnstedt I, Hemminki K. Familial testicular cancer and second primary cancers in testicular cancer patients by histological type. Eur J Cancer [Internet]. 2001;37(15):1878–85. Available from: https://doi.org/10.1016/S0959-8049(01)00172-1.
24. Dieckmann KP, Pichlmeir U. The prevalence of familial testicular cancer: an analysis of two patient populations and a review of the literature. Cancer [Internet]. 1997;80(10):1954–60. Available from: https://onlinelibrary.wiley.com/doi/full/10.1002/.
25. Grulich AE, van Leeuwen MT. Incidence of cancers in people with HIV/AIDS compared with immunosuppressed transplant recipients: a meta-analysis. The Lancet [Internet]. 2007;370(9581):59–67. Available from https://doi.org/10.1016/S0140-6736(07)61050-2.
26. Bray F, Richiardi L. Trends in testicular cancer incidence and mortality in 22 European countries: continuing increases in incidence and declines in mortality. Epidemiology [Internet]. 2006;118(12):3099–111. Available from https://doi.org/10.1002/ijc.21747.
27. Gajendran VK, Nguyen M. Testicular cancer patterns in African-American men. Urology [Internet]. 2005;66(3):602–5. Available from https://doi.org/10.1016/j.urology.2005.03.071.

28. McGlynn KA, Devesa SS. Increasing incidence of testicular germ cell tumors among black men in the United States. J Clin Oncol [Internet]. 2005;23(24):5757–61.
29. Nichols C. Testicular cancer. Curr Probl Cancer [Internet]. 1998;22(4):187–274. Available from: https://doi.org/10.1016/S0147-0272(98)90012-5.
30. Strohsnitter WC, Noller KL, Hoover RN. Cancer risk in men exposed in utero to diethylstilbestrol. J Natl Cancer Inst [Internet]. 2001;93(7):545–51. Available from: https://www.uptodate.com/contents/epidemiology-of-and-risk-factors-for-testicular-germ-cell-tumors/abstract/72.
31. Schottenfeld D, Warshauer ME. The epidemiology of testicular cancer in young adults. Am J Epidemiol [Internet]. 1980;112(2):232–46. Available from: https://doi.org/10.1093/oxfordjournals.aje.a112989.
32. Motzer R, et al. Testicular cancer, clinical practice guidelines in oncology. J Natl Compr Cancer Netw [Internet]. 2012;12(4). Available from https://jnccn.org/abstract/journals/jnccn/10/4/article-p502.pdf.
33. NCCN clinical practice guidelines in oncology (NCCN Guidelines) version 1.2019. Testicular cancer. 22 Oct 2018. Retrieved from https://www.nccn.org/professionals/physician_gls/pdf/testicular.pdf.
34. Skakkebæk NE, Rajpert-De Meyts E, Main KM. Testicular dysgenesis syndrome: an increasingly common developmental disorder with environmental aspects: opinion. Hum Reprod [Internet]. 2001;16(5):972–8. https://doi.org/10.1093/humrep/16.5.972.
35. Olesen IA, Sonne SB, Hoei-Hansen CE, Rajpert-DeMeyts E, Skakkebaek NE. Environment, testicular dysgenesis and carcinoma in situ testis. Best Pract Res Clin Endocrinol Metab [Internet]. 2007;21(3):462–78. Available from: https://doi.org/10.1016/j.beem.2007.04.002.
36. Beard C, Vaughn D. UpToDate [Internet]. Approach to the care of long-term testicular cancer survivors. 2018 [Updated 2018 Dec 20; cited 2019 May 3]. Available from: https://www.uptodate.com/.
37. Vaughn DJ, Gignac GA, Meadows AT. Long term medical care of testicular cancer survivors. Ann Intern Med [Internet]. 2002. [cited 2019 May 3];136(6):463–70. https://doi.org/10.7326/0003-4819-136-6-200203190-00010.
38. Hu GX, Lian QQ, Ge RS, Hardy DO, Li XK. Phthalate-induced testicular dysgenesis syndrome: Leydig cell influence. Trends Endocrinol Metab [Internet]. 20(3):139–45. https://doi.org/10.1016/j.tem.2008.12.001.
39. Nieschlag E. Klinefelter syndrome: the commonest form of hypogonadism, but often overlooked or untreated. Dtsch Arztebl Int. 2013;110(20):347–53. https://doi.org/10.3238/arztebl.2013.0347. Epub 2013 May 17. Review.
40. Oh, W., Overview of the treatment of testicular germ cell tumors. 2018, cited 9 May 2019. Available from: https://www.uptodate.com/contents/overview-of-the-treatment-of-testicular-germ-cell-tumors?search=nonseminomatous%20testicular%20cancer&source=search_result&selectedTitle=1~150&usage_type=default&display_rank=1#H647555688.

# Chapter 25
# Penile Cancer

**J. Ryan Mark and Danielle Squadrito**

## Introduction

Penile cancer is a rare malignancy responsible for the deaths of 300 men annually in the United States [1]. Chronic inflammation, HPV infection, and smoking are all considered risk factors, and incidence increases as men age, peaking between the 50th and 70th decades. Histology is almost exclusively squamous cell carcinoma (SCC). Management is surgical with chemotherapy used topically in noninvasive disease, systemically prior to consolidation of bulky disease, or palliation. New strategies are being tested using tyrosine kinase inhibitors (TKIs) and checkpoint inhibitors (IOs); however, their role treating metastatic disease is still unclear.

## Risk Factors and Prevention

Although penile cancer is rare, several risk factors have been clearly identified. Human papilloma virus (HPV) plays an important role in carcinogenesis. Roughly 50% of penectomy specimens for invasive penile cancer are found to contain HPV types 16 and 18 [2]. A nonavalent vaccine against HPV 6, 11, 16, 18, 31, 33, 45, 52, and 58 was approved by the FDA for use in 2016. Vaccination is 90.4% effective in

J. R. Mark (✉)
Department of Urology, Sidney Kimmel Cancer Center, Thomas Jefferson University, Philadelphia, PA, USA
e-mail: James.Mark@jefferson.edu

D. Squadrito
Department of Urology, Thomas Jefferson University, Philadelphia, PA, USA
e-mail: danielle.squadrito@jefferson.edu



E. J. Trabulsi et al. (eds.), *Chemotherapy and Immunotherapy in Urologic Oncology*, https://doi.org/10.1007/978-3-030-52021-2_25

preventing transmission in males; however, whether or not this will reduce the incidence of penile carcinoma is unknown [3].

An alternative pathway to cancer development is p53 mutation secondary to chronic inflammation of the foreskin [4]. Balanitis, an inflammatory condition of the glans, is observed in 45% of penile cancers [5]. Despite circumcision being shown to prevent HPV infection and chronic inflammation associated with phimosis, its role in penile cancer prevention is controversial.

As in other cancers, smoking has a dose-dependent relationship to the development of penile carcinoma. Men with a 45 pack-year smoking history are greater than three times more likely to develop penile cancer. Former smokers can reduce their risk in half which highlights the importance of smoking cessation in at-risk men [6].

## Natural History

The majority (61.6%) of patients with penile cancer in the United States are diagnosed with localized disease (Fig. 25.1), and 2.3% have evidence of distant metastases [7]. Without treatment, penile cancer follows a predictable pattern of spread. The tissues of the penis are drained by lymphatic channels to the bilateral superficial inguinal lymph nodes followed immediately by the deep inguinal lymph nodes and then the lymph nodes of the pelvis [8]. If uncontrolled, lymph node metastases grow and cause lymphedema, ulceration, and abscesses and can erode into the femoral vessels causing hemorrhage and death. Figure 25.2 demonstrates the devastating outcome of uncontrolled locally advanced penile cancer.

Survival is driven by successful prevention or aggressive management of lymph node metastases. pN0 men have 96% 10-year cancer-specific survival (CSS), whereas only 35% of pN+ patients are alive at 5 years [9]. There is increasing risk

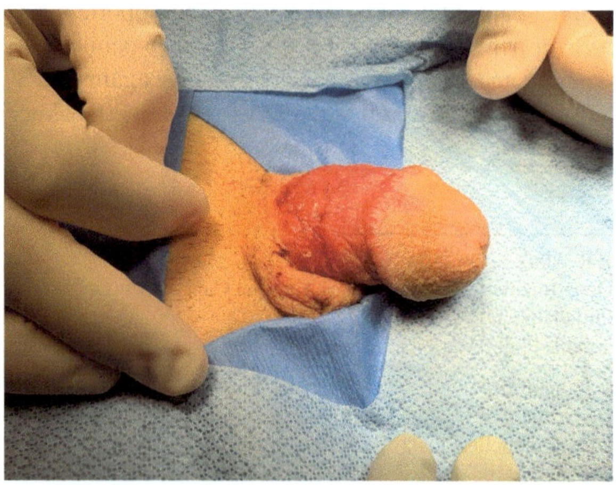

**Fig. 25.1** A 57-year-old circumcised male presenting with grade 3 pT1b basaloid penile SCC. This tumor is associated with prior HPV infection

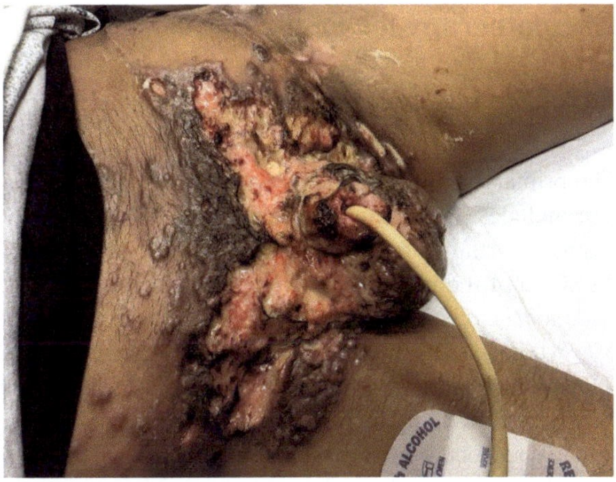

**Fig. 25.2** A 52-year-old male with G3 pT2N3M1 SCC. Bone metastases developed soon after lymphadenectomy, and he progressed rapidly on TIP, pembrolizumab, and palbociclib and died of his disease 7 months following diagnosis

of death noted with worsening nodal stage with one French study identifying 5-year CSS as 93.4%, 89.3%, 30.9%, and 0% for pN0, pN1, pN2, and pN3 disease, respectively [10]. Therefore accurate clinical staging and appropriate treatment of patients at risk for nodal progression are key to survival.

## Staging

Clinical staging for penile cancer begins with a thorough physical exam in a frog-legged position to evaluate external genitalia. The groin is then palpated to detect enlarged or fixed lymph nodes. Roughly 50% of patients with palpable disease will harbor lymph node metastases as will 20% with clinically negative groins who undergo staging lymphadenectomy. Biopsy or resection of the primary lesion is used to assess risk of metastases prior to consideration of further imaging or staging lymphadenectomy. Cross-sectional imaging is required to properly stage pelvic lymph nodes in high-risk or obese individuals where physical exam is limited. Typically, CT chest, abdomen, and pelvis with contrast is sufficient. MRI is useful in local staging of the primary tumor if corporal invasion is suspected or for surgical planning. PET-CT may also be useful.

An important consideration when staging the lymph nodes is the utility of lymph node biopsy when nodal metastases are suspected. Enlarged lymph nodes in the presence of an otherwise low-risk tumor should be biopsied to avoid the morbidity of an unnecessary inguinal lymphadenectomy. Conversely, in a patient with a high-risk lesion who has bilateral, large, or fixed inguinal lymph nodes, biopsy is an essential tool to justify the appropriate use of neoadjuvant chemotherapy prior to bilateral inguinal and pelvic lymphadenectomy.

## Chemotherapy for Penile Cancer

### *Localized Disease*

The primary tumor in patients with penile cancer is best managed with a resection that includes and adequate clean margin. The surgical excision of invasive disease requires partial or radical penectomy. For noninvasive CIS (carcinoma in situ) and Ta SCCa of the penis, topical chemotherapy can be considered as an alternative to wide local excision or laser therapy. In a study of 44 patients with CIS of the penis, 5% 5-fluorouracil applied to the lesion for 12 hours every 2 days for a total of 28 days resulted in a 57% complete response rate. Eighty percent of these patients experienced a durable response for a mean 34 months (range 12–180 months). Recurrence occurred at 5 months on average in a total of five patients (20%). Imiquimod was used to salvage these patients with a complete response rate of 44% in the second line [11]. The use of imiquimod as first-line topical therapy has also been described.

### *Locally Advanced Disease*

Node-positive penile cancer has the potential to become bulky and unresectable if ignored. For cases of bilateral disease and unilateral large nodes (mobile or fixed), the NCCN guideline recommends biopsy and neoadjuvant chemotherapy [12]. A phase II prospective study of cisplatin, paclitaxel, and ifosfamide (TIP) in 30 patients with cN2 or cN3 penile cancer has led to widespread adoption of this regimen. Twenty-three of the patients were able to complete all four cycles and experienced an objective response rate of 50% including a 10% complete response rate. Median survival was 17.1 months [13].

After lymphadenectomy, if regional metastases are detected, adjuvant chemotherapy has been shown to improve survival compared to surgery alone. Cisplatin, paclitaxel, and 5-fluorouracil (TPF) are alternative regimens to TIP that have shown benefit as adjuvant treatment. In one retrospective study, 21 patients were treated with TPF following lymphadenectomy. 66.7% of patients were pN3, and there were 23.8% and 9.5% of patients with pN2 and pN0 disease, respectively. The majority (66.7%) of patients received three cycles of TPF (range 2–4) and achieved median DFS and median of OS 22.7 months, and 85% of patients were alive at 1 year [14]. When compared to neoadjuvant TPF in cN2-3 disease, adjuvant therapy had a higher 2-year DFS (36.8% vs 7.1%); however, due to small sample size, statistical significance was not reached [15]. These studies illustrate the utility of systemic chemotherapy in addition to lymphadenectomy in the management of bulky nodal disease; however, a recent retrospective multicenter study of 743 men who underwent lymphadenectomy for penile cancer noted OS improvement only in patients with pN3 disease. There was little or no benefit on multivariate analysis to neoadjuvant or adjuvant chemotherapy in men with limited disease (N0-N2) [16]. As a result, some have argued against adjuvant chemotherapy in pN2 patients, but this is controversial, and at the time this chapter is written, adjuvant chemotherapy for men with both pN2 and pN3 penile carcinoma is recommended by NCCN and EAU guidelines [12, 17].

### *Metastatic Disease*

Metastatic penile cancer carries an abysmal prognosis. Single agent cisplatin has a meager ORR of 23% leading to the use of multidrug regimens for those that can tolerate the adverse effects [18]. TIP has favorable toxicity compared to other regimens and is often preferred in chemo-naive patients due to the 50% ORR reported in the neoadjuvant setting [13]. For patients progressing after chemotherapy, survival is less than 6 months, and multiple combinations of second-line chemotherapy have failed to demonstrate a meaningful response. Cisplatin, methotrexate, and bleomycin (PMB) have resulted in one partial and one complete response in two of five patients treated; however, this regimen has limited clinical utility as it is very toxic [19]. In a phase II first-line PMB trial, 5 of 45 patients died secondary to treatment-related complications [20]. Common chemotherapy regimens are listed in Table 25.1.

## Targeted Therapy

Overexpression of the epidermal growth factor receptor (EGFR) has been associated with a number of cancer types. It is a member of the HER family of tyrosine kinase receptors and in its normal state functions to support epithelial growth. Mutations resulting in increased EGFR activity are found in lung, anal, head and neck, and brain cancers [21]. As a result, its role as a therapeutic target in these malignancies has led to successful drug development and approval for use by the FDA. SCCa of the penis also commonly shows overexpression of EGFR. One study

**Table 25.1** Common chemotherapy regimens for penile cancer

| Regimen | Schedule |
|---|---|
| Paclitaxel, ifosfamide, cisplatin (TIP) [13] | Day 1: paclitaxel, ifosfamide, cisplatin<br>Day 2 and 3: ifosfamide + cisplatin<br>Repeat every 3–4 weeks for four cycles |
| Paclitaxel, cisplatin, fluorouracil (TPF) [14] | Day 1: paclitaxel + cisplatin<br>Day 2: cisplatin + fluorouracil<br>Days 3–5: fluorouracil<br>21-day cycles |
| Cisplatin, methotrexate, bleomycin (PMB) [20] | Day 1: bleomycin + methotrexate + cisplatin<br>Day 8: bleomycin + methotrexate<br>21-day cycles |

identified high expression in 44% and low expression in 44% of tumors examined. Thirteen had no EGFR expression [22]. This has led to interest in understanding the role of EGFR inhibitors for the treatment of penile cancers.

One of the first prospective phase II trials to test this treatment approach explored the efficacy of the irreversible pan-HER tyrosine kinase inhibitor dacomitinib. This oral medication (currently FDA approved for patients with metastatic NSCLC) was given as monotherapy to 28 men with recurrent locally advanced or metastatic penile cancer. The ORR was 32.1%, and there were eight partial responses and one CR. Overall survival was 13.7 months in all patients and 20 months when excluding M1 patients from the analysis [23]. While these outcomes do not outperform TIP in a neoadjuvant setting, the patients in this trial had recurrent and metastatic disease making them a higher-risk group. Dacomitinib was also well tolerated with no serious adverse events or discontinuations potentially increasing the number of patients eligible for systemic therapy.

## Immunotherapy

Checkpoint inhibition with anti-CTLA4 and anti-PD1/PD-L1 monoclonal antibodies has ushered a new era of systemic therapy for urologic malignancies. While these drugs have shown great utility in SCCa of the lung, skin, and head and neck, there is a paucity of data regarding their use in penile carcinoma. SCC of the penis lacks the high tumor mutational burden predictive of a robust response to these new agents, and there is still an effort to understanding the tumor microenvironment of this malignancy [24]. The rarity of this tumor and the short survival associated with recurrence following first-line therapy have likely contributed to the lack of data. At this time, the only reported outcomes for penile carcinomas treated with checkpoint inhibitors are small case reports or in trials of IO use in a mixed cohort of rare tumor types. A recent phase II study of the anti-PD1 inhibitor pembrolizumab in 127 patients with rare solid tumors has been reported. Only three patients with penile carcinoma were enrolled with one patient demonstrating at least a 50% decrease in measurable disease by 27 weeks, while the other two patients died [25].

## Conclusion

Penile cancer is a rare and potentially aggressive malignancy. Thoughtful management of regional lymph nodes has proven key to patients' ability to survive this devastating disease. As such, systemic therapy plays a vital role in those with regional metastases. Cytotoxic chemotherapy is still the preferred systemic means of treatment; however, as our understanding of the tumor microenvironment and molecular pathogenesis grows, newer agents are likely to play a more important role in modern management of this disease.

**Clinical Pearls**

- Chronic inflammation, HPV infection, and smoking are all considered risk factors for penile cancer, and incidence increases with age, peaking between the 50th and 70th decades.
- Roughly 50% of penectomy specimens for invasive penile cancer are found to contain HPV types 16 and 18.
- The majority (61.6%) of patients with penile cancer in the United States are diagnosed with localized disease, and 2.3% have evidence of distant metastases.
- Survival for invasive penile cancer is driven by successful prevention or aggressive management of lymph node metastases.
- Roughly 50% of patients with palpable disease will harbor lymph node metastases as will 20% with clinically negative groins who undergo staging lymphadenectomy.
- Biopsy or resection of the primary lesion is used to assess risk of metastases prior to consideration of further imaging or staging lymphadenectomy.
- Cisplatin, paclitaxel, and ifosfamide (TIP) are considered the gold standard for neoadjuvant and adjuvant treatment of locally advanced disease.
- Metastatic penile cancer carries an abysmal prognosis, with mortality common and quick after failure of first-line chemotherapy.

There may be a role for EGFR inhibitors for the treatment of metastatic penile cancers.

## References


1. Douglawi A, Masterson TA. Penile cancer epidemiology and risk factors: a contemporary review. Curr Opin Urol. 2019;29(2):145–9.
2. McCance DJ, Kalache A, Ashdown K, Andrade L, Menezes F, Smith P, et al. Human papillomavirus types 16 and 18 in carcinomas of the penis from Brazil. Int J Cancer. 1986;37(1):55–9.
3. Giuliano AR, Palefsky JM, Goldstone S, Moreira ED Jr, Penny ME, Aranda C, et al. Efficacy of quadrivalent HPV vaccine against HPV infection and disease in males. N Engl J Med. 2011;364(5):401–11.
4. Mentrikoski MJ, Stelow EB, Culp S, Frierson HF Jr, Canthro HP. Histologic and immunohistochemical assessment of penile carcinomas in a North American population. Am J Surg Pathol. 2019;38(10):1340–8.
5. Dillner J, von Krogh G, Horenblas S, Meijer CJ. Etiology of squamous cell carcinoma of the penis. Scand J Urol Nephrol Suppl. 2000;205:189–93.
6. Maden C, Sherman KJ, Beckmann AM, Hislop TG, The CZ, Ashley RL, et al. History of circumcision, medical conditions, and sexual activity and risk of penile cancer. J Natl Cancer Inst. 1993;85(1):19–24.
7. Burt LM, Shrieve DC, Tward JD. Stage presentation, care patterns, and treatment outcomes for squamous cell carcinoma of the penis. Int J Radiat Oncol Biol Phys. 2014;88(1):94–100.
8. Wood HM, Angermeier KW. Anatomic considerations of the penis, lymphatic drainage, and biopsy of the sentinel node. Urol Clin North Am. 2010;37(3):327–34.

9. Ornellas AA, Kinchin EW, Nobrega BL, et al. Surgical treatment of invasive squamous cell carcinoma of the penis: Brazilian National Cancer Institute long-term experience. J Surg Oncol. 2008;97(6):487–95.
10. Marconnet L, Rigaud J, Bouchot O. Long-term follow-up of penile carcinoma with high risk for lymph node invasion treated with inguinal lymphadenectomy. J Urol. 2010;183(6):2227–32.
11. Alnajjar HM, Lam W, Bolgeri M, Rees RW, Perry MJ, Watkin NA. Treatment of carcinoma in situ of the glans penis with topical chemotherapy agents. Eur Urol. 2012;62(5):923–8.
12. National Comprehensive Cancer Network (NCCN). NCCN clinical practice guidelines in oncology. Penile cancer. Version 1.2020. January 14, 2020. National Comprehensive Cancer Network. Abstract available at: https://www.nccn.org/professionals/physician_gls/pdf/penile.pdf.
13. Pagliaro LC, Williams DL, Daliani D, Williams MB, Osai W, Kincaid M, et al. Neoadjuvant paclitaxel, ifosfamide, and cisplatin chemotherapy for metastatic penile cancer: a phase II study. J Clin Oncol. 2010;28(24):3851–7.
14. Necci A, Lo Vullo S, Nicolai N, Ragi D, Giannatempo P, Colecchia M, et al. Prognostic factors of adjuvant taxane, cisplatin, and 5-fluorouracil chemotherapy for patients with penile squamous cell carcinoma after regional lymphadenectomy. Clin Genitourin Cancer. 2016;14:518–23.
15. Nicolai N, Sangalli LM, Necchi A, et al. A combination of cisplatin and 5-fluorouracil with a taxane in patients who underwent lymph node dissection for nodal metastases from squamous cell carcinoma of the penis: treatment outcome and survival analyses in neoadjuvant and adjuvant settings. Clin Genitourin Cancer. 2016;14:323–30.
16. Necchi A, Lo Vullo S, Mariani L, Zhu Y, Ye DW, Ornellas AA, et al. Nomogram-based prediction of overall survival after regional lymph node dissection and the role of perioperative chemotherapy in penile squamous cell carcinoma: a retrospective multicenter study. Urol Oncol. 2019;37(8):531.e7–531.e15.
17. Hakenberg OW, Compérat E, Minhas S, Necchi A, Protzel C, Watkin N. (2018) EAU guidelines on penile cancer. Retrieved from: https://uroweb.org/wp-content/uploads/EAU-Guidelines-Penile-Cancer-2018.pdf. Access date [4/10/2020].
18. Gagliano RG, Blumenstein BA, Crawford ED, Stephens RL, Coltman CA Jr, Costanzi JJ. cis-Diamminedichloroplatinum in the treatment of advanced epidermoid carcinoma of the penis: a Southwest Oncology Group Study. J Urol. 1989;141:66–7.
19. Wang J, Pettaway CA, Pagliaro LC. Treatment for metastatic penile cancer after first-line chemotherapy failure: analysis of response and survival outcomes. Urology. 2015;85:1104–10.
20. Haas GP, Blumenstein BA, Gagliano RG, et al. Cisplatin, methotrexate and bleomycin for the treatment of carcinoma of the penis: a Southwest Oncology Group study. J Urol. 1999;161:1823–5.
21. Liu X, Wang P, Zhang C, Ma Z. Epidermal growth factor receptor (EGFR): a rising star in the era of precision medicine of lung cancer. Oncotarget. 2017;25(8):50209–20.
22. Chaux A, Munari E, Katz B, Sharma R, Lecksell K, Cubilla AL, et al. The epidermal growth factor receptor is frequently overexpressed in penile carcinomas: a tissue microarray and digital image analysis study of 112 cases. Hum Pathol. 2013;44(12):2690–5.
23. Necci A, Lo Vullo S, Perrone F, Raggi D, Giannatempo P, Calareso G, et al. First-line therapy with dacomitinib, an orally available pan-HER tyrosine kinase inhibitor, for locally advanced or metastatic penile squamous cell carcinoma: results of an open-label, single arm, single-centre, phase 2 study. BJU Int. 2018;121(3):348–56.
24. Chen YP, Zhang Y, Lv JW, Li YQ, Wang YQ, He QM, et al. Genomic analysis of tumor micro-environment immune types across 14 solid cancer types immunotherapeutic implications. Theranostics. 2017;7:3585–94.
25. Naing A, Meric-Bernstam F, Stephen B, Karp DD, Hajjar J, Ahbert JR, et al. Phase 2 study of pembrolizumab in patients with advanced rare cancers. J Immunother Cancer. 2020;8(1):e000347.

# Index





E. J. Trabulsi et al. (eds.), *Chemotherapy and Immunotherapy in Urologic Oncology*, https://doi.org/10.1007/978-3-030-52021-2

**S**

MIX
Papier aus verantwortungsvollen Quellen
Paper from responsible sources
FSC® C105338

If you have any concerns about our products,
you can contact us on
**ProductSafety@springernature.com**

In case Publisher is established outside the EU,
the EU authorized representative is:
**Springer Nature Customer Service Center GmbH**
**Europaplatz 3, 69115 Heidelberg, Germany**

Printed by Libri Plureos GmbH
in Hamburg, Germany